HEALTH AND FOOD
Problems and Solutions

HEALTH AND FOOD

Problems and Solutions

MOHINDER SINGH (IAS)

GYAN PUBLISHING HOUSE
NEW DELHI - 110002

HEALTH AND FOOD
Problems and Solutions

Published by Gyan Publishing House
5, Ansari Road, Daryaganj,
New Delhi - 110 002
Phone : 23282060, 23261060
Fax : 011 - 23285914
E-mail : gyanbook@vsnl.com
Visit our website at : \\www.gyanbooks.com

First Published in India 2003

Rs. 595

ISBN : 81-212-0832-7

Laser Typesetting by : Varsha Graphics, Delhi

Printed by : Delux Offset Printers, Delhi-110035

Contents

Preface

The book is designed to help the reader gain a better understanding of selected aspects of health and food.

Most of all, it offers information, facts and suggestions. At least, disabuse some readers of a few myths that hamper healthful living.

The author had the benefit of receiving numerous letters and telephone calls from readers of his published articles, especially the ones appearing regularly in publications like *My Doctor and Beauty Care* (since discontinued) and *Modern Practical Psychology*. Their queries and concerns have enabled the author to give a more practical shape to the offered material.

Modern times are witnessing an explosive growth in medical knowledge. This, in turn, has given rise to a plethora of research studies and surveys, let alone discoveries and new drugs. The media is ever on the lookout for fresh findings and breakthroughs in the health field, as these make heady news. On one hand, there are frequent reports of magic cures. On the other, scare stories pertaining to foods or lifestyle are not uncommon. Well, many of these magic cures may just be in the laboratory stage, and many of the scary findings based on inadequate research or too narrow a sample.

It therefore calls for an element of scepticism and caution when one is exposed to media stories on the subject of health and food.

The book is not meant to be read like a novel, continuously. Readers can pick and choose whatever interests them.

Mohinder Singh

Introduction

The book is divided into eleven sections. Eight of them deal with matters relating to health. The remaining three discuss food in its health context.

The first section pertains to modern lifestyle approaches to health, with all that emphasis on hygiene, selective food, and moderate exercise. It discusses the current quest for happiness, the prevalence of depression, and the emerging armoury of "happiness" pills. Secrets of sleep and dreaming are spelled out and some steps suggested to combat insomnia or lack of sleep in teenagers. And a plea put in for a better understanding and adjustment of left-handedness.

The second section deals with certain specific health problems. One of the serious ailments afflicting these days is the widespread prevalence of hypertension—a known hazard for the heart and brain. Keeping high blood pressure under control has therefore become a key consideration.

The other common ailment is colds, coughs and flue. People need to know how precisely colds are caught. What's the effectiveness of the cold remedies sold commonly in the market. Somewhat similar to colds are allergies. With all the sorts of new chemicals coming into everyday use and the growing spectre of indoor pollutants, allergies have been on the rise, especially among the urban folk. Happily, with care and the new crop of drugs, allergies are not hard to tackle.

Heavy users of computer keyboards are known to suffer from RSI (Repetitive Strain Injuries) to their hands and arms. Besides pain, RSI can result in serious disability. A new area of medical research has opened up to devise preventive as well as curative measures for RSI.

Pain itself, whether the usual headache, backache or any other pain, is being subjected to sustained research. The basic approach is to manage pain in a way that it does not debilitate the body.

Similarly the rising urban phenomenon of feeling "tired all the time" is being investigated. Quite a few novel theories about it are being advanced.

The third section concerns gender-related health issues. Men's health—an area relatively neglected as compared to women's problems—is dealt at length: the enlarged prostrate, prostate cancer, and impotence. Then there's the propensity of men to take greater liberties with their health.

As to contraception, the progress of the male pill and the complexity of its use are discussed. And there's the fascinating story of the abortion pill.

IVF is blossoming. Many infertile couples are seeking donated semen or fertilized eggs, let alone measures to boost their own semen and fertilized eggs. And this is also giving rise to more of twins and triplets—whether wanted or unwanted.

How to get the good sperm? This is becoming an engaging quest, with all sorts of new possibilities. The Indian scene has yet to catch up with international standards as to the offered choice in sperm.

With donated eggs, women beyond menopausal age are in a position to bear children. This poses its own health and moral issues.

Travel, particularly air travel, is vastly on the increase. Section four dwells on health-specific aspects of travel. It gives an idea of the air in aeroplanes; the air that stays exceptionally dry and can contain pollutants. Passengers are advised to guard against dehydration by frequent drinks of water.

How to combat jet lag? Jet lag is a health hazard, more so with business travellers and airline crews who have to travel frequently across continents. And then how they can stay connected to their family while being out on travel. Women business travellers have the added concern for personal safety. And sitting immobile for long hours in crowded airline seats can cause complications in blood circulation.

Airline food, with its limitations of mass production hours before use and its re-heating, cannot be the best. Yet airlines are ever trying to improve its acceptability. They are offering choices such as vegetarian food, and other ethnic preferences. Diabetics can have special meals.

Section five deals with medicines, doctors and hospitals. Medicines, to give optimum benefit, require a well-laid regime of taking.

The changing role of doctors is discussed. Theirs is the dilemma of how much a doctor should tell his patients and the relatives. Whereas reticence was the rule in the past, some doctors may now err on the side of telling too much of frightening news, at times proving incorrect.

The use of placebos instead of medicines poses another dilemma to doctors. How much they should tell the patient?

Hospitals tend to make medical mistakes. How to minimize such mistakes remains a tough proposition. People visiting patients in hospitals have to keep a few things in mind. And then there are difficult patients. How should the nursing staff take care of them?

The story of aspirin! Its versatile use is still to be fully documented. And the overuse of antibiotics that is endangering the very effectiveness of these wonder drugs.

Section six attempts to explain the puzzle and the process of ageing. It goes into some length on how the old feel?

Aided by advances in medical science and hygiene, people are living longer and staying fitter into their senior years. The traditional image of the old as infirm and helpless is fast changing. Indeed they are growing older more slowly.

More and more seniors are enjoying money and mobility. No doubt there are ageing losses, such as impaired hearing, sight, or movement, but many of the elderly are succeeding to retain a high morale. Between men and women, women are seen to be ageing better than men.

With affluent oldsters growing in numbers—and they demanding requisite attention, the industry has to equip itself with meeting their requirements. Travel/tourist industry has to design specific programmes for them. And retail trade will have to make changes that make it easier for their older customers to shop.

Section seven dwells exclusively on eyes. What a wonder is the eye! This needs some explaining.

The commonest eye ailment for the young in modern times is myopia. Why is myopia spreading so fast? Some attribute it to the start of reading at an early age. Correcting myopia through laser surgery poses its own benefits and risks.

The two eye diseases most common to older people are glaucoma and macular degeneration. Glaucoma, which initially causes loss in peripheral vision, can now be contained from doing further damage to the optic nerve through a regime of eye drops. Newer, more responsive eye drops are coming to the market. As glaucoma calls for a long-term regime of eye drops, an opportunity is taken to show how best to put eye drops. When eye drops fail, surgery becomes the last resort.

Degeneration of the macular area—the central part of the retina that affords us clear pictures and minute details—makes the image hazy. A whole lot of research is on but as yet there's no proven cure for macular degeneration.

Section eight deals with baby behaviour and health. It starts with a few basics on babies, such as baby's hearing, smell, sight, tasting, and crawling. And explains how babies attract their mother's attention through the in-born reflexes of smiles or crying. A mention is made of some of the survival strategies that babies adopt.

Can you really spoil a baby by pandering to its demands? The answer is, no. And parents are advised how to handle the situation and not panic when the baby gets sick.

The sleep and dream pattern of babies is discussed. Babies, it seems, sleep differently. Where should the baby sleep—with parents in the same bed or in a separate cot or even a separate room, and at what stages of infancy?

And then some special problems pertaining to kids, such as hyperactive children or taking care of twins. Expert opinion favours medical intervention for hyperactive children.

The first food section explains how food is absorbed in the body, yielding various components of nutrition. And how brain signals the requirement of food—the mystery of appetite.

As to taste, people think they're getting flavour messages from the taste buds of their tongue. Yet the tongue detects only a few basic tastes—sweet, salty, bitter and sour. It is our sense of smell—10,000 times more sensitive that our sense of taste—that distinguishes various flavours.

Food adulteration has been there for centuries. Whereas the same has been largely eradicated in advanced countries through rigorous testing and supervision, the evil practice still flourishes in our midst.

Food additives give rise to certain misgivings. Yet food additives—as distinguished from cheaper substitutes that food processors use to cut costs—are now an important part of many foods we buy and enjoy; ice cream, biscuits, soft drinks, soups, potato chips, even bread. A primary purpose of additives is to make food look attractive; much of our appetite for food is based on sight. No wonder, the manufacturing of artificial flavours has grown into a major, complex industry.

Much attention is centred these days on the effects of various foods on weight. It has given rise to many unsettling questions. Are the fat at fault? Are you overweight, and if so by how much? What's more fattening: Fats or Carbohydrates? What's the role of dieting? And allied complications, such as anorexia and bulimia. The food versus fat debate goes on, with no end in sight. Possibly the only conclusion that stands unchallenged: eat, drink and be moderate.

The second section on food pertains to particular items getting reputed as healthful. Those included here for discussion are ginseng, garlic, orange, tomatoes, apples, bananas, and eggs.

And, of course, water. In this context, increasing premium is being placed on the security (from pollution and contamination) provided by commercially bottled water and water-purifying devices.

The last section on food lists a few items that have been caught in controversy: sugar, salt, coffee, chocolate, chillies.

People prone to high blood pressure are usually advised to skimp on salt; our normal diet provides more than enough salt for body's essential needs. They are especially enjoined to cut down on processed foods, such as potato chips, which contain an excess of salt.

Chocolates are presumed to be less fattening than our usual sweets, because cocoa butter in chocolate is not fattening.

Chillies are rated as friendly fire. And are said to do little harm, if one can relish and tolerate them otherwise.

One can, however, see no end to controversies about certain foods, whether it is coffee or alcohol, red meat or white meat, salt or sugar. The industry behind each of these also muddies the health debate while backing its products.

1
Health : General

Health: Back to Basics

The modern man's quest for health continues on its vigorous course. Research on new ways to head off diseases is being pursued on all fronts. Scientists are busily exploring the potential of a whole array of drugs and vitamins, various sorts of foods and thousands of herbs for prevention and cure of diseases. Lots of studies and surveys are being conducted as to what helps lower risks of developing killers like cancer, heart disease and diabetes. Even the long neglected tribal and traditional systems of medicine are being investigated in the process. And cookbooks are doing their bit by according increasing attention to the health aspect of their products.

The quest goes on relentlessly. But what's the gist of the current findings? These are coming out surprisingly simple: eat enough of vegetables and fruits, and take moderate exercise. Back to basics, that's the message.

Of course this advice is more relevant to societies which eat too much meat. And it assumes that people will stay protected against infections through clean drinking water, uninfected food, and avoidance of other infections and impurities. Surely a good deal will also depend on the quality of urban air they breathe.

How have health scientists arrived at such a simplistic approach after all that elaborate and advanced research? A few of their findings make interesting reading.

Vitamin A. Vegetables like spinach and carrots contain a compound (beta carotene) which turns into vitamin A in the body. The chemical being an antioxidant, it neutralizes the highly reactive oxygen molecules in the body. And these are the molecules that might damage DNA or protein, thereby setting the stage for cancer, cataract, even artery-clogging. Researchers also found that adequate levels of this wonder chemical make for lower incidence of lung cancer, and prevent the recurrence of the tumours of mouth and throat.

The recommended daily allowance is 6 mg, about what you get from 150 grams of carrots or sweet potatoes. Taking vitamin A directly is not the same thing, as vitamin A itself is not antioxidant. And too much intake of vitamin A can cause headaches and vomiting.

Vitamin B. Extra doses of vitamin B (folic acid) are being recommended, especially a dosage of 4 mg daily for women trying to get pregnant. This considerably reduces the chances of a malformed foetus. The best means of taking vitamin B are leafy vegetables and legumes.

Vitamin C. Vitamin C (largely found in citrus fruit) has an ever lengthening list of useful attributes. Some recent studies indicate that it lowers the risk of heart disease, through an increase in blood levels of "good" cholesterol and a decrease in the levels of "bad" cholesterol. And over 90 large-scale studies of vitamin intake and cancer conducted by California University have come to the conclusion that vitamin C protects against cancers of digestive tract, rectum, breasts and lung.

Vitamin E. Another recent US study has brought out that vitamin E, again an antioxidant, helps in reversing the immune system damage that comes with ageing. High doses of vitamin E are also observed to have delayed the hardening of the arteries. Green leafy vegetables, nuts, whole wheat, and vegetable oils are high in E. A daily dose of 15 mg for men and 12 mg for women is being recommended. That means taking adequate helpings of the above mentioned items twice or thrice a day.

The main approach is to meet your requirements of these vitamins—needed to prevent serious body deficiencies and diseases—through diet, not pills. Admittedly, some of the elderly, children, or pregnant women may require a supplement of pills to make up for their nutritional deficit. But for everyone else, the best regimen of vitamin pills can't replace a diet rich in fruits and vegetables.

In fact the more they are delving into the secrets of fruits and vegetables, the more the health scientists are discovering the wonders of these foods for the human system.

Moderate Exercise

The latest researches indicate that moderate exercise can help cut your risk of developing a range of serious aliments, including colon cancer, diabetes, high blood pressure and heart disease. The earlier emphasis on jogging or sweating oneself out in hard exercises is taking a backseat. But pronounced evidence is accumulating about the health hazards of being a "couch potato". Some of the latest findings about moderate exercise go like this.

A 20-minute brisk walk a day helps boost blood levels of "good" cholesterol that can protect against heart disease by vacuuming cholesterol deposits from artery walls.

Moderate physical activity—fast walking or active gardening—can lower high blood pressure where the diastolic readings still range between 90 to 100. Experts think that exercise somehow tones the circulatory system so blood can be pumped under less pressure. Similarly many patients with mild hypertension may not require medicine if they exercise regularly.

Evidence is collecting that even moderate exercise has some protective effect on people from developing the adult-onset diabetes. In one study, the risk of diabetes among men in the age group 39-68, dropped by 6 per cent for every 500 calories burnt in exercise per week—equivalent to a daily one-mile walk. Of course, exercise alone is no insurance against this complex disease. But you can better your odds by avoiding a sedentary life.

Exercise, it has come out in some studies, appears to prevent colon cancer by helping to speed food through the system, leaving less time for carcinogens to remain in contact with the colon lining.

Contrary to popular impression that an arthritic knee could be damaged by exercise, a suitably supervised exercise actually strengthens it. Again exercise contributing through weight loss can help prevent arthritis.

Both men and women suffer bone loss in old age, especially women once estrogen levels drop. While exercise itself cannot prevent osteoporosis, it helps pre-menopausal women build up their bone densities so as to be served better in old age.

No wonder, an expert was let to remark, "Everything that gets worse as your age improves as you exercise."

With all the advances in health and medicine, the basic formula for health is staying the same; eat enough of fruits and vegetables, and take moderate exercise.

The New Health Mantra

Over the last two decades, many of our upwardly mobile people have come to embrace the new health mantra, the "healthy life-style". The same features in the form of a strictly observed bodily regime—of regular exercise, a balanced diet (coupled with an unceasing concern for clean drinking water), a structured daily rhythm of activities, a consistently growing list of avoidances and self-denials.

The new health mantra has even spawned a political movement, with its activists wanting the state to curb smoking and discourage the consumption of things deemed harmful to health, such as paan massala or gutka. To them it is not a question of running a "nanny state" but simply practising preventive medicine.

Indeed the healthy life-style movement is setting the stage for a new explanation as to why people become ill and suffer. Traditionally, people looked to religion to understand their sufferings. Illness was often seen as punishment for some transgression in this life, or even in an earlier existence. And so the religious took a spell of serious illness rather stoically, accepting it more as a divine judgement. The not-so-religious, unable to imagine any higher purpose in their sufferings, felt helpless, confused, mostly fretting "why me?" The mental suffering that accompanied illness was often accentuated by the apparent pointlessness of it. No wonder, a serious health setback engendered intense feelings of bitterness and resentment.

Two closely related features more than any other mark the modern spirit: the ability to act and the ability to make things different—this ability limited only by the available resources and know-how. In the field of health, it means the enhancement of health and the elimination of disease. The owner of the body is now a manager, a supervisor and an operator rolled into one, with medical profession supplying him or her with ever more complex technological products to perform these functions; in way appointed by medical authorities to invigilate and supervise the piece of machinery assigned to his or her care.

The healthy lifestyle has given rise to the idea that sickness is avoidable. Information about the consequences of overeating, under-exercising, overweight, smoking and excessive drinking is available in plenty. Even governments are getting involved in spreading the good word. The underlying premise of the healthy life-style movement is that if you persist in an unhealthy life-style, you have only yourself to blame if you fall ill. Males, it's made out, happen to take more risks with their bodies than their female counterparts.

The accusatory tone can sometimes operate unfairly, based more on assumptions than scientific evidence. For example, it's still unclear whether a regular intake of fat necessarily leads to heart attack, or whether the lack of exercise causes a stroke. But in the minds of people who have embraced a "healthy life-style", what's important is the association, say, between butterfat and heart attack. Some of them can't escape a feeling of guilt even after consuming one fatty meal or smoking a few cigarettes. Scientific medicine does not support such fears because the offending agent is not of sufficient quantity to cause trouble. But in the healthy life-style movement, the understanding of disease becomes more a matter of faith than science. The movement puts so much emphasis on self-control and self-discipline, people become scared to indulge in as much as some simple transgression. People have never been healthier before. And, if you still fall sick, possibly you didn't read the right newspaper articles.

Whereas the lifestyle movement tells patients that getting sick is their own fault, it also helps focus their attention in a positive, promising manner. By ascribing illness to a cause like bad living habits, patients are able to regain a sense of balance that comes from associating a complex problem with a single factor. They feel a sense of empowerment, believing that health and sickness are under their control. They see their efforts to get better as another form of self-improvement.

Health Mantras: Now and Then

When I was a kid in the 1940s, staying healthy seemed simpler. You went for foods liberally garnished with desi ghee; ghee not only the hallmark of taste but the most glorified source of strength. As a hostel student, you commonly brought your own tin of ghee, kept it under lock and key, and took out a tablespoon of it at every meal. You gorged happily (no troubled conscience then) on sweets whenever given a chance. The thick buffalo milk was the thing, preferably with a creamy crust on top. Of course, you walked a lot those days; riding anything except a bicycle was exceptional.

When you fell ill—everybody suffered periodic bouts of illness—the family doctor had little trouble finding out what was wrong with you. Often his first question: how are the bowels moving? And then he felt your pulse, asked you to stick out your tongue, tapped your chest with two fingers, or flashed a torch inside your throat. And then you got a bottle of some bitter mixture to speed your way to recovery.

One's doctor those days had usually been through at least a few personal episodes of illness on his own and had a pretty good idea of what it was like for his patient. Today's young doctors hardly know what patients feel; for them the nearest thing to a personal education in illness is the common cold. That possibly makes a good case for the continuance of common cold.

In the fifties, most successful people developed stomach ulcers. The assumption was that ulcers were caused by tension in top jobs. There were only two classes of people then—those who had ulcers and those who gave them. In recent years, the heart attack has replaced the stomach ulcer as the medical badge of the overworked male; anybody with normal blood pressure these days just isn't paying enough attention to his job.

Another medical problem seemingly on wane is broken arms. In my days you saw quite a few schoolboys with arms in sling. Now an arm in plaster cast is a rare sight. Is it all from the new techniques in bone-setting, or is it that today's children don't climb trees the way we did?

Medical science is now at the cutting edge of high technology. They're performing miracles of surgery. They're so advanced they can determine a baby's developments in the womb and undertake remedial surgery. Indeed, with so many health stories of miracle cures coming up, it is not the fear which hurts most, it's the hope.

With killing or near-killing illnesses largely reserved for one's advancing years, medical science is busily inventing many new health risks that include hormones in chickens, antibiotics in mutton, dyes in lipsticks, mercury in fish, radiation from TV, cancer from cell phones, even glue on postage stamps.

We're told, a long airline flight in crowded Coach class could bring on blood clots, and jogging can cause heart problems in the elderly. Staying in sun gives you cataract. Eggs clog the arteries, coffee can lead to gout, tea to constipation. Tap water is deemed non-drinkable, and the normal city-air non-breathable. The wine-bibbler is headed for cancer of the larynx, and the nondrinker less protected against heart attacks.

Specialization has reached such a state, patients have to learn to diagnose themselves before they know which specialist to call. Anyway hardly any doctors are left, all have turned specialists. Today when you visit one, you are likely to be given an elaborate list of tests to undergo. And when you see him again with all those test reports, he could well spend more time reading the reports than looking at you.

The writer Wilbur Cross understood it all. "Caution!" he cried. "Living may be dangerous to your health!"

How Happy Are You?

Am I happy? Why can't I be happy? Shouldn't I be happier than I am? Questions like these are often uppermost in our mind.

We've never had it so good, and yet we seem to stay less happy than our parents or grandparents. That's the paradox. Those worthies anyway kept their feelings to themselves while we talk all the time about our happiness. Are we pursuing happiness too hard?

In his book *Britain on the Couch: Why we are Unhappier Compared with 1950, despite being Richer*, the author makes the point that more of his countrymen are depressed now than 50 years ago, even though they are markedly better off. Similarly Robert Frank in his book *Luxury Fever: Why Money Fails to Satisfy in an Era of Excess* claims that decades of rapidly increasing affluence and lavish spending in America has not made anyone happier.

How many people are happy—and why? Can social scientists measure something as hard to pin down as human happiness? Most researchers in this field have to content themselves with simply asking people to reflect on their happiness with life—or what psychologists call "subjective well-being".

American psychologists, David G, Myers (author of *The Pursuit of Happiness: Who is Happy and Why*, William Morrow, 1992) and Edward Diener are in the forefront of what they term the Science of Happiness. For over twenty years they have been examining the life patterns of happy people; asking through researchers more than a million people across the world—a representative sample of the human race—to reflect on their happiness and life satisfaction. The idea is that some of the patterns discovered in the research may offer clues for transforming circumstances and behaviour that work against well-being into ones that promote it.

Based on these self-reports, the two psychologists have arrived at a few findings of human happiness.

No time in life is notably happier or unhappier. The common impression that times of "mid-life crisis" or declining years are unhappier doesn't seem to hold true. In fact the old as a group may have more "life satisfaction" than the young—"the minds of the young are full of the things they want to achieve and have not, whereas most of the elderly have either achieved what they wanted or made their peace with the fact that they never will".

Gender again gives no clues to subjective well-being. Neither men with their higher earning power nor women with their greater capacity for intimacy register any happier than their opposite-sex counterparts.

Does wealth predict happiness? Wealth, it seems, is like health. Although its utter absence can breed misery, possessing it is no guarantee of happiness. As a person's income rises towards the middle-class level, his or her sense of well-being rises as well. But once basic material needs are met, income decouples from happiness.

A survey among Forbes' 100 wealthiest Americans showed them "only slightly happier" than the average American—-some kind of "nature's revenge" law that denies extra contentment to the wealthy. And several studies have revealed that big winners of lotteries were not appreciably happier after a year or two of their win. The sort of lifestyle you expect drifts upward, without necessarily a corresponding rise in happiness levels.

In fact a booming economy minting new millionaires creates a psychological climate in which, ironically, everybody suffers. The "have-nots" lose, since they are seized by envy for a happiness they never knew they lacked until they happened to peek through the hole in the wall and spied the elites enjoying unimaginable riches. The "haves" lose in a different way: "sudden wealth syndrome" afflicting the newly rich with a sense of isolation and uncertainty, as if they have been teleported into an alien world.

Marriage seems to prevent people from becoming unhappy as well as actively promoting their happiness. And the association of marital happiness and overall happiness is even greater for married women than for their husbands.

Religiously active people report greater happiness. There seems to be a positive link between faith and well-being.

Stable extroverts seem to have the best chance for happiness. Their sociability and enjoyment derived from the company of other people generates much positive effect.

And while existence of a "happiness gene" has yet to be established, happiness seems modifiable only within limits imposed by our genetic leash.

Why so many people stay unhappy for no ostensible reason? Some attribute it to the spread of godlessness. Once life used to have God at its centre. A setback or deprivation was accepted as a part of the divine purpose. A lot of people no longer have that kind of faith. Indeed few worry about heaven any more; we all want to be happy here and now.

Another explanation: far more people are now without work, either through rising unemployment or long periods of retirement. When you're busy working you have less time to feel unhappy. Take the retirees. With lengthening life span and better health standards, many more people with fairly active minds and bodies are living out decades without purposeful work.

Some blame it on rampant individualism, which causes us to think that our setbacks are of vast importance, and thus something to be depressed about.

Or it could be runaway consumerism. Like a narcotic drug, materialism requires more and more to produce the same brief high. Consumerism also causes people to spend rather than save, which does trigger a certain anxiety in daily life.

And now recent research at Carnegie Mellon University brings out that extended Internet use could cause a decline in psychological well-being. Researchers are puzzling over the findings. They had expected that the Internet would prove socially healthier than television, since the Net allows users to choose their information and to communicate with others. The fact that Internet use reduces time available for family and friends may account for the drop in well-being, researchers hypothesize. Another possibility is that exposure to the wider world via the Net makes users less satisfied with their lives.

Happiness, it's said, is more a question of *disposition* than *position*. We may feel euphoria or misery over an event, but soon we revert to our usual self: the discontented remain glum; the sunny-natured continue cheerful. The change in circumstances merely causes a blip in the predictable graph of our lives.

And this disposition may have something genetic or it could be influenced by our upbringing. Recent research on the interaction between depressed mothers and their newborn babies shows that a baby becomes aware when a mother does not respond in the way the baby wants. After repeated attempts to attract the mother's attention, the baby gives up trying and becomes distressed.

At one time, women were constantly being enjoined to keep their men happy. Women's magazines devoted chunks of space to instructing women how to keep their husbands happy. Now magazines overflow with advice how women can achieve happiness for themselves—unhappiness deemed unacceptable.

A couple of things that clearly militate against happiness are excessive anger and prolonged grief. "For every minute you're angry, you lose sixty seconds of happiness," someone said. It is extremely important to ask ourselves whether the strength of our anger is really justified; you could get wildly angry over something you would ordinarily find mildly irritating. Again an attitude of forgiveness promotes happiness; bitterness only harms the person who harbours it.

Some persons grieve over a death too long. According to one professor of psychiatry, the appropriate length to mourn over one's parents or a spouse is two years. Any longer mourning is the symptom of depression known as "irrational grief".

What can you do to promote happiness? Experts are agreed that the best recipe is to keep busy. When people say they are happy, they are almost always busy, and caught up in activity—they are too busy to be miserable. "To fill the hour—that is happiness," says Emerson. Busy people have less time for introspection and it's introspection that often chases away happiness; more so the kind of introspection that slips into self-deprecation. That way getting interested in others instead of focussing all the time on one's own problems is a sure help. People obsessed with their own happiness seldom find it.

For phases of mild depression, brisk exercise is likely to be more effective than pills and therapy.

"No man is happy who does not think himself so," said Marcus Aurelius, the philosopher-emperor many centuries ago. Myers and his colleague go a step further. In their view, acting happy is likely to make you happy.

Better feign happiness if you don't feel like it. Fake it. Pretend self-esteem. Feign optimism. To some the whole thing may sound phoney but the phoniness should gradually subside. You're in a testy mood but when the phone rings you feign cheer while talking to a friend. Strangely, after hanging up, you no longer feel so grumpy.

Dwelling too much on whether you deserve to be happy or don't is one sure way of not being happy. You must see yourself as valuable. Constantly criticising yourself or making impossible demands on yourself can ruin your chances of happiness. In short, be your own best friend.

Martin Seligman at the Chicago University is teaching his students "learned optimism". According to him, a positive psychological outlook not only improves "life outcomes" but enhances health directly. Emotions are said to play a role in regulating the immune system—the more positive your sense of well-being, the better your white blood cells function.

Happiness here has to be distinguished from pleasure. Pleasure is momentary, a biological reflex, a fleeting reward. Happiness, partly an abstract thing, is not a passing state of mind but something more basic, largely a condition of life.

Psychologist Mihaly Csikszentmihalyi (author of *Creativity: Flow and the Psychology of Discovery and Invention* dwells on the link between creativity and happiness. He calls this feeling "flow" that people experience when engaged in work or activity which absorbs them and gets the best out of them. In many ways, the secret to happiness is to learn to get the flow from almost anything we do, including work and family commitments, says Csikszentmihalyi. The more flow we experience in daily life, the more likely we are to feel happy overall.

Economist Richard Easterlin (author of *Growth Triumphant,* University of Michigan Press, 1996) discusses the debatable link between happiness and wealth.

Living standards have soared during the twentieth century, and should be rising for decades ahead. Are human beings getting happier? Not necessarily, says he. And explains the paradox that people become less satisfied over time with a static standard of living. Money can buy happiness but only if the amounts get bigger and other people are not getting more. We feel rich if we have more than our neighbours, poor if we have less.

The belief that once people's basic material wants are satisfied they seek to achieve non-material or spiritual goals doesn't seem to be holding good. Easterlin's evidence anyway points to the persistence of materialism. Each step upward on the ladder of economic development merely stimulates new economic desires that lead the chase ever upward. Needs are limited, not greed; and science has developed no cure for envy, laments the economist.

And he sums up his pessimistic diagnosis: "In the end, the triumph of economic growth is not a triumph of humanity over material wants; rather, it is the triumph of material wants over humanity."

Yet science has opened a new way of happiness—the happiness pill. There are now hundreds of mood-altering drugs, both legal and illegal.

Chemically, electrically, or otherwise, science may eventually provide a technical solution to the problem of happiness. Whether this way of achieving happiness or banishing melancholy is good for the human race is open to question.

Depression or Everyday Unhappiness!

> "You have only a limited number of days on this earth; the fewer spent wishing you weren't, the better off you are."
>
> —Andrew Solomon in his book *The Noonday Demon* (2001)

Andrew Solomon is "fabulously well connected, fabulously social and fabulously rich".

Born rich, graduated from Yale and Cambridge, he's the author of three successful books; his latest one *The Noonday Demon* netting him an advance of $1.3 million. He lives in an enormous mansion, with its constant stream of guests—the powerful, the chic.

Yet at 37 (looks 27, he jokes) Solomon stays depressed. He suffered three breakdowns in five years. And travelled all over the globe in search of treatments—traditional, alternative, fantastical. *The Noonday Demon*, largely an autobiographical account, offers a wealth of detail about depression, its causes and cures.

"What's he got to be depressed with?" one is tempted to ask. But anyone who knows anything about depression will recognize the futility of the question.

Julian L. Simon, the distinguished University of Maryland economist, describes his 13-year-long depression: "When I say that I was depressed I mean that, except for some hours when I was working or playing sports or making love, I was almost continuously conscious of being miserable, and I almost continuously reflected on my worthlessness. I wished for death, and I refrained from killing myself only because I believed my children needed me. Endless hours every day I reviewed my faults and failures, which made me writhe in pain. I refused to let myself do...pleasurable things...because I thought I ought to suffer."

There are several similar components to almost all depressions. Three of these are relatively familiar:

1. Our energy is radically reduced. We feel flaccid.
2. Our enthusiasm is also radically reduced. We lack interest in others, whether family, friends or colleagues, and in those activities which were the day-to-day agenda of our lives.
3. Our hope is gone. Actually, we are profoundly pessimistic, even preoccupied with death. All depressed people share a sense of dread. Almost all the time it feels that the worst hasn't yet happened. Bad as it is, more is coming down, and soon. Only we don't know what it will be.

Once called melancholia, depression is no modern discovery; it was clearly known to ancients. But depression now figures in epidemic proportions, afflicting an estimated one in five in advanced societies. According to Dr A.K.Sharma, the psychiatrist who offered consultations at a recent mental health check-up camp organized in the capital, one out of every four persons in Delhi is suffering from depression, even children as young as 3-4 years old. Dr Sharma attributes it more to all sorts of pollution, overcrowding, and intensified competition for living standards. The demon of depression, unlike the demon of hunger and want, dwells largely amidst the more affluent and sophisticated sections of society.

Depression is often seen by unsympathetic pragmatists as self-indulgence, but there's such a thing as clinical depression, the turning-in of anger on the self for some loss or failing. Whereas grief is depression in proportion to the loss, depression is grief out-of-proportion to the circumstances. And one's failings can be real or imagined.

Severe depression can be quite disabling, almost as disabling as arthritis. Depressed individuals may be spending more days in bed than those with chronic gastrointestinal problems.

Happily for the depressives, medical science has been coming up with a number of effective anti-depressant drugs, offering prospect of relief to a majority of sufferers. Another thing that has helped the treatment of depression is the growing public openness on the subject. Those who have sampled depression's dark offerings are speaking out and seeking help. Styron's book *Darkness Visible* where he mostly discusses his own ordeal of depression has become an important landmark.

The new generation of drugs allows a sophistication and flexibility in treatment that was not possible in the past. And, of all these drugs, Prozac retains its premier position. What's so different in Prozac from the other anti-depressants used for years? The basic principle of all is the same: to bolster the action of serotonin, one crucial chemical that transmits impulses between nerve cells. Shortage of serotonin, scientists believe, is a major cause of depression.

The traditional anti-depressants did the job in a scattered fashion, thus needing larger doses and causing serious side effects like dizziness, blurred vision, constipation and weight gain. They even caused low blood pressure and heart disturbances—real hazards for the elderly. Prozac is more narrowly focussed; it manages to maintain higher levels of serotonin, but with low toxicity.

Introduced in 1987, Prozac, called "the Pill of Pills" has been the hottest psychiatric drug in history. The green and white capsule contains white powder. The recommended dosage is commonly one capsule at breakfast. Prozac is usually taken for not less than 18 months. Till now no serious adverse effects have come to notice among its users; Prozac low toxicity goes in its favour.

Of course, this medical breakthrough is not free from controversies. Peter Kramer in *Listening to Prozac* cites a number of cases where long-term users underwent marked personality changes. One of his patients is now feeling less serious about life. Another woman patient overcame lifelong shyness and began to date regularly. Kramer finds these changes vaguely disturbing.

The unprecedented success of Prozac has given rise to several similar formulations, such as Wellbutrin and Anafranil. And quite a few others are on the way.

The pharmaceutical breakthrough has, however, given rise to a novel phenomenon: the medicalization of unhappiness. Doctors, particularly in the USA, are prescribing "happiness" pills more often to more and more people. This raises the question: Are doctors getting better at diagnosing depression, or are they simply diagnosing "everyday unhappiness" as a variant of depression?

These questions are now at the centre of a debate within the medical community over who the new patients being treated with antidepressants are and what treatment guidelines are being used. There is a suspicion among some doctors that it is not the sickest persons who are being given psychotropic drugs but those patients who complain the loudest about being unhappy. Apologists, in turn, are quick to point out that it is hard to know where everyday unhappiness ends and clinical depression begins, especially borderline depression (i.e., low spirits with no physical symptoms)

In the past, medical science cared for the mentally ill, while everyday unhappiness was left to religious, spiritual, or other cultural guides. Now, medical science is moving beyond its traditional border to help people who are bored, sad, or experiencing low self-esteem.

Evidently, it cannot be a change in life that causes the uplift in spirit, since for the people taking these drugs, life does not change. Generally, most people calculate their happiness by external circumstances. But these drugs enable people to feel better even though their external circumstances remain unchanged. There often develops a lack of congruence between outside circumstances and a medicated patient's good feeling. The outside world becomes, in a way, detached from their inner life. Its influence decreases.

Psychoactive medication, much like alcohol and narcotics, causes a disconnect between the inner and outer life. This is the problem with using it to treat everyday unhappiness. The disconnect caused by medication is very different from the state of thoughtful detachment encouraged by many cultures and religions for the purpose of isolating people from everyday disappointment. The latter contributes to wisdom, stability and maturity; the former creates a state of mind that is somewhat stuporous.

So Many So Depressed

Depression is now the hottest topic in the world of mental health. So many stay so depressed these days. Doctors in turn usually diagnose any complaint of tiredness and lethargy as depression.

Anyone howsoever settled can suffer from depression. Even the fat and jolly are not immune. In a recent bestseller, *Prozac Nation: Young and Depressed in America: A Memoir*, Elizabeth Wurtzel remains terminally depressed and evades suicide with the aid of Prozac, an antidepressant drug. Wurtzel the 28-year-old journalist has everything going for her: glamour, beauty, intelligence, money, success. Here is "a new, groovy kind of depression for a new, groovy kind of people".

Depression can even be a contagious condition in a close relationship, says Thomas Joiner, a psychologist at the University of Texas. In a study of 96 pairs of college roommates, it was observed that roommates of depressed students tended to become more depressed themselves. The other person may become depressed because the originally depressed person is no longer available, having withdrawn into himself/herself from depression.

One bright spot in Joiner's report: "High reassurance seeking roommates of non-depressed targets became somewhat less depressed." In other words, the lowering of depression may also be contagious.

The very act of admitting one's depression makes things easier. No wonder self-help groups such as "Depression Alliance" are springing up in many countries, in the manner of Alcoholics Anonymous. And Samaritan slogans: "Whatever you're going through, we'll go through it with you" or "Defeat Depression".

There is however criticism in some quarters that depression is being "oversold" medically to the elderly. Oldness itself is a reason to be sad if you dwell upon it. Depression in old age is often less a clinical disorder than a natural response to the predictable losses of the elderly: deteriorating physical faculties, loss of friends, all the more compounded for the widowed.

Severe depression can be quite a disabling phenomenon. A few recent studies have shown that depression can be as disabling as arthritis, with depressed individuals spending more days in bed than those with chronic gastrointestinal problems.

Depression is no longer viewed as a simple case of character flaw or lack of self-control. It is now recognized as a disease. And there could be a hereditary disposition to it—depression runs in families. The hereditary vulnerability is then triggered by environmental stress.

Depression can affect children, too—now progressively at a younger age. But it mostly starts from puberty. Women are two to three times more likely to suffer depression than are men; women have to mask their misery under the corset of duty and family. And people under forty are three times more likely to suffer depression than their elders.

What exactly is causing this rising incidence of depression? No one knows for sure, more so when the phenomenon involves both societal factors and the personal-cum-economic problems of individuals. It is however surmised that the diminishing role of the extended family could be to blame. Another could be the lessening reliance on religion as a moral support. Then there's a huge increase in the pressures and expectations which society places on individuals, especially the young. The changing roles between men and women can also be causing confusion and stress.

Women and Depression

Simi often stays depressed. There are days when depression brings on deadening lethargy or bouts of self-loathing. These spells of despondency interfere with her appetite and sleep, perhaps her sexual drive, too.

Simi and her architect husband Mohan, live in a well-appointed flat of their own. They have two kids, a girl of three and a baby boy 2 months old. To their relatives and friends, Mohans are a happily married couple, enjoying good income, and with no particular worry in the world.

Simi isn't exactly sure what makes her so depressed? Is it because she has put on hold a promising career in textile designing to rear a family? Is she envious of her counterparts working at interesting jobs? Or, was she getting jealous of Mohan himself—smartly groomed every morning and busily driving away to work, while she in her nightclothes was left changing nappies and dusting sofas? Or, is it something genetic—her mother was definitely depressive?

Simi, sharp and sensitive, would love to shake off this shadow of sadness. She has tried more of reading novels, more of serial watching, and more of elaborate cooking. Yet the depression descends on her whenever she's free from work.

Simi's dilemma: should she call attention to her mental unrest or should she simply soldier on in silence? She doesn't seem inclined to seek professional help.

Depression is defined as an emotional state marked by melancholy, inactivity, and self-deprecation. The depression may be fleeting or chronic, mild or severe. What is central to depression is the element of self-loathing, a sense of one's worthlessness or abject failure. Sometimes these feelings are strong enough to produce suicidal urges. This self-denigration, psychiatrists say, often stems from a sub-conscious disappointment or anger or hatred towards another person or even a circumstance.

And, unlike the demons of hunger and want, the demon of depression largely dwells among the affluent and the sophisticated sections of a populace. With rising living standards and competitive pressures, depression has become a common scourge in advanced societies, afflicting an estimated one in ten.

Happily for the depressives, medical science is fast coming up with a number of effective anti-depressant drugs. Whereas a mild depression may respond to talking therapy alone, most cases call for a combination of drugs and psychotherapy.

One thing that has helped the treatment of depression is the new-fledged openness on the subject. Those who have sampled depression's dark offerings are speaking out and seeking help. Styron's book *Darkness Visible* where he mostly discusses his own ordeal of depression has become an important landmark. In Styron's case, the depression lifted, burned off by drugs and psychotherapy, and stay in a hospital. However people who come out of it have to watch against a recurrence of the same—the way reformed alcoholics do.

The new generation of drugs allows a sophistication and flexibility in treatment that was not possible in the past. And, of all these drugs, Prozac retains its premier position.

But no drug is ever perfect. Some side effects are always there, such as constipation and dry mouth. Medicines can't gift happiness to mankind without exacting some price. The sorrow of a broken love affair, the death of a dear one, or the loss of a job or money or position can't be simply overcome by medicines.

One important development in dealing with depression is the emergence of gender-sensitive psychology. It is being increasingly recognized that women require different medication and behavioural therapy than men because of their different hormonal surges, especially progesterone's ebb and flow with the menstrual cycle. Many women also fall prey to postpartum depression, a minor or major depression that overcomes them in the weeks after a childbirth; sometimes lasting as much as a year. The same can be occasioned by hormonal changes as well as the added stress of a newborn child. With quite a few women, the birth of a child also marks the start of marital violence.

"It's a common misconception among psychiatrists and psychologists that the risks and causes of depression in men and women are the same, so treatment should be the same," says Ellen McGrath, chairwoman of the 30-member US expert panel on female depression and disorders. "But none of that's true. Paying attention to gender differences is an essential part of therapy for depression." Besides biology, men and women are brought up differently.

The expert panel found that the incidence of depression showed up twice as often in women as in men, and for a far wider variety of causes, including violence and sexual abuse against them, excessive focussing on depressed feelings, hormonal effects of the menstrual cycle, birth control pills and childbirth, body dissatisfactions, marriage strains, pressure of parenting, and weaker economic position.

Psychotherapists are therefore counselled to look carefully for those underlying factors to choose from an array of therapy approaches that are especially effective with women's problems. For example, group therapy is considered more useful for women than men. The latter tend to lack confidants, while women open up more easily to close friends.

What about the children off depressed women? A barrage of recent studies conclusively proves what was suspected: the children of depressed parents particularly mothers—like the children of alcoholics—can suffer significant psychological damage. Their emotional scars, starting as early as the first few months of infancy, can last deep into adolescence and possibly beyond. Many deficits and disturbances have been observed in these children such as low birth weight and excessive crying in newborn babies whose mothers were depressed during pregnancy (detailed in the book *Gloom in the Womb*; inability to smile starting at 3 months of age; lower concentration in school; hostile behaviour or a withdrawal in adolescence; and increased depression as time goes on.

Depressed mothers are emotionally "flattened" and are thus able to give less encouragement and affection to their children. At some moments she may be sharp and angry at being bothered, at others she may become intrusively involved in her kids. An "overcontrolling" depressive mother might sit for hours clutching and stroking a four-year-old. Middle-class mothers with postpartum depression may even tend to display far more irritability and volatility with their infants during the first six months than non-depressed mothers. Their infants in turn often become withdrawn, refusing even to look at them, what to say of smiling at them. For a child, the first six months are crucial for learning social interactions, and the same get retarded in these kids.

In adolescence, the troubles of children with depressed parents mount up. Either the child becomes wild, out-of-control, or overtly obedient and sensitive. These are the strategies a growing child usually adopts to gain the attention of the preoccupied depressed parent. In both ways it hurts the adolescent's personality.

The point of all the current research on parental depression isn't to aim an accusing finger at the parents for their children's problems. The basic aim is to help depressed parents, particularly mothers. She has to examine the hard facts of her life to identify the cause of her depression, whether it's from being deprived of the satisfaction of an outside job or from a destructive marriage.

Meanwhile experts offer a few tips to depressed mothers when dealing with their children.

Avoid talking your problems to your children; it will only undermine their sense of security. Instead, talk to your spouse, a friend, a therapist.

Never criticize your child; only criticize specific behaviour. Say "That was selfish," not "You're a selfish girl".

Don't malign your parenting skills to your children. Learn these skills if you are deficient.

Our Phobias

What a paradox are phobias? They are common but kept hidden; they are curable but left untreated. It is estimated that one person in 15 suffers a phobia. These can develop at any age, though the incidence of phobias is higher in young and women.

The essence of phobia is fear out of proportion to any threat involved—an unrealistic fear, seemingly inappropriate and unreasoning. For instance, it's understandable to fear snakes while walking in a snake-infested area. But to freeze on seeing snakes in a zoo snake-pit or even ones appearing on television is something entirely different.

Sources of perceived threats are well-nigh numerous: flying, heights, hospitals, needles, closed or crowded spaces, snakes, spiders, lizards, dogs, cats, cows, horses, bacteria, dirt, darkness, water, fire, thunder, lightning, strangers, flowers, even specific numbers like 3 or 7. It's an endless list. And each one of these phobias has been duly given a scientific name. The word phobia itself comes from the Greek word *phobos*, meaning dread or panic.

Irrespective of the source of phobia, their effects on phobics are almost identical. They provoke apprehension, a pounding of heart, tenseness, and a feeling as if one's going to faint. Panic attacks can be severe enough to make a person lose control, opt for a reckless escape, even grow berserk or drop dead.

A phobia impels you to avoid the feared thing, which in turn makes your fear greater when you have to face it next time. That way steering clear of what terrifies you is no real answer to an irrational fear.

And such escape could be impractical too. A sufferer of aquaphobia (fear of water) could avoid going into or near deep water. But avoidance isn't easy against agoraphobia (fear of public places). Life can become quite restrictive for phobics who fear to venture out into crowded streets or buses, negotiate busy railway stations or mingle with large public gatherings.

What causes phobia is still incompletely understood, despite much research on the subject. Many theories have come and gone. Psychoanalysts blamed it on unresolved sexual conflicts—a teenage girl's spider phobia (arachnophobia) stemming from the hairy sexuality in those arachnid legs. Behaviourists say that all fear is learned, mostly in childhood, like a childhood experience of being nudged by a cow or nearly getting drowned in water. Others believe that many of these fears are basically genetic; we inherit them in our genes. To it is added the parental example. If, after you are bitten by a dog, your parents panic whenever you are near one, then according to theories of observational learning you are likely to acquire a fear of your own.

Approaches to treatment of phobias also differ, reflecting the different theories about their causes. In some phobias drugs that augment the action of serotonin are found helpful, drugs like the latest anti-depressive Prozac. However the mainstay of most treatment plans is exposure to what is feared, a reversal of the previous avoidance. This is usually done gradually, starting with smaller doses (not unlike injecting a controlled, safe element of a disease through vaccine to confer immunity). Exposure levels are increasingly raised, allowing time to learn relaxation techniques and counter fearful thoughts.

Here are a few common phobias, of which I happen to have some personal experience.

Claustrophobia: I don't know how and when I became claustrophobic—the fear of closed places. But it has dogged me for years. And this I know that my mother was highly claustrophobic, though my brothers are not.

Claustrophobia often grips me when travelling alone in a small lift, or when the doors of a plane are ordered shut. Lying at night in a train carriage with lights off can trigger the same. At times I just can't help sitting up and switching on the light, unmindful of what my fellow passengers might say. My worst experience was when visiting the Kolar Gold Mines, the lift took a party of us down to a mile. Nearing the bottom I was seized with such a panic of being closed in that only the exercise of utmost self-control kept me from shrieking.

The standard treatment is to expose the claustrophobic to what he or she fears most. If you're afraid of lifts, they'll make you go up and down in one repeatedly, till the fear is gone. In the beginning someone may come along but soon you go alone, briefed with some facts about how safe are modern lifts.

Aerophobia: My fear of flying has both an element of claustrophobia—being packed in a narrow metal tube with all exits barred, and the scare about plane safety. I'm assailed by images of birds flying into the jet intake, mechanics with hangovers forgetting to tighten bolts, pilots in poor shape from fatigue, or a hijacker with a hand grenade.

The very idea of something as heavy as a huge plane—loaded with so much luggage and packed full with passengers—lifting up in the air and staying there is never fully convincing. The landing manoeuvre is supposed to be the riskiest of all but I, for one, am most frightened at the time of take-off. Suppose the plane fails to lift; it will end up crashing through the boundary barrier. I keep gripping the armrests tight till the aircraft actually comes off the ground. The fact that runways have the requisite extra space for halting the 180mph speeding plane if the take-off aborts, hardly makes any dent into my apprehensions.

Maybe, I should take the kind of course a friend of mine recently took in London. Run by the British Airways, the one-day course cost him £ 129. His aerophobia, he says, is now a thing of the past. Indeed he has started enjoying air travel.

His account of the *Aviatours' Fly with Confidence* course runs like this. It began by a senior pilot—with a calming trust-me-smile—explaining the triplicated safety devices fitted to the vital equipment of every aircraft, the extensive tests a plane undergoes before flying, the rigorous training standards that all pilots must satisfy which can often take up to 20 years to complete. "No other job, no matter what it is, is examined so thoroughly and regularly as that of a pilot," he stressed. Things like aircraft noise, banking, wing movement and the physics of flying were explained. And answers given to people's misgivings on lightning striking the plane or it getting buffeted in wind turbulence.

The psychologist on the course clarified how our fears could be made to vanish with some understanding and knowledge about flying. And he taught various relaxation techniques like self-talk routines and breathing exercises.

After lunch—soft drinks only; the dehydrating Dutch courage firmly frowned upon—there was an hour's flight in a Boeing 757. Participants were encouraged to walk about in the plane, visit the cockpit or otherwise feel relaxed. The captain and the crew chatted and laughed with the participants and everybody got into good spirits.

Trypanophobia: It is difficult to explain how the world appears to someone who's afraid of needles. A grown-up person showing obsessive fear of an injection is more a laughing matter than a subject for sympathy.

Yet I've suffered from trypanophobia since my boyhood. Lucky, we now have more oral medicines than injections. It's not only the pain of the prick, I nurse the notion that needles have the knack of breaking in the flesh and travelling into the body. And now the additional fears of a needle being contaminated with AIDS.

I can't look at my arm when taking a prick; in fact, I turn away my gaze even when someone dear is getting pricked. Of late, a friendly doctor has been trying to help me overcome my fear of needles. And he seems to be succeeding.

Phobias, psychiatrists tell us, are curable. Yet it does involve a good deal of motivation on the part of the phobic and competent expert intervention. Many of us, it seems, go on living with our phobias when energetic steps could see us getting rid of them.

Secrets of Sleep

"Most people overeat 100 per cent, and oversleep 100 per cent, because they like it. That extra 100 per cent makes them unhealthy and inefficient."

The man who wrote these words in his diary was Thomas Alva Edison, the man who invented the electric bulb. Once the bulb banished darkness, the average person's sleep time of 9 hours each night came down by 1 ½ hour.

How much sleep do we need? All of us sort out this question for ourselves. Society lauds those who are known to cut down on sleep for work. In fact, during the 1980s sleep became somewhat unfashionable—with the attendant belief that those who couldn't function without their nightly eight hours were soft, flabby, and weak. Mrs Thatcher crowed on needing only fours hours of slumber. Mrs Indira Gandhi was said to be doing well with five hours of it.

Can we really alter our sleep requirement or otherwise change our sleep habits? Veteran sleep researcher Dr. Wilse B. Webb of the University of Florida answers: "I spent five years of my life trying to prevent nocturnal rats from sleeping during the day, and they spent five years teaching me I was rather foolish." Human beings can alter their sleep pattern temporarily, but they return to a sleep budget that seems genetically fixed.

First the fundamental question: what is sleep? Why should we spend one-third of our lives at this unproductive activity—in a state which imitates death? A sixty-year-old person, for example, has spent at least twenty years asleep.

Sleep is a process that is so important to the physical and psychological well-being of living things that nature has gone to inordinate lengths to allow sleep. Some birds can sleep while in flight. Some fish can sleep while swimming. A giraffe takes up to a minute to get up, uncurling those lanky legs. During this time the animal is completely unprotected. To place the giraffe in such a position of vulnerability each day, sleep must be very important indeed. "If sleep does not serve an absolutely vital function, then it is the biggest mistake the evolutionary process has made," says Dr. Allan Rechtschaffen, a sleep researcher at the University of Chicago.

Many theories have been formulated; yet why we sleep remains an enduring mystery. In small mammals, sleep may save precious energy (in lowering the thermostat sleep conserves energy and the need for food) when the prospects for foraging are not good, but in other species this explanation is not satisfactory. In despair, some have suggested that sleep may simply have kept our ancestors out of trouble at night.

Poets, artists, and common folk alike have always assumed that sleep is rest for both the body and brain—welcome period of recovery, whether from physical or mental exertion.

> "O sleep! O gentle sleep!
> Nature's soft nurse. . ."
>
> Shakespeare in *Henry IV.*

Yet, a simple observation suggests that sleep is, in its essence, for the brain. If we lie awake but immobile for an entire night, in the morning our muscles may be relaxed but our mind is not, and our sense of well-being is lost. A waking brain is conscious. Sleep, or perhaps certain phases of sleep evidently offer the blessing of unconsciousness or at least liberation from the tyranny of memory and thought.

"Some people think they don't move at all in sleep," says Dr. J Allan Hobson, professor at the Harvard Medical School. "They swear to you that they go to bed and never change position. Not true. My studies show that everybody makes at least 8 to 12 major posture shifts at night. Insomniacs may double or triple that." In fact, on average, we change positions every 12 minutes while we sleep.

Too many sharp movements constitute "tossing and turning" and make for poor sleep, but too few shifts–sleeping like a log—may be worse. Alcohol, for one, inhibits movement. Someone drunk to stupor risks paralysis in sleep. You can kill a nerve in one night just by lying on it—for example, the radial nerve in the upper arm.

People in their 60s and beyond start to feel sleepy earlier in the evening—as if the brain had moved forward a few time zones. And they wake up correspondingly early. That way, late nights aren't the thing for older folks.

After the common cold, difficulty with sleeping is perhaps the most prevalent health complaint, ranging from transient insomnia to dreaded narcolepsy. There are more than 50 sleep disorders, the prominent ones: head banging, sleep walking, nightmares, SIDS (Sudden Infant Death Syndrome), teeth grinding, restless legs syndrome, apnea, snoring, and other breathing disorders.

The largest complaints, of course, are about insomnia, a mask for many conditions. Insomnia itself is not an illness but a symptom of some other disease or problem. The leading contenders are anxiety, drug or alcohol dependency, or psychiatric disturbances. Often, the difficulty begins during a time of stress but lingers after the crisis has passed.

The worst thing about insomnia: the world appears hopeless to an insomniac around 4am. F. Scott Fitzgerald, the noted American writer, observed in his autobiographical pieces *The Crack-Up*: "In the long dark night of the soul, it is always three in the morning".

The despair is primarily physiological. The body's blood sugar is at its lowest point in the wee small hours of the morning, which in turn, means that the brain is more prone to depression and general gloom. Experts advise, better munch on chocolates, if you aren't inclined to get up for work at that hour. Chocolate does send a rush of sugar into the blood stream—life always looks better after chocolate.

For double-bed couples, every sleep disturbance is a shared one and, if you add duvet wars, the disruptions of small children, different body temperatures (fit people are hottest), not to mention snoring, groaning, scratching, lip-smacking, nose-whistling, clucking, kicking, the case is unarguable: whosoever sleeps alone sleeps best.

The night is prime regenerative time for your skin, especially in the wee small hours of the morning. With a surge in collagen the skin repairs some of the DNA damage sustained by it during the day through exposure to Ultra-Violet rays.

And the skin stays more porous at night. That way any skincare used on the face or the body before retiring for the night is likely to be more effective at getting to the lower levels of the skin where it's actually needed.

On average, we lose about half a litre of fluid from the body each night. This dehydrates the skin—another good reason to moisture the skin well before bed. "If the skin is dehydrated, creasing on the face (from the weight of the head in some sleeping positions) won't bounce back and you'll actually create a permanent line in the skin," says an American dermatologist Professor Mary Lupo. That is why those who sleep with their face down get more wrinkled than those who sleep with face up. A satin pillowcase is some help, if you can't sleep face up.

And you can do your heart a favour if you don't jump out of bed too suddenly in the morning. The circulatory system, otherwise at relative rest, has to work much harder to cope with the sudden movement; and this can't be good if there is a weakness in the heart.

Incidentally the levels of testosterone in men and progesterone in women are significantly higher in the morning hours than at any other time of the day or night. That way the best time for lovemaking would be morning, not the usual nighttime before retiring to bed.

Strategies Against Insomnia

Do you have trouble sleeping? And, worse still, do you *worry* about having trouble sleeping? You've got plenty of company. Countless adults complain about insomnia—insufficient or unsatisfactory sleep. And no medication is used more widely than sleeping pills.

How much sleep do we need? The correct amount of sleep for you is more a personal thing, depending on how you feel the next morning. A few historical figures— Leonardo da Vinci, Napolean, Goethe—are said to have managed with with something like 4 hours of sleep. The accepted norm for adults is currently around seven and half hours.

Researchers have determined from diaries and other evidence that the typical person in the eighteenth and nineteenth centuries slept a total of nine-and-a-half hours each night. By 1950's it had dropped down to eight. And the average has been declining since then in urban, industrialized societies.

It is commonly believed that the elderly need a lot less sleep. Yet a man of 75 needs only half an hour less than a 35-year old. Some busy people follow the strategy of under-sleeping on weekdays, to be made up by sleeping longer hours on weekends. But this ability to accumulate sleep—to have a long period of sleep without arousal—seems to lessen with age.

But then what's the whole point of sleep? Despite all the accelerated research on the subject in the last fifty years, huge gaps in our knowledge persist. No one really knows why we need sleep. It can't be just to while away the sunless hours. Consolidating all sleep into a single block is again a peculiarly human trait. Most animals catnap, take their sleep activity in smaller doses.

"The only known function of sleep," says Seidel, director of Stanford's Centre for Insomnia Research, "is to promote wakefulness for the next day."

What do you do if you're having trouble sleeping? What are the self-help techniques, and when has one to seek medical intervention?

The latest trend in insomnia treatment is the recognition that there's no single answer to how to sleep better. It's important for physicians and sufferers alike to focus on precisely what the nature of the sleep problem might be. That way treatment can be targetted to the specific problem.

One person may struggle to fall asleep but sleep like a baby once he does. Another person may have no trouble falling asleep but may be unable to sleep restfully through the night, waking up time after time. Yet another might easily fall asleep, sleep like a log, but always wake up too early, unable to get back to sleep.

Here are a few self-help strategies you could profitably employ if you happen to suffer from any of these symptoms.

Trouble Falling Asleep: First of all, don't worry too much about having trouble falling asleep; the worry itself can start to interfere with your ability to fall asleep, even when the initial cause of sleeplessness is gone. "Trying to sleep is the worst thing you can do," cautions Peter Hauri, director of the insomnia programme at the Mayo Clinic in Rochester, Minnesota in his book *No More Sleepless Nights* (John Wiley, 1990), "because the more you try to sleep and focus on sleeping, the harder it will be to fall asleep."

And he adds, "The clock in the bedroom is poison in most cases. It puts too much pressure on you to fall asleep." Better stick your alarm clock in a drawer, hide your wristwatch, and throw a towel over the VCR clock, too.

Relaxation techniques, such as meditation or controlled breathing with relaxed muscles help. You have to find what you are most comfortable with. Feel your body relax. Counting sheep isn't as silly as it sounds.

Learn to associate your bedroom with sleepiness, not tossing about in frustration. Better retire to your bedroom only when you're sleepy Don't make yourself go to bed at a certain time if you aren't tired. Some sleep experts even go as far as to say that you shouldn't read, or eat or watch TV in bed. If you're having trouble falling asleep, get up and go to another room until you're sleepy again.

Almost everybody is agreed that caffeine—over three cups of strong coffee a day—can delay sleep. Your body's tolerance of caffeine can also be dramatically altered as you grow older. And caffeine is much longer acting than people appreciate. Heavy smoking is still worse for insomniacs.

Many people use alcohol to help them sleep. While alcohol may induce sleep, at the same time it lowers the quality of your sleep; often wakes you up four hours later in a state of gloom. Similarly sleeping pills like Valium get people to sleep 15-20 minutes earlier for the first few days, but after that they do no good—and increasing amounts of harm.

Unsound Sleep: The body's temperature normally goes up during the day and down at night, often by as much as 2 degree F. But insomniacs have less variation. They don't get as warm in the day or as cool at night, and their sleep stays shallow and fragmented.

The link between exercise and sleep was known. But new sleep experts are more specific about *when* and *why* of exercise. You should heat your body with exercise about six hours before bedtime. Thus you'll start cooling down just as you want to go to sleep. While exercise—walking, running, cycling—three times a week will help your heart, but it may not be enough to promote sleep. Half an hour five days a week is a good target. If you really want to sleep naturally, live naturally.

If you tend to get distracted by outside noises, better mask these with the neutral noise of a room air-conditioner, or cooler, or fan, or hot air blower. A backgound of The New Age rainforest music has helped many overcome distracted sleep.

A room too hot or too cold can awaken you. And so also a heavy, spicy dinner. The latter increases production of stomach acids which are disruptive of sleep.

Awaking Too Early: Many people have no trouble falling asleep or sleeping soundly through the night. But they cannot remain awake beyond the early morning hours and they cannot manage to sleep till sunrise. They're suffering from *advanced sleep phase syndrome* (ASPS), which is essentially the opposite of delayed sleep disorder. Whereas the latter is prevalent in young persons, often from tensions of work, ASPS is common in old age. People under depression get awakened too early in the morning, often preceded by unpleasant dreams—we dream more towards the early morning hours.

While depression has to be taken care of separately, a good strategy is to delay sleep. Fortunately there is a solution: bright light—4 to 5 times brighter than ordinary indoor lighting. Bright light, especially when falling on the face, helps to reset the body's circadian rhythm, or internal clock, which has been found to control hormone levels, body temperature and arousal.

Gradually as you delay falling asleep with the help of bright light, your waking time will shift accordingly. Choose a sensible and practical time to get up, and get up then.

Sleep specialists advocate a nap in daytime, something that the young and busy often deny themselves. According to brain wave tests and other studies, human beings have an inherent tendency to sleep "twice" a day—an urgent need to sleep for many hours at night and a less urgent need to sleep briefly in the afternoon. Such naps are rated as proper sleep and contribute to the total daily sleep requirement. An afternoon nap is particularly useful in warding off an undesirably early onset of night sleep.

Your sleep disorder could also be due to some physical condition like apnea or narcolepsy, or milder ones such as the restless legs syndrome or teeth grinding.

Apnea, which is marked by heavy snoring, is very common. But serious cases call for treatment, and here drugs or surgery are quite effective.

Narcolepsy whose symptoms are excessive daytime sleepiness and at times, sudden, uncontrollable sleep attacks is again amenable to treatment.

Similarly medical science can successfully intervene to alleviate restless legs syndrome and teeth grinding.

Sleepy Teens and Schools

Stop waking up teenagers at the crack of dawn, and they just might make better grades in school. That's the latest word from sleep scientists and education experts.

By the early 1990s, researchers began to find, surprisingly yet consistently, that the sleep patterns of adolescents in high school are discernibly different from those of younger children as well as from adults. Their circadian rhythms, determined by the release of the hormone melatonin and other factors, were telling them to stay up later and to get up later. Teenagers often feel alert into late hours of the night—well after their parents have collapsed into bed.

From age 12 to 18, we see a steady pushing back of time at which young people go to bed, especially socially-active urban teenagers. And that's not only for studies; it could be television, hobbies, or "partying". Anything important or interesting is good enough to push back their bedtime. On the other hand, schools are sticking to their traditional regime of starting early; some even starting earlier than before.

Parents often experience considerable difficulty in waking up a teenager. While the pre-adolescent children tend to wake up easily and seem eager to start the day, teenagers usually need several reminders and much prodding to get up. Parents even tell you of times when they actually pushed a teenager out of bed, only to find him asleep on the floor. Sleep-deprived teenagers can be as cranky as tired three-year-olds and even less fun to deal with. The countervailing belief (it's the early bird that gets the worm) that this was largely laziness on the kids' part is rather misplaced.

Researchers have also come to the equally unexpected conclusion that teenagers as a group need *more* sleep than pre-adolescents—that their bodies and minds require additional unconsciousness to grow best. Studies worldwide indicate that the optimal sleep time for most teenagers was around 9 hours a night.

It is in this context that William Demant—the world's leading sleep specialist who discovered REM—makes out that "very early high school start times are not only misguided, they're inherently 'abusive' to many high school kids." Education experts believe an early start best for the needs of younger children, while the later start seems best for high schoolers.

No wonder, many a teenager with early school timings— further compounded with long bus rides or long travel time—has been observed to reach school with his or her brain essentially in sleep-mode. Subjected to prolonged commuting time, high schoolers often have to get up as early as 6. In one recent American survey, half of early-rising 10th graders were found to be in the "pathological" range of sleepiness at 8 a.m. "The students may be in school, but their brains are at home on their pillows," says Mary Carkskadon, editor of the book *Adolescent Sleep Patterns*, 2002.

Researchers have also observed that sleep-deprived kids can't learn as well, and display impaired ability to pay attention, to remember and to do calculations fast. Indeed it has been found that sleep-debt in teenagers leads to impulsive behavior, losing control of the moment, and that's when really bad things can happen. And loss of sleep also increases teenage drivers' already elevated risk of car accidents.

In the light of these findings, efforts at Congressional level have been made in USA to change the commonly prevalent high school timings of 8.00-8.30 and 3.30-4.00 to 9.00-9.30 and 4.30-5.00. This would not only give the teenagers an extra hour of sorely-needed sleep but will help keep them off the streets from 4 to 5 p.m., peak hours for juvenile delinquency.

The voices of change include many students (though not all), some parents, medical and sleep experts. But then any such change is opposed by most teachers (worried it would lengthen their work day), transportation officers (it would raise transport costs), and coaches (fearing shrinkage of extracurricular activities).

As a result the move has made little headway, except for some selected schools taking it up on an experimental basis. Nobody seriously challenges the strength of arguments advanced by sleep researchers, whereby teenagers would gain an added hour of sleep as well as get to school when they are 'most ready to learn'. Yet, vested interests and practical difficulties in implementation make the switchover rather daunting.

The subject of school timings vis-à-vis the sleep pattern of teenagers has yet to trigger a serious debate in our country. In fact there has been a trend towards opening of high schools earlier than before, while commuting time has been steadily rising in big cities. On top, teenagers are going to bed much later than before.

The result: many a youngster gets up fighting his biological clock and reaches school carrying a sleep debt. The consequences for students losing sleep by early rising are clear; they lose a significant ability to learn, especially during the beginning teaching periods.

New Approaches to Dreaming

Everyone of us dreams. As grown-ups we regularly dream for about one-and-half hour every night. And now we know that dream sleep occurs to most mammals, even birds, with unfailing regularity.

Research into sleep made a major breakthrough in the middle 1950s with the discovery of REM sleep. There are actually two different kinds of sleep: REM (the rapid eye movement phases) and NREM (the non-rapid eye movement periods). When we fall asleep we start with 70-90 minutes of N R E M sleep, followed by some 15 minutes of REM sleep. And this NREM-REM cycle goes on through the night, with REM phases getting longer as the night proceeds.

REM sleep is distinguished by the appearance of rapid eye movement behind the closed eyelids. Periodic twitching of facial muscles is common. There is marked increase in heartbeat and blood pressure. Brain temperature goes up, indicative of heightened brain activity. Sleepers have vivid dream experience during REM phases.

Wake someone during REM sleep, and he or she may be able to recall bulk of what was being dreamed. But if the sleeper isn't awakened, most of the dream will be lost. Dreams melt quickly; perhaps 95 per cent of what we dream is never remembered. No wonder some people claim they never dream.

On the well-tested principle that nature rarely does something for nothing, we can easily assume that dreams serve some important function. Volunteers deprived of REM sleep by experimenters developed symptoms of psychological disturbances. When later allowed to sleep without interruption, they gave evidence of dreaming intensively as if to compensate for previous deprivation.

What is the exact function of dreaming? This is now an area of much scientific research, aided by advances in neurobiology and instrumentation. Far more is getting known about the human brain; that it contains between 20 billion to 100 billion nerve cells. And that the brain's nerve cells communicate in chemical messages called neurotransmitters, with each nerve cell or neuron in simultaneous communication with upwards of 10,000 others. Each cell sends between two and a hundred messages every second, ceaselessly, day and night.

Freud, making his brilliant psychoanalytical interpretation of dreams, didn't have the advantage of all this neurobiological knowledge. According to him when the inhibitory demands of wakefulness are diminished in sleep, our repressed wishes, particularly those associated with sex and hostility, are released in dreams- the basis of his "wish fulfillment" theory. And these wish impulses are apt to come in disguised form; a person dreaming of slicing a melon (manifest) rather than hacking an enemy (latent). Freud's exposition and the elaboration to it from others following him, stayed supreme till the new era of dream research began with the discovery of REM.

A hardheaded scientific attitude is crystalizing that dreaming, rather than revealing our repressed yearnings, may be carrying out vital maintenance work for our minds. Free of the stimuli of waking hours, the brain may be catching upon its filing, assimilating, categorizing and storing in memory.

To Allen Hobson, a Harvard psychiatrist and neuroscientist, dreams are caused by electrochemical signals darting helter-skelter around the brain, like untied ballons released in a room. That's why dreams are so bizarre. He disagrees with Freud's view that dreams are obscure and require analysis to know their import. To him, dreams are transparent, uncensored, only unedited, and dreaming is a process as automatic as breathing. If dreams had any special meaning or information to convey, how do we explain that ninety-nine messages in every hundred are lost before they are delivered.

Two neuroscientists, Crick and Mitchison, have advanced the "theory of elimination". According to them, dreaming is the way by which we rid ourselves regularly of those accidental or inefficient files we accumulate in our brains during daily lives. The nightly acts of dreaming send charges through the memory networks not to illuminate but to eliminate from the brain information we don't need to remember. Dreaming keeps the computer from getting overloaded, they say. To them, remembering a dream indicates that the brain did not satisfactorily accomplish its nighttime housekeeping chores. But then the critics of this speculative theory ask the question: if the brain is ridding itself of an unnecessary load, what determines what's to be kept?

Dreaming, some say, may be offering a repeated opportunity to rehearse important strategies for surviving in the waking world. For an animal it could be search for a prey or a concern for one's own safety. For a human being with the more complex world, it may be ambition, jealousy, love, hate, insecurity, sexual activity and other social interactions.

Supporting evidence for the premise is forthcoming in laboratory experiments. For instance Dr Michael Jovet of France has shown that during REM sleep cats seem to be acting out "predation strategies". By clever neurosurgery, Jovet linked brain and muscle in his laboratory cats so that, during sleep, they would be able to move their bodies in accordance with what was going on inside their heads. As soon as they went into REM, the cats would crouch and spring at imaginary mice. Incidentally cat and human brains are roughly similar in design, and for a student of sleep a better subject would be hard to find.

Bert O. States, Professor of Dramatic Art at the University of California, has advanced another theory of dreams in his book *The Rhetoric of Dreams* (Cornell University Press, 1988). Far from censoring unacceptable thoughts, States says, the dream is one of the most direct of psychic functions, processing experience in patterns of association. He thus regards the dream as a means by which the mind "thinks" images out of feelings and attitudes and then converts these images into other images along the path of the dream narrative. A parallel is drawn between dreaming and art-making. In States's view the dreamer, like the poet or painter, is an image maker with a unique capacity to be alive inside his own images. Though the book draws heavily on the insights of psychology and neurophysiology, the theory is unlikely to attract serious scientific attention.

And now comes another book *Crisis Dreaming* by Rosalind Cartwrig and Lynne Lam (Harper Collins, 1992). The book is about what we dream when suffering a crisis, and what strategies could be adopted to alter bad dreams, even use dreaming for positive support in waking life. Here's a brief account of what the authors say.

During the day we may fool ourselves and others by putting on a good front, by denying the excitement or fear that any major change may bring, but our dreams show what is really going on inside. Night after night they reflect the ever-changing circumstances of our daily lives. In our dreams we connect today's experiences to earlier ones that involved similar feelings. Each night, our dreams help us get ready to face tomorrow's demands.

Some people think that dreams burst forth, fully formed, in seconds. They don't. They last from 10 minutes at the beginning of the night to as long as 45 minutes just before we wake up. The first dream usually states the theme for those that follow, drawing on a recent experience, usually one involving some feelings of anxiety or uncertainty. The next harks back to a similar earlier experience, and the rest integrate the old and the new. Dream stories become "crazier" in each succeeding REM phase, more complex in story structure and more remote from present reality. It is from the last one, the one that is often the most fantastic, that we usually wake up.

Dreams of men and women are remarkably different. Studies indicate that men and women in the same college courses or in the same profession dream differently—despite social changes human nature has not changed.

Women have more friendlier characters in their dreams than men do. While women usually dream of home and families, shopping and doing things with kids, men's dreams relate more to travelling and fixing things, working or competing with others. Women's dreams are more likely to take place indoors, and men's outdoors. Whether you are a male or female is a far more potent determinant of nature of your dreams than whether you are young or old.

Dreams are designed to help maintain our self-identity, our sense of who we are, as our life circumstances change. We need a good self-image to ride successfully the bumps of everyday life. Those whose dreams suggest that all is not well should not be content to shrug them off as unimportant. A bad dream, like an elevated temperature, is a symptom that something is wrong—a sort of emotional thermostat. It is a distress signal, a message from our sleeping mind to our waking mind that is risky to ignore. Studies also show that the mind-set we have during our dreams affects our attitudes and behaviour the following day. After a bad dream, we awaken more discouraged than we were at bedtime. After a good one, we feel more optimistic.

Although bad dreams are more common than good ones, most bad dreams do not wake us. But nightmares, the frightening heart-pounding ones, do propel us from sleep. Nightmares are actually a cry for resolution, for finding a way to incorporate the terrible experience into our lives.

When our daily lives fit well into our established sense of self, our nightly dream work runs on automatic pilot. Our dreams do their work silently whether we pay attention or not. But in times of crisis dreams go into action.

The crisis dreaming method aims to change hurtful dreams to positive, healthy ones. It enables people to stop bad dreams while they are in progress and rewrite the scripts. In this way we can redirect dreaming to perform its proper function: to reinforce our sense of identity—first by recognizing those aspects of our present crisis that are negative, and next by finding images of strength already filed in our memory banks. Thus we can activate those images to change our waking attitudes.

The crisis dreaming method has been used to restore self-confidence to people with life-threatening illnesses and victims of rape and other demoralizing assaults. The technique can be undertaken alone or with the help of a therapist. It is said that to negotiate one's way adroitly through stormy times, one needs four things: good friends, good genes, good self-image, and good dreams.

If you currently are wrestling with a major life crisis, the first step is to pay more attention to your dreams. Of course the conventional wisdom says that most of us can only recover from a crisis by changing our waking lives, not our dreams. Yet changing the endings of your bad dreams can be a giant step towards recovery.

Under the crisis dreaming method people are encouraged to recall as much of their dreams as possible. They are advised to keep a dream diary, as well as a day diary. When admitted to a sleep laboratory, a technician monitors the recording chart and watches the sleeper on a video monitor. He knows that a dream is hatching each time the brain waves speed up and the eyes begin to move rapidly. Accounting for the average dream span of various REM phases, he wakes the sleeper closest to when the dream is ending, but before it is ended. Then the awakened person, lying in the same sleeping pose, is asked to recall his dream on a tape recorder. People are known to recall bulk of their dreams when assisted in this fashion.

The premise of dream therapy is that if bad dreams make you awaken discouraged and downhearted, rewriting the scripts to improve the endings should lead to better moods. The four steps are: to recognize when you are having a bad dream; to identify what it is about the dream that makes you feel badly; to stop any bad dream; and to change negative dream dimensions into positive ones. Most people are amazed to be told that a bad dream can be stopped and that you don't have to let it continue. Again with practice you should be able to instruct yourself to change the action of your dream while remaining asleep. Altering the outcome of a dream appears to be a tall order, but it's an achievable goal, usually with some assistance from a therapist.

To authors of *Crisis Dreaming,* dreams can become the core of our ability to assimilate major changes in our lives, good and bad, successes and failures.

Any Bad Habits to Declare?

Have you any bad habits? Habits such as hair-twirling, nail-biting, throat-clearing, foot-jiggling, doodling, teeth-grinding, and a host of similar ones that loom annoying to those around us.

A recent study at North Dakota University failed to find one person without any bad habits. In fact the average number of bad habits per person was found to be seven.

Why exactly do we develop these habits? Psychologists ascribe it mainly to our anxiety reducing behaviour. And they break down bad habits into two broad types: nervous habits (when one is anxious), and boredom habits (doing something to pass the time).

Nervous habits essentially focus on the body: nail-biting, teeth-grinding, throat-clearing, twisting/pulling hair. Boredom habits usually revolve around an object, such as fiddling with a pencil while speaking to someone, doodling while on phone, tapping a pen on the desk, or lighting a cigarette.

When we come under stress, we get a rush of adrenaline. This is nature's way to give the energy either to run away or stay and fight when the life is in danger. This helped when primitive man hunted for survival.

Now most of our stressful situations arise from work and here the "fight or flight" scenario has little relevance. As a result, the adrenaline-produced nervous energy in the body manifests itself in bad habits—usually by making our feet restless, but also by making us play with our hair, bite our nails, and so on. In extreme forms of such nervousness, sufferers are known to pull out their hair. All this activity is meant to assuage the excess nervous tension generated in stressful work.

Boredom habits arise when someone is bored, impatient, and wants to get things over quickly. A typical example is the interviewer who taps his pen on the desk because he is impatient with the ramblings of the interviewee. Again, these habits surface up when someone is stuck in a boring situation, such as being unable to leave a dull meeting for fear of appearing rude.

According to the Dakota study, the average length of time that each habit lasts is eight years, although for some people a habit can last a lifetime.

How to kick a bad habit if you wanted to? The first step is to acknowledge that you have one. Then find out what triggers it: anxiety or boredom? And are there any practical means of easing out that anxiety or boredom? Anyway when you catch yourself indulging your habit, stop it by doing something else with your hands or feet, to dispel the nervous energy or the feeling of boredom.

Psychiatrists work by first raising awareness of the bad habit and then asking the sufferer to do just the opposite of the original habit—like asking a nail-biter to sit on his hands. People are usually placed in front of a large mirror so that they can see how unattractive their habit is.

Of course, the long-term solution is to get rid of the anxieties that cause the bad habits. Asking yourself whether your anxieties about all the things, you imagine could go wrong in future, are really realistic. Holidays are possibly the best time to break bad habits as one is more relaxed and less burdened with work stress.

Our Sweat is Nothing to be Ashamed of

The toiletries industry has spawned a host of body deodorants, antiperspirants and other products to counter sweat. And keeping oneself dry is sweaty conditions is deemed chic, more so for women.

Yet our sweat is nothing to be ashamed of; it's pretty wholesome stuff. Human sweat is 99 per cent pure water, with traces of salt and potassium.

What's more, a talent for sweating is an indicator of a body in good working order. A fit person sweats about twice as much as a sedentary one, and sweats at lower temperatures. An athlete can lose something like 5 litres of water exercising for a couple of hours on a hot day. And in an acclimatized body this salt loss is easily recouped.

Men sweat more than women. A woman's body has to reach a temperature one degree higher than a man's before she begins to perspire. Nature has blessed women with a higher threshold for heat.

The main mechanism for cooling our body are the sweat glands. When the internal temperature rises, over 2 million eccrine glands start secreting water—an odourless one, contrary to common belief—to the skin surface. This is the sweat that cools the body as it evaporates.

The trouble arises when humidity climbs close to 100 per cent. There's no way for the sweat to evaporate. Our consequent discomfort is evident. Even in lower humidity, nearly half of our sweat trickles down our body in salty rivulets instead of evaporating forthwith.

But then why has sweat earned a bad name? Actually, in addition to countless eccrine glands, we also possess apocrine glands. The latter, far fewer in numbers, are found in the armpits, the genitals, and anywhere we have hair. These are the stinkers. They produce a milky stuff that gives out a pungent odour when acted upon by the skin bacteria.

The apocrine glands have another characteristic. They continually secrete a concentrated fatty sweat into the gland tube. When we are under severe emotional stress, these glands contract, expelling the thick sweat out. The smelly liquid that way broadcasts our inner turmoil to the outside world.

Hairy people tend to sweat more because their numerous hair follicles provide home to more apocrine glands. East Asians have fewer apocrines than people of Caucasian origin, and therefore sweat less. And their sweat is much less smelly.

It's only in the sanitized modern age that human sweat and its smell often figure as embarrassing and unwelcome. At one time sweat was even regarded as an aphrodisiac. Elizabethan lovers were known to exchange peeled apples they had worn under their armpits. And Napolean, in a letter to Josephine, indicated his pleasure in her natural aroma. "I will be arriving in Paris tomorrow. Don't wash."

Left-handers: How Different?

Recent researches are showing that left-handedness is more than a minor difference. Evidence is accumulating that left-handedness has significant social, educational, and psychological implications, and affects many aspects of health, even longevity. That way, left-handers are truly different.

What is left-handedness? People commonly equate it with writing and/or eating with left hand. Yet true left-handedness involves the preferred use of left hand in various skilled actions requiring a dominant hand, such as using a hammer, throwing a pebble at a target, swinging a racquet or bat or fly swatter, holding a match to strike or thread when threading into a needle, holding a knife for cutting things or a toothbrush for use.

Around 10 per cent of people are left-handed and that is common to every society and culture over the globe. And everywhere more men are left-handed than women.

It has however to be remembered that right-handedness is a genetically fixed trait in human beings. This is something unique to Homo Sapiens. All other animals—dogs, cats, rats—seem to be equally split between right-and-left pawedness.

What makes a certain percentage of every population left-handed? Despite much research on the subject, no fully convincing explanation is forthcoming.

Surveys show that if your mother was left-handed, your chance of being left-handed was approximately doubled. Father's handedness didn't seem to matter that much. If both mother and father are left-handed, your prospects of being left-handed rise between three and four chances out of ten; with both parents right-handed, the odds are about one in ten.

Evidently all left-handedness cannot be traced to inheritance. Even identical twins sometimes don't share common handedness. There must be other causes of left-handedness, and nobody is yet sure as to what exactly are these.

Surveys indicate that in groups of individuals with known or suspected brain injuries, the number of left-handers is much greater than is found in groups of normal individuals. The presumption is that the pathological condition associated with their brain injuries probably also altered their handedness. It could often be an injury sustained in stressful birth. Children with a history of difficult delivery show a higher incidence of left-handedness. Again prematurely born children have been found about five times more left-handed or mixed-handed compared to normally-born children. The likelihood of left-handedness also increases in children born to older mothers.

Handedness becomes well established between three and six years of age. Some scientists surmise that slower development in some children, especially of the left hemisphere of their brain, does not allow the dominance of the right hand to develop.

Stanley Coren, a Canadian authority on handedness, carried out a detailed study to verify whether the left-handed actually suffered from any retarded growth. He found that left-handed women in North America were 59 per cent more likely than right-handed women to have their first menstrual period after they were fourteen. Similarly left-handed males were 57 per cent more likely to fall into the delayed growth group—as measured by the age of appearance of adult-pattern body hair—than were the right-handed males.

Indeed, Stanley Coren came up with the astounding finding that the average life span of American left-handers was 9 years shorter than the right-handers, as borne out by the reliable statistics available on league-level baseball players. What had led him to undertake the study was the alarming discovery that the left-hander percentage of 13 in 20-year-olds fell drastically to 5 in 50-year-olds and there were less than one per cent left-handers left among 80-year-olds.

Of course, this relates to averages. Surely there have been long-lived left-handers. A few famous ones are Pablo Picasso (92), Charlie Chaplin (88), Benjamin Franklin (84), Queen Victoria (82). And there's Ronald Reagan.

Anyway one thing is obvious. The left-hander is at greater risk of accidents than is the right-hander. And it's not because the former is necessarily clumsy or less coordinated. Certainly a tennis star like John McEnroe, a golf hero like Arnold Palmer, or a great cricketer like Wasim Akram can't be accused of being clumsy. It is largely because left-handers have to operate in a right-handed world.

Available statistics show that left-handers are more prone to accidents at home or at work, in playing games and using implements. Especially in industrial settings such as factories, mills and machine shops, the environment is rather badly designed for the left-hander. Sawing and drilling machines are designed for use by right-handers. Portable power tools are meant to be held in the right hand, with the safety switch to be operated by the right thumb. And most controls in machinery are located on the right side. All this can lead to greater industrial injuries for the left-handed.

Even otherwise the left-hander is subject to numerous difficulties and inconveniences in everyday life.

Take schooling. The left-to-right writing is set up for a right-handed writer; the most comfortable and controlled hand movement is a pull across the body. For a left-hander it operates in reverse. Even with languages with a right-to-left script such as Persian or Urdu, the curve of letters favours the right hand.

A commonplace school item like the ruler has a bias. For the ease of the right-handed user, the numbers are lower on the left and increase as you move right—thus facilitating line-drawing from zero to the length required. A left-hander, whose natural inclination is to draw a line from right to left, has to contend with the complication of starting at higher numbers.

In classrooms and lecture halls where seats have fixed arms for writing, all these arms are invariably positioned on the right. Left-handers end up twisted to the side as they attempt to take notes.

Most important of all, teachers should be trained into instructing left-handed children to write properly. Often, even a well-intentioned teacher ends up giving left-handed children inappropriate writing instructions.

Many kitchen utensils and gadgets are designed for the right-handed. The pouring spout of pans and ladles is positioned for the right-handed. Doors of microwave ovens and washing machines open from right to left, making the use awkward for the left-hander.

But presumably the worst tool for left-handers is the common scissors. The blades are tapered for right-hand use. And many scissors, particularly industrial ones, have specialised holes for inserting the thumb in one and three to four fingers in the other. Inserting the left thumb and left fingers in them is difficult, even hurtful to the fingers.

Telephone receiver, held in the left hand, seems suited to left-handers. But it has actually been designed for right-handers. While the left hand is holding the receiver, the right hand is left free to take notes. For a left-hander to perform these tasks, the user must shift the receiver to the right hand, which causes the cord to drape itself across the dial and in front of the body in an annoying and interfering manner.

To be a good hunter or fisherman one must be right-handed. Bolt action rifles have the operating lever on the right side. And the typical fly-casting rod has the winding lever on the right. The simplest solution attempted by left-handers usually involves turning the fishing rod upside down. But that makes the rod to rotate in the hand and is tiring to hold.

While left-handers seem to suffer no evident disadvantage in racquet and bat sports (indeed they enjoy a certain advantage in boxing and fencing) but they just can't play field hockey or polo left-handed. Even ballroom dancing is designed to have a right-handed man dance with a right-handed woman. It is based on the right-handed bias to "veer" right.

What can be done to make life easier and safer for left-handers in our right-handed world? Unfortunately, one solution that first springs to many minds—to change the left-hander into a right-hander—is not the correct one. Training in early childhood may improve the ability of the right hand to use a pen or spoon; here girls do better than boys. But changing handedness from left to right is an effort doomed to failure—let alone the ethics of interfering with the freedom of choice. Left-handedness is not a simple movement preference that has developed into a habit. It probably reflects differences in the pattern of neural circuitry in the brain.

The modified left-hander will still have the left-turning and counterclockwise-rotation tendencies of most left-handers. And in times of stress or when rapid action is necessary, will still revert to the use of left hand.

As over 10 per cent of the world's population is left-handed, it should be feasible for certain mass-produced items to have an alternative version for left-handed use. Kitchen utensils, scissors, drawing instruments, hand tools and corkscrews can be candidates for such special designs.

Other tools can be redesigned as to be amenable for easy use by either hand. For example, you can have grips with finger grooves that can be used by either hand. Doors of microwave ovens or washing machines could open up instead of sideways. Control panels in many machines could be shifted in front instead of on the right. Or a duplicate panel provided on the left, at least an extra safety switch on the left.

A whole lot of things can be improved for left-handers, once designers, engineers, managers and others in authority become more alive and sensitive to the difficulties of left-handers.

The main problem is that left-handers largely remain an invisible minority. People often fail to notice left-handedness in colleagues and acquaintances, what to say of strangers. Indeed, most right-handers never bother to think about left-handedness at all.

And this is further compounded by the fact that left-handers also seem to want to remain invisible. Possibly they are afraid of snide remarks against them, or their job prospects getting prejudiced, or even their health insurance rates going up. Happily the age-old prejudices against left-handers are on the wane, yet condescension from right-handers almost always peeps through.

Eventually left-handers have to make themselves more visible. They have to organize to gain better recognition of their problems and set in motion an active movement to modify tools and equipment for their use.

Left-handers are different and so are their requirements. On the credit side, left-handers are often blessed with better spatial ability, and figure significantly well among musical and sporting prodigies.

Age-old Prejudices Against Left-handers

Lefthanders International is there and so also a bimonthly *Lefthander Magazine*, but left-handers have virtually no politically-active organization anywhere to gain support for attitudinal changes in the majority and the needed modifications in tools and equipment.

Around 10 per cent of people in every society happen to be left-handers. And studies from tools, fossils and cave paintings reveal that this percentage has remained relatively constant over the last 50,000 years.

This sizeable minority of left-handers has been a persecuted minority throughout the ages in every culture—for no evident fault of its own. It has been subject to prejudice, humiliation, and discrimination.

Take language itself. The word *left* comes from *lyft*, which means "weak" or "broken". The Oxford English Dictionary defines *left-handed* as "awkward", "clumsy", "ill-omened", "inauspicious". A *left-handed compliment* is actually an insult. A *left-handed honeymoon* is with someone else's husband. And left-handedness in prevailing sexual parlance hints at homosexuality.

While the words *right* or *right-handed* always carry a positive connotation, *left* or *left-handed* invariably imply something wrong or unwelcome.

And it is the same in every language. In French the word for left is *gauche*, meaning "crooked", "ugly", and "uncouth". The German word for left-handed is *linkisch*, also meaning "awkward, clumsy, maladroit". And similar situation obtains in all of our languages.

Possibly the worst scenario is in Latin, where the word for left is *sinister*, meaning evil.

In all cultures, left is deemed unlucky. Various sayings and signs associate the right side with good luck and the left side with bad luck.

If your right palm itches, you will receive money; if your left itches, you will lose money.

If your right eyelid twitches it means that some absent member of your family will return. A twitch from your left eyelid may foretell a death in the family.

If your right ear buzzes you are going to hear some good news. If your left ear rings it means bad news is coming.

Itching in the sole of the right foot augurs a successful journey, whereas itching of the big left toe spells trouble.

Simply put, something that happens on the right means good fortune, something that happens on the left means misfortune.

Even a mole on the left side of the chest is a sign of a wicked person, while a mole on the right side of the chest indicates a talented individual. This mole business looks too trivial but in medieval times of witch-hunting it could become a matter of life and death. A standard procedure in trial of an accused witch was the public examination of her naked body. Among the possible "proofs" of witchcraft was a blemish or mole on the left side, which was always interpreted as a mark of the Devil.

The notion that the right side is blessed and left side cursed manifested itself in many practices. For example, there was the Roman tradition of entering a friend's house with the right foot first. Romans were so particular about it, when entertaining they would post a slave next to the door to be sure that every guest entered with the right foot first. From this foot-watching slave comes the term *footman*.

Weak and potentially at risk, the left side is protected through amulets: in shape of bracelets, arm bands, rings. Presumably, arising out of this belief, developed the custom of wearing a ring on the fourth finger of the left hand. Circling the weakest finger on the weaker hand, it is intended to protect the wearer from bad things and temptations.

Both the Jewish and the Christian traditions are strongly right-handed in their nature and practices. The Bible is particularly strong in its damnation of the left. Only the right hand can be used for priestly benedictions. The Devil alone baptises his followers with the left hand.

And the same prejudices prevail in virtually all other religions.

When Buddha expounds the path to Nirvana, he describes a road that divides into two paths. The left-hand road, the wrong way of life, is to be avoided, while the right-hand road is to be followed as a path to enlightenment.

A ritual in Islam involves washing before prayers. First the right hand and arm are washed, up to the elbow, and then the left hand and forearm. While washing the right hand the devout worshipper says, "Oh my God, on the day of the judgement place the book of my actions in my right hand and examine my account with favour." When he washes the left hand he says, "Place not at the resurrection the book of my action on my left hand." Here the right hand signifies salvation, the left hand damnation.

In many oriental countries, people are forbidden to eat with their left hand, which is considered "unclean" because it is used for cleaning after defection. The practice can claim some hygienic merit. But the right-hand bias is obvious; the "unclean" act is to be performed by the left hand while the right hand is used for a wholesome activity like eating.

These are just a few examples of the age-old bias against the left hand. It's a whole long list. Left-handers are not only discriminated against by the language and attitudes of society, but also in overt and explicit ways by custom, superstition and religion. And all this merely because certain people use their left hand instead of the right for things like writing, eating food or brushing the teeth.

Till recent times, children were rapped on knuckles if they tried to write with the left hand. Particularly girls came in for strong corrective measures as left-handedness in girls was deemed a significant liability in the marriage market.

The age-old prejudice against left-handedness is happily waning fast in developed nations and among educated sections in developing countries. This has also resulted in a rise in the numbers of left-handed. In Britain, for example, left-handers now account for some 11% in women and 13% in men. Research suggests the number could rise further as women's average childbearing age increases. Older mothers are more likely to have left-handed children.

The average right-hander today could feel that the bias charge is overplayed; he or she may deny any feelings of superiority or disdain. Indeed, many right-handers hardly notice left-handedness in others, even in their colleagues and acquaintances. Yet when we scratch the surface of the right-hander's mind, an element of condescension towards left-handers often peeps through. And this could take some time to disappear completely.

Exercise for Desk Workers

Take a short break if you have worked continuously at your desk for a couple of hours.

First get into the relax mode. Draw half a dozen deep breaths—inhaling through your nose and exhaling through your mouth. Stretch your arms and legs.

And then the following exercises.

Strengthen Back and Buttocks

- Bend your knees slightly as you stand with hands at your sides.
- Tilt your upper body forward as you push back your arms and buttocks.
- Raise your head and shoulders.
- You'll feel it in your back down to your legs.
- Do this three times.

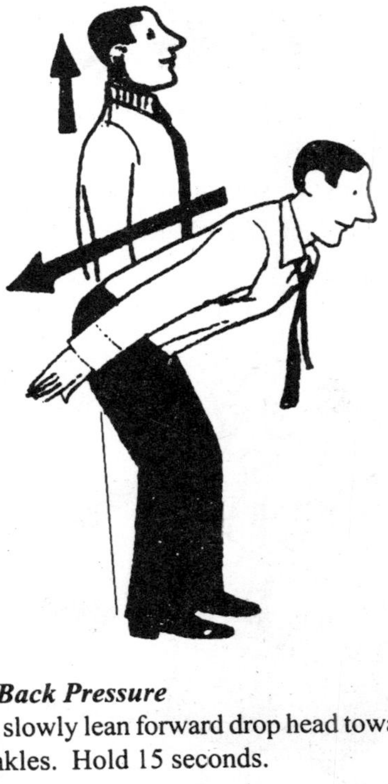

Relieve Lower Back Pressure

- Exhaling, slowly lean forward drop head toward knees, and let hands drop at ankles. Hold 15 seconds.
- Inhaling, unwind, slowly bringing up the head.

- Exhaling, stretch arms toward ceiling.
- Do this five times.

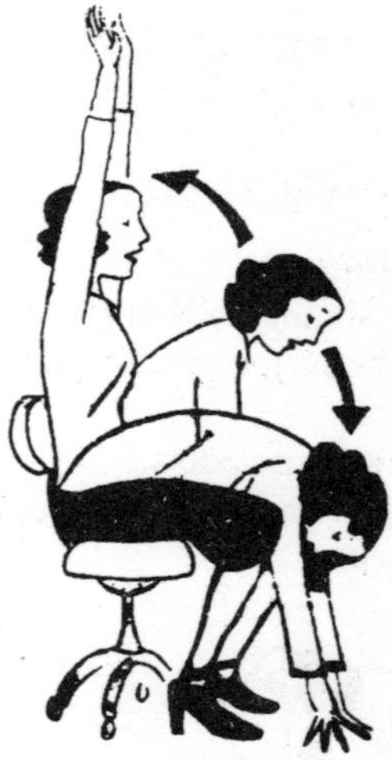

Strengthen Upper Back and Shoulder Muscles

- Lift hands to shoulders.
- Keep elbows down as you push shoulders back with your arms.
- Hold this position for 15 seconds.
- Do this three times.

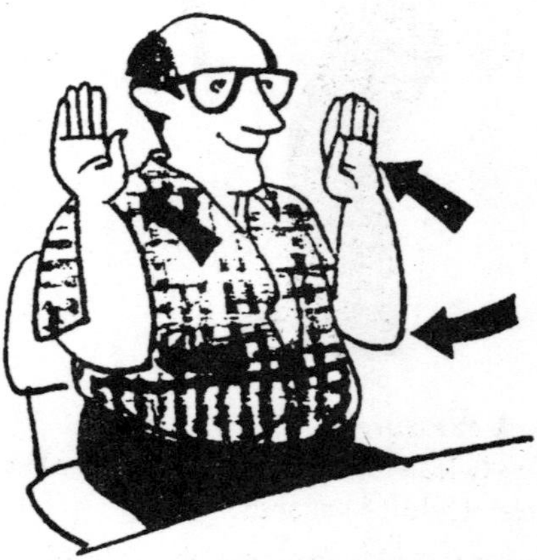

Relieve Back Tension and Stretch Hips

- Stand with feet apart and knees bent.
- Crouch your body as low as you can without pain.
- Hold this position for 15 seconds.
- Do this five times.

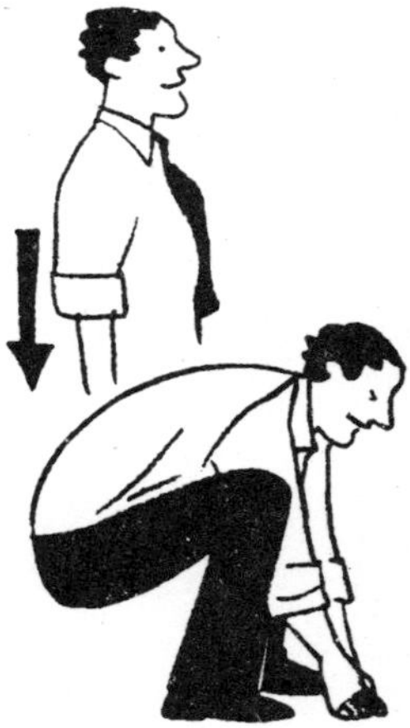

Stretch Abdominal and Chest Muscles

- In a standing or sitting position, place your palms on your lower back.
- Stretch back your upper body.
- Hold this position for 15 seconds.
- Do this three times.

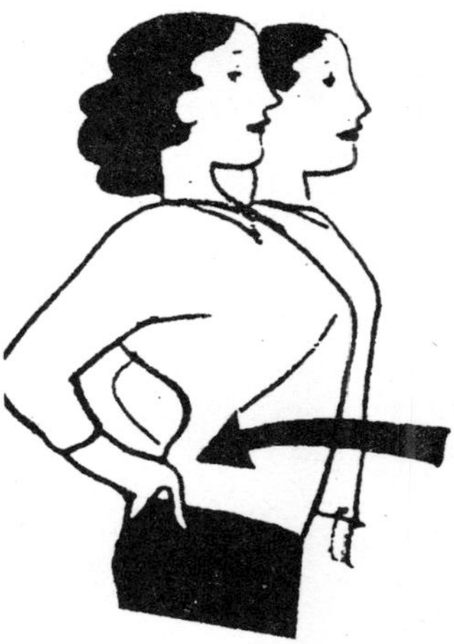

2
Some Specific Health Problems

Hypertension

Possibly no adult medical condition is more rife these days than high blood pressure. Twenty per cent of the world's population has "mild" hypertension (the medical term for elevated blood pressure). Only fifty per cent of the sufferers know about it and only twenty-five per cent are being treated—half of them effectively.

Generally speaking, the lower the pressure, the better. Forget about such myths as 100 plus your age is normal for the systolic reading or that as long as diastolic number is not high, the systolic figure does not matter. We now know that an elevated systolic figure (when the heart is pumping) and normal diastolic number (when the heart is resting) is associated with a significantly higher risk of stroke, especially in the elderly.

Your target should be 120/80, how so old you are. 130/85 is acceptable. If your pressure is always above 140/90, it should be lowered. Insist on treatment even if you feel perfectly well.

Blood pressure does increase with age as blood has to be pumped with greater force through blood vessels grown less elastic with age. As many as 50 per cent of people over 65 suffer from elevated levels of blood pressure.

Nobody knows exactly what causes hypertension. Several factors are said to be implicated. For one, high blood pressure runs in families. But how this genetic trait is transmitted from generation to generation, no one has a clue.

Certain personality traits are being associated with high blood pressure, such as the sort of aggressiveness and competitive spirit that makes it difficult to relax, impatience and irritation with delays, a disposition to get angry quickly, or worrying excessively over one's failures.

Some blame it on the stress of modern life: meeting deadlines at work, tensions of commuting, even high levels of noise at workplace. Of course, some people are more susceptible to stress than others; individual thresholds of stress vary enormously.

Nature, as a safety measure, raises our heartbeat and blood pressure when a physical threat is perceived so as to heighten our preparedness for it. As problems in modern living go on and on everyday, our muscles stay tense and hearts beat faster over extended periods. In the process the blood pressure stays high for far too long.

Monitoring Hypertension

Stephen Hales, a British bishop, was the first person to measure blood pressure. He sliced into his patient's artery, joined the vessel to an 11-ft-tall glass column, and saw the blood pushed up to the 8-foot mark. The year: 1711. The patient: a horse.

As high blood pressure is often symptomless, it becomes particularly important to have periodic check-ups, so that the condition could be dealt with before any damage is done to the body.

For anyone with hypertension, a home monitor can be a valuable tool. Home monitoring is especially useful for people with "white-coat hypertension"—those whose blood pressure is driven up by the stress of having a doctor measure it. A regular record of blood pressure is a distinct help to the doctor for fine-tuning the treatment.

All sorts of home monitors are now available in the market: mechanical units, electronic ones that are pumped by a squeeze bulb, self-inflating electronic models, even finger units that have a tiny cuff for the index finger. In self-inflating models, blood pressure reading and pulse rate come up in the shape of digital display.

With practice and possibly a little coaching, you can manage quite accurate readings with simple electronic monitors, within a margin of one or two mm HG. Better take blood pressure reading at the same time of the day as BP varies with different times of the day. And occasionally have the home-reading cross-checked at the doctor's.

Controlling Hypertension

A change in personality traits is problematic; bulk of these traits are already formed by the age of 20. Lifestyle changes, however, can be brought about if there is the requisite motivation. Recommended measures commonly include a regime of physical exercise, weight control, cutting down on foods rich in cholesterol and fats, and moderation in daily intake of caffeine (not more than three cups of coffee) and alcohol (not more than two standard units). Indeed two drinks a day is said to protect the coronary arteries from the buildup of atherosclerotic plaque. Regular exercise is not only essential for weight loss but by itself, lowers elevated blood pressure.

Around 50 per cent of those with high blood pressure are salt sensitive. For these people, lowering the salt intake, even to a modest degree, will help lower their blood pressure. While it may not bring blood pressure to completely normal, it will help to control it.

Yet a third of people with high blood pressure are known to be salt resistant. Lowering their salt intake wouldn't benefit them. With simple tests a doctor can find out whether a particular person is salt resistant or not.

A recent study by DASH researchers in USA (*The DASH Diet for Hypertension* by Thomas Moore, M.D. Free Press) has come out with the finding that a diet high on low-fat dairy products and vegetables could reduce blood pressure independent of salt consumption, exercise and weight. They believe that a low-fat diet rich in three minerals (potassium, magnesium and calcium) could be doing the blood pressure lowering trick (synthetic supplements aren't as much a help as actual food).

It's common knowledge that blood pressure level rises in morning hours. The body gets a rush of adrenalin to be ready for day's activity (no surprise, more strokes and heart attacks occur between 6 a.m., and 10 a.m., than in any other 4-hour period of the day). Now there are medicines that specifically target early-morning rise in blood pressure.

Despite their best efforts to improve lifestyles, most hypertensives will eventually need anti-hypertension drugs. Pharmaceutical companies have responded by bringing out a host of new drugs besides the old standbys of beta blockers and diuretics. It is for the physician to choose among the various therapies, picking up the drug that fits each patient's particular needs.

All in all, the good news is that a change of lifestyle, backed by suitable drugs, can keep high blood pressure under control. And there is no reason why persons suffering from mild hypertension should not take advantage of it. Hypertension is a major cause of life-threatening vascular diseases, especially effecting the heart, brain, eyes, kidneys and circulation in the legs.

The Cold War

If you're like most people, you'll "catch" cold 2-3 times in a year. For children it's about six times.

A cold is an inflammation of your upper respiratory tract and it happens when one of two hundred odd varieties of rhinoviruses takes residence in your rhino, a doctor speak for "nose".

Rhinoviruses find the human nose a near-perfect environment in which to grow. The nose has a temperature of 32-33 degrees Celsius (optimal for growth of viruses) which is a few degrees cooler than the body temperature (37° C), and an abundant supply of oxygen.

Upon infection, your body becomes a "virus-making factory" for a day or two as your guests replicate by the millions—this is also the period when you're most contagious.

On the first day of illness, you typically notice that your throat is sore or scratchy. On the second and third days, the membranes of your nose and sinuses thicken to the point of obstruction. A thin, clear secretion flows freely from the nasal lining, with inflammation turning the edges of nose raw and red. As the cold persist, the secretions become dense and gluey.

Many people also develop a cough. A hacking cough can torment you by day and drive you mad at night.

The initial infection is followed by the body mounting its defences: coughing, aching, sneezing, and low-grade fever. Crucially, fever slows down the virus that prefers to operate at cooler temperature. That way any drug taken to bring down fever actually has the effect of prolonging the cold.

Sneezing is good for you. Every time you sneeze you make a million germs homeless. And these can only survive outside the body for a few minutes, unless they find another host in the meantime.

Once infected by a particular cold virus, you gain immunity from it. No wonder, older people get less colds, as they tend to develop immunity to many rhinoviruses through exposures over the years. Women get colds oftener than men, more from handling children suffering from colds.

What sets a cold apart from flu (influenza), is the absence of high fever. Your temperature typically stays below 101 degrees Fahrenheit. Pity, people still use the terms 'flu' and 'cold' synonymously; the two are quite different.

People harbour all sorts of notions about colds; both false and true.

Damp, Cold or Drafty Weather Causes Cold

In Hindi, the word *sardi* denotes both being made cold and a cold itself. And colds are curiously seasonal. Yet colds depend not on the weather but on human contact. Hand-to-hand transmission of virus-contaminated nasal secretions spread most common colds. If you have a cold, you're especially likely to touch your infected mucous membranes, contaminating your hands, and then touch and infect others.

You can Easily Catch a Cold from Someone Sneezing or Coughing without Covering the Mouth

This is not exactly true. Coughing, talking, and sneezing don't send viral particles very far and the particles contain only a low concentration of rhinovirus. Controlled experiments have shown that even kissing rarely transmits a cold.

Alcohol is an Effective Cold Remedy

False. Consuming alcohol does not destroy cold viruses, nor improve cold symptoms.

Fatigue Makes you more Susceptible to Colds

There's no proof that fatigue or "feeling tired" makes you vulnerable to colds. Of course, it can make you feel worse once you have the infection.

You're More Likely to Catch a Cold or Flu in the Winter than in the Summer

This is partially true. But it's not directly due to the weather. Winter season brings people together indoors, which leads to more person-to-person contacts. Most of all, the infection is acquired by children in school and then transmitted to adults at home. Children are the warm and welcoming hosts to many a virus.

Try Not to Stifle Coughs

This is correct. Coughing helps you get rid of phlegm and mucus that can clog airways and accumulate in the lungs.

Thorough and Frequent Hand-washing Helps Protect Against Transmission of Colds and Flu

This is absolutely true of colds. Rhinoviruses can live for hours on hands. If you have been touching other people's hands or any inanimate surfaces on which viruses have just been deposited, a soap hand-wash can help you stave off the virus contamination. There are reports of new anti-septic skin cleansers being developed that, unlike most soaps, would not only kill viruses on people's hands immediately but continue to do so for hours afterwards.

Popular misconceptions abound about the role of medicines for colds. Virtually every product marketed for relief or treatment of colds is of dubious value.

Take coughing. Despite the nuisance and sleep disturbance, research into coughing is one of the slowest-moving areas of medicine. Treatments have changed little in the last fifty years. Almost every remedy—and medicines are on offer to suppress dry coughs, soothe a tickly throat, or to loosen phlegm—is based on opiates such as codeine. A detailed study recently concluded by Knut Schroeder and Tom Fahey in Britain (*British Medical Journal*, Vol. 324) finds that there was no good evidence that common cough medicines worked.

Coughing is a part of the body's natural defences, so suppressing it completely isn't necessarily a good thing. Consider what would happen if you failed to cough when a bit of food got lodged in your windpipe. But then dry cough —-which expels nothing—has no apparent benefit and can safely be suppressed.

Of late, research is on to understand the exact mechanism of coughing. The same is proving a far more complex phenomenon than was assumed. The eventual idea is to produce a drug that could deactivate the over-stimulated sensory receptors in the respiratory tract, causing cough. Or, even something for the brain to numb down its reaction to sensory over-stimulation.

As to cold remedies, there is a lack of evidence for the efficacy of various zinc preparations. Aspirin may alleviate headaches, but has been blamed on increasing a runny nose. Antihistamine drugs do reduce the volume of secretions from the nose but they induce drowsiness, and so better taken at sleep time. Throat lozenges and nose inhalers again have a marginal effect.

There is some evidence that vitamin C can slightly reduce the duration and severity of cold symptoms if taken in large doses—around 2,000 milligram a day (something contained in two to three dozen oranges), as compared to the recommended dietary dose of 60 milligrams. Such a high dose can have possible complications for some in the shape of diarrhea.

A good strategy is to lie in bed until the illness has passed, while fortifying yourself with a lot of warm fluids. In isolating yourself you also minimize the chances of infecting others.

In the absence of a "magic bullet", perhaps the best, and certainly the cheapest, cure is steam inhalation. Steam not only helps unblock the nose, the higher temperature generated by it in nose region retards the growth of the virus.

There are those who, in their anxiety to get well quick, ask their doctors for antibiotics. And nurse a sense of disappointment, at times edging on frustration, if their doctor sends them away empty-handed. We are all, to a varying degree, hypochondriacs.

Attempts to develop antiviral drugs have largely failed because of the wide variety of viruses responsible. Antibiotics do not work

against tiny viruses (about hundred times smaller than bacteria). In fact the over-prescription of antibiotics for colds is contributing to the emergence of bacterial resistance to various antibiotic drugs.

The old adage about the cold germs still seems to ring true: "Whatever you do, we're three days coming, three days here, and three days going." So better wait restfully while your body makes enough antibodies to destroy the virus; what doctors call the "tincture of time".

Lately there have been reports of medicines being developed that offer actual respite from common cold. One is a nasal spray to be inhaled several times daily. The other is a pill. The two remedies in the pipeline claim to prevent replication of the viruses by attacking a large group of viruses at the same time.

The world watches with interest, tinged with a certain skepticism, whether this will herald a breakthrough in the Cold War.

Men, Women and the Common Cold

The common cold is really common. It infects the poor and the rich. The virus infects a mansion as readily as it will infect a slum. That way the common cold germs are the true democrats.

And it infects men and women equally. Indeed it effects women more as they come more in contact with their cold-infected school children. Yet amazing, how men and women differ so widely in their typical /response to an attack of the common cold.

A woman struck down with cold—the works: running nose, sneezes, coughs, aches and fever—is likely to take the visitation stoically, somewhat uncomplainingly. Coping with childbirth and menstruation, she's possibly acquired a higher threshold of discomfort. If unable to do household work any more, she simply slumps in bed—inwardly amused at others floundering without her to run the household. And usually takes no pills or cures except periodic mugs of tea (for relief there isn't anything like a hot liquid, to soothe the throat, loosen up congestion, and keep the kidneys flushing away wastes).

And when the worst is over, she rises and tries to function again, as if the whole thing was more a nuisance than an illness.

Small children are luckier still; they don't even know they've "come down" with cold. Their leaps and frolics continue as long as they aren't laid low.

Many a man is apt to treat an attack of common cold as a personal attack on him, and on his work schedule. In anger and frustration, he may well swear at everything in sight: at himself (for skipping his vitamin C, standing in draught or neglecting his exercise), at the lousy weather, at city authorities (for unsanitary conditions), at his colleagues (as a possible source of infection), and at the doctor (for not fully appreciating the gravity of the attack).

And every man, it seems, has devised his own method of "fighting" his cold, a sort of manual of tactics. You can possibly make a good guess about a man's character from the way he tackles his cold.

Busy executives often opt for intensive medical intervention. Large doses of vitamin C, zinc lozenges, antihistamines, and antibiotics. They take alarming doses of heavy drugs with gusto. Pressurize their doctors for some knockout drops or even an injection.

Then there are the whimperers. Feverish in bed, they set up a steady moan, "Hai Ma", while their wives are massaging their chests with Vicks, and otherwise dancing attendance. The whole household stands alerted to their woe.

Whereas a woman is generally defensive about her cold, a man talks. Talks how bad this one is compared with the one he had last winter. How the last one was in the head while this one really does seem to be (cough, experimental cough) in the throat. He talks how his back hurts and his chest is stuffed up with bilge. He wonders if he got it shaking hands with strangers or playing bridge. And he talks interminably about the relative merits of various pills and nasal drops.

Allergies

Are you prone to sneezing, coughing, wheezing, itchy eyes or nasal congestion? Most people associate allergy with pollen in the spring season or with food allergens. Yet dust and dust mites indoors are the single greatest cause of allergy.

Once the bane of a small, sniffling minority, allergic rhinitis now counts its victims in millions. To many of us, an allergy attack means a minor inconvenience, causing just a few days of discomfort. But to some others, this can lead to a disabling asthma attack.

People harbour a whole lot of vague or misleading assumptions about allergies. Here are a few allergy myths.

Allergies are Mainly Caused by Pollen from Flowers

This is not exactly true. Weeds, rather than brightly coloured flowering plants are most likely to trigger allergic reactions. Pollen from roses and many other fragrant flowers tends to be heavy, waxy, and sticky. These pollens are not spread by the wind. Instead, insects such as bees transport pollen from flower to flower. Accordingly, allergies from these plants are relatively rare—unless you happen to be a florist or gardener.

Only long-haired pets cause allergies, not the shor-thaired ones

This isn't correct. An animal's fur is not the culprit in allergies; the real villain is a protein produced by glands in the animal's skin or in its saliva. Cats actually cause more allergy problems than dogs, because they spread the protein over their coats through repeated licking.

Hay fever is caused by hay

"Hay fever" is a misnomer because this condition is not caused by hay but by the usual pollen. The term was coined in 1828 by a British physician when he noticed that his allergy symptoms worsened during the British haying season.

Allergies are psychosomatic

To say that an allergy is "all in your head" is not correct. An allergy is a specific immunological reaction to a normally harmless substance, such as pollen, mould spores or foods or insect bites or dust mites. As the allergens come in contact with our specialized cells that act as soldiers of the immune system, the protective cells release chemicals such as histamine. These chemicals cause allergic damage, especially swelling and inflammation. Thus our immunological defences, meant to protect us against bacteria, sometimes harm us through causing allergic reaction. Happily, an allergy is not infectious.

As I am allergic to something, so would be my kids

This is partly true. The tendency to develop allergies does seem to run in families. A child's chances of developing allergies are about 25 per cent if one parent has them. This goes up to 75 per cent if both parents have allergies. But sometimes people develop allergies when neither parent has them.

Despite their ubiquity, allergies remain mysterious. Scientists still don't know why human body mounts a scorched-earth defence against harmless substances and wounds itself in the process.

Many culprits have been proposed, including pollution. But some researchers are now hinting at a startling possibility: with modern life becoming progressively more hygienic, the human immune system has run out of things to do. It attacks allergens, and the body itself, as if it was bored.

The main rationale for this view is that almost half the people in the developed world are now allergic to something. People in developing countries like China, India or Indonesia have much less trouble with allergies. Again among people in any country, those in the upper strata with higher standard of hygiene suffer significantly more from allergies and asthma than the poor with greater exposure to infections. At the merger of Germany, it came as a revelation that the cleaner West Germany had much higher incidence of allergies than the soot-blackened, air-polluted East Germany.

What can you do if you have become prone to allergies?

It is important to remember that no one need be miserable during the grass, tree and weed pollen seasons, considering the host of available treatments.

Among the strategies for avoiding pollen: remain indoors between 5 a.m., and 10 a.m. when pollen counts are the highest; not to hang clothes outside to dry as they will collect pollen; and wash your hair every night.

Houses and apartments are the favourite resting places for dust mites, moulds, fungus, animal dander, and other allergens.

Rugs and carpets provide a natural resting place for airborne allergens and irritants such as dust and bacteria. Carpeting is also home to millions of dust mites. The scales your pet dog or cat sheds also tend to adhere to carpets. While regular vacuuming certainly helps, the best bet is to have tile flooring with only scatter rugs, which could be deep-cleaned once or twice a year by professional cleaners. As dust mites thrive in humid conditions, air-conditioning with its dehumidifying property keeps mite population down, while water coolers do the reverse.

Avoid heavy drapes on windows as these collect dust and mould. Using lightweight curtains which can be washed periodically in hot water is a good strategy.

Leather, vinyl, and plastic-coated fabrics for furniture help control the growth of mites as compared to cloth coverings.

Dust is not usually a big problem in the kitchen, but mould is. Mould grows rapidly in damp environment, of which there is plenty in the kitchen. The effected places need to be wiped with soapy water.

Bookshelves should be dusted periodically as dust is likely to settle on books stacked on shelves.

Dust mites are found in abundance in most beds, where they feed on the dead skin cells the occupants shed while they sleep. It's the fecal matter—a dust mite evacuates around 20 times a day—that really cause allergies. Covering all mattresses in airtight, washable plastic fabrics is a good idea. Bed sheets should be washed weekly in very hot water to get rid of mites and their droppings. And better keep pets out of the bedroom.

Anti-allergen sprays are now available in India to deactivate dust mites and their droppings. And these are quite safe. For one, an anti-allergen spray called "Mitey" should be able to take care of dust mites if sprayed once in two months.

Beauty products, such as hair dyes, hair sprays, sunscreen, nail polish, makeup can cause allergic reactions. And it is not easy to determine the trigger, as many women use 25 or more beauty products. Physicians often advise women to eliminate all cosmetic products, then add one item back at a time and observe whether symptoms return.

Of all the allergies, those from food are deemed most dangerous. This calls for much care, especially with young children, to avoid those foods or their ingredients.

Some people are allergic to smog; their eyes feel heavy and runny. With smog a common phenomenon during winter, especially in cities like Delhi, sufferers are advised to wash their eyes repeatedly with clean water, even wear protective glasses.

Once antihistamines had a major drawback: sedation. People required to drive were reluctant to use things like Avil. Today, a new generation of non-sedating antihistamines, such as Allegra and Claritin, has come up. These are effective at drying out membranes in the nose and sinuses, and subduing bouts of sneezing and itchy, watery eyes.

People allergic to pollen can acquire long-lasting relief through allergy shots. However those allergic to dust mites or animal dander don't respond quite as well to the shots.

Allergy shots work like vaccine. At each visit the patient receives a slightly more concentrated solution of the allergen vaccine. Admittedly allergy shots ate time-consuming but to some serious allergy sufferers these often prove the best remedy.

Hypochondria

My mother, it seemed, developed into a hypochondriac around the age of 50, though she was loathe to admit the same. To us she looked fairly fit, but began showing signs of obsessive worry about her health.

Her worst hypochondriac phase was when for several years she feared she had a glandular cancer. It all arose from a small swelling in the neck, which she possibly exacerbated by constant touching. Thrice she was examined by various specialists, x-rayed, even a biopsy done. And all these tests showed no signs of cancer. Her own brother, a noted surgeon, gave her a clean chit but her fears about the cancer just wouldn't go away. The resulting anticipation and apprehension affected the quality of her life; she continued anxious and depressed.

Eventually mother died peacefully at the age of 84, suffering a stroke in sleep.

A hypochondriac is defined as one who suffers from an excessive preoccupation with his/her own health and has a tendency to find evidence of disease in insignificant signs.

Admittedly most of us suffer from a degree of anxiety about our health—health is very important to most people. For the majority of us, however, these feelings of anxiety about our bodies malfunctioning are replaced by other preoccupations soon enough. And even when we take our health concerns as far as a trip to the doctor, most of us are reassured by their diagnosis or opinion, and we quickly move on to worrying about other things: work or money or marital relations. For some people—hypochondriacs—this isn't the case; their feelings of preoccupation with a disease, real or imagined, start to dominate their thinking.

Hypochondriacs tend to fall into two groups: those who have a medical illness but are plagued by constant worry about it even if their condition has stabilized; and those who perceive themselves ill despite all diagnostic tests and examinations to the contrary.

At times apprehensions about ill-health may not just come from physical sensation but also from something seen on television or read in a magazine. For those with severe health anxiety, such information could trigger feelings of hyperawareness of the body which are very real.

Hypochondria is an affliction its victims suffer in silence—and shame. Whereas the sick usually attract our sympathy, hypochondriacs are sneered at, joked about. To those of us who have never experienced it, hypochondria may seem comical, a non-disease. Yet, the malady is responsible for much human misery and vast expense in doctor's fees and unnecessary medical tests.

Men and women happen to experience it equally. And, surprisingly, hypochondria most commonly surfaces in one's twenties and thirties, otherwise deemed the healthiest stage in life. Luckily, parents who have suffered from health anxiety don't seem to pass it on to their children.

Hypochondriacs, especially of the mild variety, do manage to function all right, a few even achieve great things, but often at the cost of happiness. Some notable hypochondriacs in history were Charles Darwin, Leo Tolstoy and the French novelist Marcel Proust. The English poet laureate Alfred Tennyson was particularly worried about going blind, though he lived into his eighties with tolerable eyesight. James Boswell, Samuel Johnson's biographer, had an obsessive fear of venereal disease. He actually chronicled his lifelong struggles with hyp in seventy essays called *The Hypochondriack.*

The tragedy is that most hypochondriacs are painfully aware of the irrational nature of their fears about their bodies and health. Yet they feel powerless to dismiss them. These fears are largely associated with the working of internal organs, and with cancers, brain tumours, heart attacks, and now even AIDS. "It is easy for people to say don't think about it. But no matter how remote the chance that my headache is a brain tumour, the thoughts won't leave my mind," admits one sufferer.

Surely the world has witnessed a remarkable progress in health and medicine in the last fifty years. One result: our expectations for diagnosis and treatment are high, far too high, say some medics. We seek quick relief for every discomfort. Indeed we live in an era of activist medicine, where drug companies and doctors have made us hungry for "magic bullets".

Feeling well is no longer a good enough reason to put ideas about illness out of mind. If you don't have a detectable disease, you may worry about harbouring hidden risk factors. Most illnesses, especially the major ones, are actually blind accidents, but this doesn't stop the hypochondriac from being always on red alert.

Do the media have a hand in the spread of hypochondria? Researchers report findings in medical journals. The media select the most important stories to report to the public. Much of what the media gives out serves people well.

Yet journalists are always on the lookout for newsworthy stories. Alarming stories get patronized, as alarm makes news. Or reporting the advent of a "wonder drug"—of course, with a cautionary note. People don't hear the cautionary notes when these involve their health. If media coverage has raised the level of our health consciousness, it has, unwittingly, also raised the level of health anxiety in many people.

Amid the welter of health studies, health news, health tips, and health warnings, medical consumers are exposed to much that is confusing and contradictory. One study finds that vitamins boost the immune system, another doesn't. Health-conscious consumers give up mutton for fish only to read that this "heart healthy" food may drive up cholesterol, too. The public fixates on endless reports of what to do and what to avoid, unmindful that some of these studies are nowhere definitive.

The media has actually helped generate the new health mantra, with all its emphasis on healthy lifestyle. The same features in the form of a strictly observed bodily regime—of regular exercise, a balanced diet (coupled with an unceasing concern for clean drinking water), a structured daily rhythm of activities, and a consistently growing list of avoidances and self-denials. The underlying premise of the healthy lifestyle is that you have only yourself to blame for your ill-health if you persist in unhealthy practices.

Despite its widespread prevalence, few hypochondriacal patients ever receive a true diagnosis—or assistance. Physicians are reluctant to get involved; it's a touchy subject and hardly the diagnosis most patients want to hear about. For the average general practitioner, who is trained to spot and treat those with genuine physical illlness, dealing with someone suffering from hypochondrosis is very difficult.

Hypochondriacs accordingly would do well to stop "doctor shopping" and see someone trained to deal with this complex mental-health problem. Pity, hypochondriacs generally shun psychiatrists; they prefer to go to mainstream doctors who have no time, inclination, or expertise to deal with this condition.

For physicians, whose self-esteem is deeply rooted in their ability to cure disease and dispel symptoms, hypochondrial patients can be a nightmare. They are difficult and demanding; they solicit assurance only to reject it; and they switch doctors frequently. In fact, the hypochondriacal patient, like a whiny child, is skillful at getting doctors to do what he wants, or thinks he wants. Doctors are pressurized to prescribe repeated diagnostic tests and procedures.

Yet things may now be changing. The malady has begun to emerge from a long period of disregard and neglect. During the last two decades, a small but growing group of psychiatrists and general practitioners has been attempting to unravel the mysteries of hypochondria. One common conclusion they are reaching is that hypochondriacs are not malingering or pretending to be sick. Their pain and anguish is genuine as well as intense.

Psychotherapy alone had proved rather disappointing in curing hypochondria. But when combined with some modern drugs, such as Prozac, the results are promising.

This suggests that hypochondria, like depression, may have a bio-chemical origin, which essentially means low serotonin levels in the brain. And so amenable to treatment through drugs like Prozac which raise serotonin levels. That's good news to hypochondriacs.

And now there is even a website for help and advice: http/healthanxiety.com.

Risks of RSI

The term RSI (Repetitive Strain Injury) rests on the premise that tissues that would normally be able to withstand the stresses to which they are exposed during a work activity, eventually sustain injury because they experience *repeated exposure with insufficient time in between exposures to heal properly*.

Hands, wrists, and shoulders are the prime RSI targets as it's the hands that are mostly used in any work activity. And, while such injuries can occur in professions as diverse as dentistry, music making, calligraphy and carpentry, most RSI these days is traceable to prolonged typing on computers. Data-entry clerks are known to have a high incidence of RSI. And perhaps the incidence of RSI is underreported in journalists.

We take our hands for granted—indeed, people are very surprised to discover that the hands could be crippled from overuse.

Real-life scenario may well be different. Day in, day out, you arrive at your office, log on to your computer, and spend most of the following eight hours sitting, making tiny hand movements while staring at the screen. Sitting immobile for long hours—the usual feature of such work—is in itself the unhealthiest of all the prolonged postures. And more so if you sit in a chair with a poorly designed back.

In standard typing, a typist is obliged to make many diversionary movements: taking out papers for typing, interfacing these with carbon sheets, inserting them in the roller, often physically moving the carriage return after each line of typing. At the end of every page the arms are lifted to take the papers out. In contrast, the computer keyboard operator keeps on stroking keys without any relieving body movement. It is estimated that a data entry clerk averaging 10,000 strokes an hour could generate more than a ton of pressure at his finger tips during the day.

With hour after hour of such work over years, tiny microtears mar the soft tissue in various limbs involved. The muscles tighten, a reaction to the damage, and now work less efficiently. The muscles that work the hands and arms become weaker and weaker, but this weakness is usually not noticed until after pain develops.

Among the most prominent warning signals are pain, numbness, tingling, stiffness, shaking, and loss of sensation—especially in your thumb, index or long finger—or feelings of heaviness in shoulders, arms, hands, or neck. Yet many people don't take this body's warnings seriously or want to rough it out. But the longer you ignore your symptoms, the more pain you're likely to experience later on.

Some feel they have recovered when the hands become pain-free on vacation. But the symptoms often recur within hours of returning to work.

People tend to keep their condition a secret or take recourse to self-medication. Getting massages, using splints, or buying ergonomic aids may even worsen the situation by prolonging the early stage of RSI.

Your best bet is to consult at the earliest a good doctor, someone specially trained in treating RSI. RSI is not like garden-variety aches and pains that come and go. The injuries developed over years will take time and patience to go. There is really no simple or magic "cure", whatever some sufferers may come to believe.

The commonly prescribed remedies of anti-inflammatory medication or repeated cortisone injections, often don't cure the problems. And these drugs have serious side effects. RSI calls for a highly specialized treatment, tailored to individual cases. A host of new remedies have come up in recent times to choose from. One of the latest books on the subject is *The Repetitive Strain Injury Recovery Book* by Deborah Quilter (Walker & Co. 1998).

Experts are agreed upon a few tips that help minimize repetitive strain injuries in computer-based work, especially to those already suffering some symptoms.

It is advisable to minimize computer use to the extent possible. You could, for instance, stay off relatively inessential computer use such as video games or even prolonged surfing the Internet.

Look for ways to reduce keystrokes, such as using macros and quick keys. Keys can also be reconfigured to perform other functions.

Frequent, regular breaks are critical to preventing re-injury—something like a 5-10 minute break after every 20 minutes. At least change focal point after every 10-15 minutes by staring at something else than the screen. Anyway stop typing—even if you can't stop working—when you feel fatigued or experiencing pain.

The ideal break is to get up and walk around. A variety of low-cost software programmes can be customized to flash a reminder about your need to take a break.

Closing one's eyes or cupping them with hands helps, and so also raising and lowering of outstretched arms.

To counteract the adverse effects of sitting, stand as often as possible during the day. Get into the habit of standing when talking on telephone.

When the computer is taking its time to download graphics, use the opportunity to get up out of your chair and move, instead of sitting frustrated. Incidentally drinking lots of water helps.

Don't underestimate the importance of a proper workstation.

The most critical item is the chair—safe, adjustable, and comfortable. Your feet should rest flat on the floor. If not, use a footrest. Tilt the seat so your hips are slightly higher than your knees. Position the backrest to support your lower back. The front edge of the chair should slope slightly so it does cut into your thighs. And there should be enough room for you to put a loose fist between your knee and the front of the seat. Some people prefer chairs without armrests for freer movement, but armrests actually support the shoulder, allowing you to relax the muscles around the neck.

Lower the keyboard tray until your forearms form a 90-degree angle. Place the monitor an arm's length away from your torso, your eyes level with the top of the screen. Holding your elbows close to your sides is no good.

The mouse was introduced to make computer software easier to use. But the mouse presents its own problems in RSI. It overworks the dominant hand, and so also the click finger. Many people grip it too tightly while others err in keeping it at a different level than the keyboard. Again most people plant their wrists and forearms on the desk while they position the cursor with waves of the wrist. This action bends the wrist upward and sideways at the same time, placing much strain on the forearm muscles.

Given the dangers of the mouse, it is much better to substitute keystrokes for click commands. Plenty of scope for this exists. Best is to keep the mouse at elbow level and to hold it gently.

While computers are coming into widespread use in the country, our authorities have yet to lay down safety guidelines for occupational health. Most workplaces have a computer environment which ranges from the inadequate to hazardous. And there are no prescribed standards which ensure the safety of computer-based workers.

A nationwide survey of such workers was conducted by the Centre of Research in Environmental and Biological Sciences (CREBS), Hyderabad. Nearly 2 lakh people were medically examined by a team of over 200 eye specialists and other doctors. The survey found a high incidence of eye problems, such as chronic eye fatigue. While concentrating on the screen the blinking rate drops. This in turn produces a certain dryness in the eye and consequent excessive strain 20 per cent.

You can take advantage of a number of websites relating to RSI. A few are given as follows.

General RSI Help Sites and Computer Ergonomics

http://www.rsihelp.org
http://www.mumze.com/rsi/
http://www.bilbo.com/rsi.html
http://www.ergaerobics.com/links.htm

Managing Pain

What's pain? Surely everyone of us has experienced pain, associated with injury or some type of damage to the body. Yet the phenomenon of pain is turning out quite a complex one, as researchers delve into its mysteries.

Our pain experience actually has four dimensions: nociception, pain, suffering, pain behaviour.

Nociception is the physiological impact of something averse on specialized nerve endings. Our skin and other tissues contain billions of microscopic structures called free nerve endings. These are widely distributed to internal and external body surfaces. When triggered by injury or irritation, they send warning signals through nerve fibres to the brain, where these are interpreted as pain. Besides pain, they send other signals such as of heat and cold.

Pain is the perception of nociceptive stimulation. And sometimes there is a mismatch between what is perceived and what actually exists. For example, people can feel a numbing pain in phantom limb; a limb that's no longer there, having been removed through surgery or accident. Conversely, an injury can occur without the perception of pain, as when a soldier in combat is unaware for a period of time of a wound.

Suffering is the individual evaluative or affective response to the perception of pain. Suffering can be without physical pain, such as the loss of a loved one.

Pain behaviour is the observable behaviour of individuals subjected to physical pain or psychological disturbance. Pain behaviour can be influenced by circumstances, like the presence of a solicitous spouse.

What's the purpose of pain? Pain acts as nature's warning against potential dangers to the body, a signal to take precautions against something threatening. In sick and post-operative cases, pain also secures the rest that is needed for healing. There is a very small number of persons who are born without the ability to feel pain or else very little. They run high risk of burns, fractures and accidents. And their life expectancy is shorter than average.

In a way pain is a symptom rather than a disease. In certain circumstances an astute physician will hesitate to prescribe pain-killing drugs for fear of masking a diagnosis that may point towards life-saving measures.

Acute pain is now managed mostly by administering pain-killers. And modern medical science has an ever widening range of drugs that allow doctors to relieve, at last temporarily, every form of pain we are heir to. Dental treatment should be pain-free, and so also medical procedures and tests. You see football or hockey players writhing in pain on the field afforded instant relief by their medical attendants.

No wonder, people are now advised not to put up with pain that stays more than three days or even continues unabated for a full day despite an intake of aspirin or similar pills. This sort of pain calls for medical investigation.

Chronic pain is different; its management still posing many challenges. Often physical therapy is combined with psychological approaches. Recourse is being taken to measure such as hypnosis, acupuncture, adhesive strips, and PCAs (Patient Controlled Analgesia). Acupuncture works on the principle of anaesthetizing the painful part of the body with precision needle pricks, as well as releasing pain inhibiting body chemicals called endorphins. A stick-on patch, such as Fentanyl, an opiate, can deliver a continuous dose for three days; especially useful for chronic pain.

PCA is based on the idea that the patient is the best judge of how much pain he feels and so the best judge of the analgesic dosage. PCAs use a digital pump, with a ceiling on the amount of drug that can enter the body, but its actual release controlled by the patient himself. People generally experience less pain if they can exercise a degree of control. It has also been found that under self-control conditions of PCA, most patients use less analgesic medication than they would otherwise.

That brings in the psychological element in pain. It is widely accepted that pain is worse when anxiety is high, and that pain can be controlled to an appreciable degree when anxiety can be diminished. Depression and anxiety magnify chronic pain more than they do acute pain, and traditional medical remedies seldom work.

Contraction of neck and scalp muscles as a result of anxiety build tension in those muscles, producing pain, typically headache. Relaxation and the easing of anxiety frequently brings relief. Such pain can be called psychosomatic, i.e., it seems a bodily effect stemming from a psychological disturbance.

And it's because of the psychological component in pain that placebos play a significant role in pain relief. Placebo refers to the improvement based on expectations of gain rather than on the operation of a specifically effective therapeutic remedy. There is some evidence that placebo-based improvement in pain perception has a biochemical basis: expectation of benefit triggers a greater release of endorphins by the brain.

Promoting normal activity reduces pain perception in other cases. For example, in many cases of chronic back pain, doctors often recommend cognitive therapy; teaching patients to accommodate life's negative experiences better. Doctors know that the track record of existing therapies for chronic back pain is rather poor. So they seek the antidote of work; both men and women who are busy in their work record a decrease in back pain intensity during the day. Of course there are some patients who seem reluctant to give up the rewards of their pain, such as attracting sympathy or evading the rigours of life.

Yet there are many others who suffer from incurable pain that has no immediate cause. Here is pain making their lives a misery for decades, with drugs doing little good. As the pain has no obvious and immediate cause, there is always the unspoken charge that the pain is imaginary.

Recent researches indicate that the cause of this inexplicable, unpredictable pain could be crossed wires deep within the nervous system. A disease or accident (even suffered years back) could stimulate the production of chemicals that encourage nerve growth—nature's way of regrowing damaged nerves. Sometimes these crossed wires link nerve fibres carrying everyday messages from the body's surface with the pain pathways to the brain.

In some patients this type of pain is known to disappear suddenly of its own accord. But in many others, chronic, untreatable pain plagues them for years on end.

Doctors hope, someday they would have therapies that tackle this enigmatic pain by attempting to prevent cross-wiring from occurring in the first place, or at least undoing the cross-wiring. They are now searching for the chemicals that stimulated the nervous fibres to sprout because blocking these chemicals could prevent the spectre of cross-wiring and consequent pain. Someday there would be drugs that will either block the production of these nerve fertilizers immediately following a severe injury at the actual sites where rewiring is likely to occur or they will undo the rewiring once it has happened.

Till then, these victims have to put up with their enigmatic pain. Their only consolation: it's not an imaginary pain they suffer, but from actual crossed wires in their nervous system.

No One Now Need Suffer Severe Pain

Most of us suffer occasional pains—usually headaches or backaches or an injury—which, while we have them, can make us less efficient in our work and more irritable.

Yet many of us choose to "soldier on" without taking a pain reliever as if that would signify some sort of a weakness. The present-day medical practice views this approach as rather misguided. Continued pain itself is debilitating, let alone the problem causing the pain.

Medical science can now supply you with effective pain relief whether your pain be severe or niggling, acute or chronic.

That's the good news to emerge from the technological advances in recent years. Modern medical and dental treatment should be pain free. If you find it isn't, you should ask why—and don't accept an excuse for an answer.

Similarly medical procedures, tests and investigations should involve no real pain, and you need not avoid them for fear of it. Indeed, with the current advances in pain control, all those diseases traditionally associated with suffering and pain have had their sting removed.

In the last twenty years there has been a great expansion in our knowledge of the biochemical mechanism through which pain is produced. In particular, two processes have been unravelled which are helping medical science to manage pain.

Billions of microscopic receptors exist in the skin and in most organs. They are the front-line defences, sensitive to any potential harmful stimulation. When triggered by injury or irritation, they send warning signals along nerves to the brain where the signals are interpreted as pain.

Recently scientists have discovered that, when the receptors are stimulated, cells around them release chemicals—the best known are prostaglandins. When these chemicals reach the brain through the bloodstream, they bring on pain, by lowering the body's threshold of pain.

Pain relievers like aspirin or ibuprofen don't act directly on the brain; they inhibit the release of the prostaglandins, thus indirectly reducing pain.

The second discovery is that powerful pain relievers like morphine work by attaching themselves to special sites in the brain. Clearly nature did not provide such sites in the brain in anticipation of man-made drugs. The receptors are now understood to be intended for naturally-occurring brain chemicals with which the body protects itself against pain. These chemicals have been identified and named endorphins.

Acupuncture is thought to ease pain by activating the brain's pain-relieving endorphin system. Self-activation of endorphins may also be responsible for the "placebo effect"—the pain relief that one in three people experience when given a dummy pill which does not actually contain a pain reliever.

Coping with Serious Pain

Never put up with pain which stays on for more than three days or continues unabated for a full day despite your intake of aspirin or similar pills. This sort of pain calls for medical investigation.

On the pain front, the welcome news: the ever widening range of modern pain killers and a vastly improved knowledge of methods of pain control allow doctors to relieve every form of pain that we are heir to. Even incurable diseases should no longer produce severe pain.

For doctors these days it's a routine procedure to mount a double attack when treating an illness: against the disease and against the pain.

Pain, or fear of pain, is even being taken out of dying. Hospice doctors and nurses have now so refined their skills that they can give drugs in just the right measure and just the right times to relieve pain without "drugging" the senses.

It's somewhat unfortunate that medicine's achievements in the control of pain are not more widely known because they have removed one of the great fears that people have about illness.

No one now need to suffer prolonged or severe pain. That's the gift of science, something that Homo Sapiens had never enjoyed since their existence on this earth.

Your Aching Back

In adults back pain is rated as the third commonest symptom after headache and tiredness. Indeed four out of five people will fall victim at least once in their life to backache. It is the leading cause of lost workdays.

Women outnumber men in back pain problems, let alone the backache associated with pregnancy.

And there is little doubt that with sedentary habits, poor computer posture and a longer span of life, we'll experience more back problems.

Some make out that backache is the result of poor anatomical design; human spine not yet fully adapted to the upright posture. However our spine is a miracle of design and a wonder of engineering which researchers are just beginning to unravel. Scientists know more about the inner workings of molecules than about what happens to your back when you bend over to tie your laces.

The anatomy of human back is coming out incredibly complex. The 33 vertebrae, though made of calcium, are full of blood, with cells endlessly repairing cracks. Each vertebra is attached to a whole range of ligaments and muscles. The ligaments act as check reins; bend too far and they stop your spine from curling over. The muscles controlling spinal movements are in layers, and it's hard to know which layer is contracting. Studies of backache concentrate on muscle functioning—what can go wrong with muscles and what to do about it?

Possibly the most practical and advanced work on back pain is currently being done at the Vermont Back Research Centre, University of Vermont. Researchers there not only generate scientific papers, they also produce usable gear.

For instance, the Centre has designed Virtual Corset for back pain sufferers. This electronic gadget, the size of a pocketbook, is worn over the shirt, harnessed to the chest. It monitors how the torso moves throughout the day; recording not only flexion and lateral bending but also twisting. Virtual Corset even gives a warning beep if the wearer bends his back beyond a certain degree—tailored to each individual's back condition. The data recorded in Virtual Corset is periodically unloaded onto a computer for study by the physician. This is useful information as a doctor doesn't see a patient's movements in normal life. Often the patient himself fails to notice many of his own back movements.

The Centre has invented a laboratory tool, Lordosimeter, to measure the curvature of the lower back. This helps researchers to evaluate how the sitting posture affects pressure on spine's disks. Spinal stenosis typically afflicts people in their 60s and 70s. Their ageing vertebrae's bony protuberances enlarge, pressuring nerve roots and constricting tiny blood vessels, triggering back pain. People are educated into safer sitting postures on the basis of problems revealed by Lordosimeter.

For sitting long hours on chairs, a BackCycler has been developed. It looks like a backrest cushion, wired to a power point. The gadget keeps your spine moving as you sit, and so shifts the weight on muscles. Some airline seats and executive chairs are already being fitted with a BackCycler. Of course, the best antidote still remains getting up frequently, especially in computer-based work involving much sitting.

For people working in factories and warehouses who commonly lift loads, the Centre has designed a Liftbox. It's a cardboard carton containing 16 pounds of stuffing, with wires snaked to a computer. When someone lifts the Liftbox, the accelerometer in it relays the box's velocity changes to a computer. Liftbox is being used as a research tool to determine the safest lifting techniques. And workers are trained into lifting goods at the least risk to their backs. Researchers there however concede that nobody really knows the rules for safe lifting—that's what they are still figuring out.

The Centre's studies have shown that drivers of heavy trucks, buses, surface-mining trucks, and helicopter pilots have four times the normal incidence of low back pain. One hypothesis is that shaking beats up the back and its muscles. Modern trucks and buses have improved suspension, yet the constant vibration inflicted on the back takes its toll.

The Centre has designed a machine called The Shaker that can mimic the vibrations of any vehicle, from a delivery van to a helicopter. It tests the impact of vibrations and jolting on the spine. Experiments are being conducted how to dampen vibrations with an air-filled cushion. Computer readings on The Shaker are showing promising results about the damping effects of an air-filled seat cushion.

What can be done for the persistent sufferer of back pain? Certainly there is no lack of palliative measures which include oral medication (analgesics or muscle relaxants); injections (steroids or anaesthetics); physical intervention such as manipulation, massage, local heat application, and use of corset; counter-stimulation with electrical nerve stimulation and acupuncture; and as a last resort, surgery. Often a "slipped disc" is diagnosed in the absence of sufficient evidence.

The Vermont Centre, however, still lays emphasis on lifestyle changes than medicine. To prevent back pain people are advised to keep trim, not to slouch, and exercise muscles that support the back. Long bed rest for back pain is not recommended as more than a day or two in bed actually weakens the back muscles. Instead, slowly and steadily resume normal activities. Only at first, avoid heavy lifting, repeated bending and twisting, and long periods of sitting still.

There are some tasks that may be safely attempted by the chronic back pain sufferer, and others that should be delegated to their more fortunate brethren. This is not a matter of evasion but of prudent avoidance—keeping a curb on any "injudicious burst of activity".

Work is a good antidote against chronic pain. People at work record a decrease in pain intensity. Even after returning from work they seem to experience less pain than the group that stayed home all day.

The track record of existing therapies for chronic back pain is rather poor. Surely medical research such as at the Vermont Back Research Centre is busy finding ways to alleviate and prevent chronic back pain. Yet a magic cure is proving disappointingly elusive. Sufferers perforce have to learn to live with it. And more successfully they do so, the better they cope with their affliction.

Having a Headache

"Two-thirds of us have a headache at least once a month, and only 2 per cent of people never have one," says Dr Andrew Dawson, the director of the King's College Hospital Headache Service in London.

It is estimated that at any time one in five of the adult population in the country has a headache. No wonder headaches are the most common complaints heard by doctors.

Headaches cause such a lot of suffering as well as loss of productivity, yet surprisingly little is known about them. Even what happens in the head during the most obvious of headaches, the hangover, is not clear. It is assumed that the intake of alcohol produces chemical damage, but no researcher has ever detected or located this damage.

Admittedly some headaches are the symptoms of an underlying problem, such as a brain tumour. But these constitute a tiny fraction; the vast majority of headaches occur for no known physiological reason. Some people tend to attribute headache to eye strain. But often, eye strain is not the culprit. In many cases it is more likely that the headache comes first, and that in turn gives rise to a feeling of eye strain.

And no one is sure whether a particular headache can be blamed on work stress or family problems or road rage or a difficult neighbour. People are known to develop headache from a poor sleeping position, smoking, traffic fumes, even job interviews.

That way, almost everything one eats or does can lead to a headache. For example, there's the ice-cream headache, much debated over by scientists. Some people get a pain in the head within minutes of consuming something cold.

You can get a headache if you miss your usual cup of coffee. And eating too much of chocolates can trigger a headache. Reaction to quite a few foods, such as too much meat or cheese, could also give rise to headache.

Photophobia headaches are brought on by a reaction to bright light, and phonophobia to loud noise.

There's even a phenomenon called coitus headache—though, happily, not so common. It usually comes on during sexual intercourse, and is thought to be triggered by changes in blood pressure or hormones.

Indoor Pollutants

Our exposure to most toxic pollutants could be several times higher in indoor environments than it is outdoors. But, whereas there's much public concern with city air pollution, precious little attention is focussed on indoor pollutants.

Take a typical household with small children. A toddler mouthing anything that comes to hand, crawling under the dining table, or sucking its soiled fingers. A bigger kid hugging the dog, playing with stuffed toys, or rolling on the carpet.

And it's small children who are most exposed to indoor pollutants, whether from dust mites in carpets or pesticides sticking to toys, or contaminants carried by pets. That way, kids are little guinea pigs testing the toxicity of whatever pollutants are in the home.

Children are more at risk than adults, because they have a higher metabolic rate and their organs are still developing. Weight for weight, they inhale much more than adults, while their lungs can be irritated by relatively lower levels of air pollution.

To a housewife, dust settling on sofas and beds, carpets and clothes is more of a nuisance than anything else; something to be dusted off regularly. Hardly a thought is given to the fact that house dust is host to millions of germs. And the most prolific of all are the dust mites.

If these bothersome creatures would only manifest themselves like flies or mosquitoes, a housewife could swat them or train a flit gun at them. But these eight-legged cousins to the spider and the tick are less than one-half millimetre long, and mostly invisible. And then dust mites play safe by sneaking into carpets, bedclothes, stuffed furniture, and similar soft objects.

Dust mites, one of the 20,000 species of mites, are running no risk of extinction, though they die by millions each day. Female dust mites make sure of this by laying over 50 eggs before passing out.

What do dust mites feed on? They are meat eaters, and curiously enough, their only diet consists of flakes of skin that humans constantly shed.

Each dust mite produces about 20 fecal pellets a day. And it is these waste particles that trigger allergies in people, even asthma. Infants are particularly vulnerable to dust mites.

Affluent homes with wall-to-wall carpeting, heavy curtains, and cushioned sofas prove an excellent habitat for these invisible devils.

Besides dust mites, plenty of pesticides are found deep inside carpets—often deep among the fibres and the backing, and beyond the reach of vacuuming. Pesticides, whether sprayed in rooms or on the lawn, cling to shoes and pet's paws, and then get rubbed off the carpeting. A typical sample of household carpet dust sent to a lab would disclose significant presence of heavy metals and toxic chemicals, such as lead, mercury, cadmium, pesticides and hydrocarbons.

Real thick doormats do help. Better still, if people leave their shoes at the door. Weekly vacuuming of carpets becomes a must. And the necessity of more passes over the area of rugs near the entrance, and other areas that receive a lot of traffic. A vacuum cleaner with a power head is more effective as it picks up three to six times as much dust as one without power brushes. Anyway vacuuming is vastly superior to using dusters or brooms; the latter becomes more an exercise in rearranging the dust.

For people with small kids or with adults allergic to dust mites, tiled floors with scattered rugs prove more environmental friendly than wall-to-wall carpeting. Luckily, as a people, we are given to washing our floors or wiping them daily with wet cloth. As to floor rugs, experts recommend deep-cleaning once a year by professional cleaners.

Dust filters in air-conditioners do remove much of airborne particles of dust. But then these filters have to be cleaned frequently.

People who use pesticides indoors may inadvertently expose small children to significant contamination, even if they're careful to keep kids and chemicals apart. Chemicals evaporate, drift from place to place, precipitate back onto carpets, toys and other soft household objects, with which children come in contact. And pesticides persist for months indoors because they are sheltered from sun, rain and other forces that quickly degrade them outdoors.

Lately anti-allergen sprays have come into the market. One such brand called "Mitey" from Allergy Free Inc. does deactivate dust mites and their droppings if sprayed once every couple of months. And it is deemed quite safe.

Bald Pates

It is paradoxical that, as a middle-aged man's crowning glory recedes, his beard, just a few centimetres away, is still increasing in range and luxuriance. He might well be forgiven for wondering whether the one is growing at the expense of the other, though this is not true. And what about all those wiry hair sprouting on the torso, crowding eyebrows, even coming out of ears and nostrils.

Each hair follicle has a destiny of its own which is influenced by hormones. Hairs are actually programmed according to the specific surface they are growing on. Some grow faster and thicker and longer than others. That's why grafting isn't the answer—follicles from the chest or armpits, for instance, will still produce short, curly hair when grafted on the pate.

Science has started studying the genes that are responsible for the striking differences in body hair. Successfully tracked these could someday lead to new treatment for hair growth and hair removal. Then balding and shaving could become things of the past.

The human scalp has 1,00,000 to 2,00,000 hair follicles with their cyclical production of hair. We lose 100 to 150 hair daily as a part of natural shedding. And balding gradually sets in when daily loss goes up beyond that without a corresponding increase in the replacement rate.

Hair grows an average of 1.25 cm a month. Each day, a young adult produces about forty metres of hair on the head. Hair grows faster in summer and slower in winter. Rubbing speeds hair growth.

Women too suffer hair loss. But baldness only starts to occur after the menopause; till then women are buffered by female hormones. Anyway their testosterone levels being low, hair attrition is far slower than in men.

Why some men lose their scalp hair while others don't is a mystery that has puzzled mankind for centuries. No wonder, it gave rise to a flourishing quackery business in hair. Everything imaginable or unimaginable is said to have been tried. Cleopatra gave Caesar a mix of deer's marrow, horses' teeth and bear oil to counter his bald spot.

Science now knows of the link between DHT (dihydrotestosterone), a derivative of testosterone, with balding hair. DHT is understood to interfere with the growth cycle of scalp hair, thus not allowing the hair loss from natural shedding to be made up.

But why do we have DHT receptors in the scalp is still a mystery. And why hair follicles on the front, top and crown behave differently from those on the sides? One explanation is that only the scalp hair carry DHT receptors, not the side hair. But why this should be so begs an answer.

There is the popular theory that balding men have higher levels of testosterone. These men commonly attract "the sexy" label; being blessed with a surfeit of the male hormone. Recent studies have spiked this consolation. It seems all men have roughly the same amount of circulating testosterone, regardless of the state of their hair.

Baldness is often seen to run in families. The genetic influence is obvious. Recently a hair gene has been identified. As this is a dominant gene, balding requires only one copy present to be effective, and it therefore does not tend to skip generations as commonly happens with recessive genes. A quick scan of the heads of older male relatives gives a young man a rough guide to his chances of keeping his hair.

Some experts have been advocating the lifestyle approach to combat baldness. Admittedly men are balding earlier these days. You sometimes see men who are 30 have the same level of hair loss as their dads had at 50. This quicker balding is attributed to increased stress in modern living. Stress hormones, such as adrenalin and prolactin, raise levels of testosterone and consequently DHT.

Medical experts aren't much impressed with the lifestyle approach. They argue that changing diet or reducing stress won't change hair follicles genetically programmed to fail.

That leaves the field largely to drugs. Some men taking Minoxidil for high blood pressure reported hair growth. Now rubbed down as a lotion, it can slow down hair loss. But then only a small percentage of users are known to get real hair growth.

The latest treatment licensed by FDA (the Federal Drug Authority of USA) is once-a-day pill called Propecia. It contains a low dose of finastride, a drug originally developed to counter prostate enlargement. Finastride has the effect of blocking the conversion of testosterone into DHT. About 80 per cent of its users in USA report a stoppage in hair loss, while some 30 per cent claim to have regained a significant element of their hair.

The new pill however is no magic bullet. It has to be taken every day all the time. And its long-term effects are unknown. A few regular users report a noticeable drop in sex drive. That way the only sure safeguard against going bald is castration; castrated men never go bald.

What are the chances of restoring hair once lost? A bald pate is not quite as lifeless as it seems; it conceals an army of tiny hairs lurking in little holes. The great challenge of hair research is to find ways of bringing these out. With the medical advances taking place this may well be feasible before the follicles have receded too far. But there is a point of no return.

Male-pattern baldness carries no known health risks. But the so-called good head of hair represents vitality, beauty, and youth, and is a token of the qualities of parts of the body that cannot be seen. The lately fashionable Mohican "plumage" sported by some youth is a slap in the face of any middle-aged man because this is the site on which he has greatest difficulty keeping his hair.

And baldness is a bigger blow to pride than going grey, and more difficult to hide. Hair "greys" because pigment cells fail to invade its roots. No one knows why this happens. There is a silver lining, however, because men with dark hair who grey early tend to be spared balding. The puzzling link may have something to do with the greater wiriness of unpigmented hairs.

Restless Legs Syndrome

Many of us may not have heard of the Restless Legs Syndrome (RLS). And yet this disorder is the mysterious robber of sleep. RLS is an important cause of insomnia.

The main symptom is recurrent, unpleasant, peculiar creeping sensation in the legs, occasionally in the thighs or feet. The arms and hands are rarely affected. This discomfort (seldom a true pain) worsens when we turn in for the night. And RLS—sometimes lasting only a short period, sometimes for hours—is invariably relieved when we walk. But it can reappear after the patient returns to bed.

Restless legs (a seemingly frivolous term) give rise to a sensation that is hard to describe. Some sufferers describe it as ache or pinpricks. Others have a crawling feeling like you have worms in your legs. Some experience a slow annoyance like a feather duster skimming over the legs.

No wonder doctors often think, it's simply a cramp or loss of blood flow in the legs. Or it could be arthritis. But then with RLS you get instant relief when you move or walk; the same doesn't happen with arthritis.

Perhaps the most troublesome aspect of RLS is the speed with which an urge comes to move. And this urge can sometimes become uncontrollable; leading to risky night walking. RLS specialists have drawn up a few tips for coping with the panic.

Patients are always advised to remember that though the momentary feelings and symptoms may be frightening, these are neither dangerous nor threatening. Best is to take a dozen deep breaths, as deep as you can make them and hold them as long as you can before exhaling.

Your need to move your legs is real but it is also temporary. The bothersome sensation soon goes away with walking.

Not to dwell on the fear that your RLS might get worse.

When an urge to move comes, better keep your brain active with a manageable task, such as reading, working in the kitchen or doing other odd household jobs. Keeping the brain active helps to wear out the anxiety itself.

A soak in a tub of warm water can do good.

How exactly RLS originated is not known, but now the incidence is significantly large. It is estimated that around 5% of the population throughout the world may be suffering from it in various degrees of intensity, from occasional annoyances to daily attacks. Most cases of RLS are diagnosed in people aged sixty or older.

Restless legs syndrome is usually inherited. RLS follows an autosomal dominant type inheritance pattern. This means that males and females are equally affected. And RLS keeps being passed on from one generation to the next as opposed to a recessive pattern where a particular disease will skip some generations only to return in later generations. Again, only one parent has to be affected with RLS for the children to get it. If RLS runs in your family and you are not affected, your children will never get it. Surely all children of an RLS parent don't contract it. However, statistically it is likely that half of all children of an RLS parent will someday be affected with RLS themselves if the parent has the inherited form of RLS.

Of late restless legs syndrome has been attracting a great deal of medical attention and research. One leader in the field is the Restless Legs Syndrome Foundation, Inc, 304 Glenwood Avenue, Raleigh, North Carolina 27603. It also issues a newsletter *Night Walker*. And possibly the best book to come out recently on the subject is *The Mysterious Robber of Sleep: Restless Legs Syndrome* by Virginia N. Wilson (Galaxy Books, 1996, pages 316).

According to Wilson, one of the greatest aggravations suffered by RLS victims is the lack of proper diagnosis. Too many physicians either don't acknowledge the existence of RLS or fail to recognize the symptoms, though this requires no expensive sleep disorder testing. Other doctors make all type of conjectures: hypochondria, stress, depression, allergies, muscle tautness, and imaginary ills.

RLS sufferers sometimes wonder why the medical world has not been made aware of this disorder that can ruin lives mentally and physically?

RLS is often confused with Periodic Limb Movements in Sleep (PLMS). The jerky movements of PLMS are generally too gentle to wake up patients but some sufferers kick very violently, and may injure themselves or their bedmates. Most patients with RLS have PLMS, but PLMS may occur by themselves in non-RLS patients as well.

According to Dr Wilson, the finding of the proper medication to alleviate RLS symptoms is not easy. Each patient seems to respond differently, and so he or she should find a doctor who knows RLS and is willing to devote considerable time and attention to the case.

Wilson does not favour medication where patients can make their symptoms tolerable by the correct amount of sleep and exercise, avoiding caffeine, or a simple thing like a hot shower before bedtime. But if your RLS occurs most days (nights), then you probably will need a medication that is taken on daily basis.

RLF Foundation gets numerous letters of magical cures. The Foundation's policy is not to discourage experimentation or beliefs as long the methods employed are not harmful. People however are cautioned that often such hopes prove misplaced. The problem with RLS is that it can go away on its own (while a patient ascribes it to some magic remedy) but then it can recur after some time.

By now there are tried and tested medicines for RLS. The primary ones are sedatives like benzodiazepines (Klonopin, Restoril, Halcion, Valium). All are usually taken before bedtime and are relatively safe. Another group is the Dopamine-related medications. These are useful for treatment of both RLS and PMLS. And in many cases a combination of the two medications has proved beneficial. It's for the physician to make a choice, balancing the benefits against the side-effects or other drawbacks.

According to the latest medical opinion, RLS is treatable. And serious sufferers should seek proper treatment, instead of letting RLS ruin the quality of their life.

Tired All the Time

"I am doing everything right. I eat well. I sleep well. I exercise. I don't smoke or drink. Why am I tired all the time? Why, why, why?" asks my lawyer friend in exasperation.

Yes, he has every right to ask that question.

In medical terms, feeling tired all the time is called Chronic Fatigue Syndrome (CFS). The disorder poses a puzzle to doctors. It has no identified cause and no specific diagnostic tests. CFS is more common among persons in the 20-40 age group, and more among women than men.

If the feeling of fatigue persists over months, accompanied by symptoms such as dizziness, dry eyes, nausea, earaches, chest pains, bellyache, chronic cough or weight loss, doctors usually look into patient's medical history and undertake a detailed physical examination. They run a few standard tests to eliminate the presence of any specific ailment. In the absence of the same, they tend to treat CFS with mild medication, coupled with any recommended behavioural changes. Patients are often advised not to overdose themselves with medicines; not a pill for every ache and pain. Treated competently, CFS is deemed as totally reversible.

Now, the cause of chronic fatigue could be one or a combination of several factors listed below.

Hormonal problems
Sugar imbalance
The foods you eat

The environment, especially the air you breathe
Moulds, mites, allergies
Sleep and relaxation
Exercise
Depression

Dr Ronald L. Hoffman in his book *Tired All The Time* (Poseiden Press, 1993) discusses these factors at length. But then he comes out with a few surprising findings about chronic fatigue—-secrets that fly in the face of our conventional wisdom.

His first and most important: Energy begets energy. There are people who attack their day with a gusto that seems to increase with each passing hour. They appear to be made of different stuff from the ordinary person. But they're not. People who put in tremendous energy are energized by their very activity. Physical activity oxygenates all parts of the body, including the brain. The result: more energy. According to Hoffman, once you've corrected any flaws in your lifestyle or diet or environment that may be contributing to your fatigue, then you'll find that energy begets energy.

His second finding: Life is not a steady downhill process. While a certain decline in vitality is a natural consequence of ageing, your energy quotient can be sustained at high levels well through middle age and into your senior years.

His third finding: Efforts to conserve energy can leave you more exhausted. Most people think resting a lot will cure their fatigue—yet it often makes it worse. Someone asking another to post a letter a few blocks away, because of being too tired to walk up to the letter box, is the most fatigued. Hoffman has even discovered that when he was tired, sleep wasn't always the answer.

One more secret: Stimulants may give you a short-term boost, but over the long run they can deplete you. Guzzling umpteen cups of coffee can keep you alert—but leave you ultimately depleted.

Another fact of fatigue: Fatigue can sometimes be contagious—just like a yawn. When you sit long with someone who is depressed and fatigued, you may find yourself overcome by a draining ennui.

And Hoffman cautions people who actually use sugar as medicine for the feeling of fatigue or depression. Sugar does indeed change the brain chemistry, and could impart a sense of momentary wellbeing. But then sugar becomes a form of addiction—somewhat akin to alcoholism.

Hoffman advises a switch to a diet of protein and carbohydrates, which provide the body with slowly released and steady levels of sugar, thus reducing reliance on items rich in sugar.

Here is a guide to sugar content of some common foods (grams of sugar per 100 grams of food). While raisins and dates reach 64, bananas, apricots, grapes and apples range between 16 to 12, and oranges 9. Vegetables mostly stay below 9, with onions at 5 and cabbage at 2. Jams and chocolates touch 65, ice cream 23, and Coca-Cola 11.

Favour Your Feet

In a lifetime your feet will walk, run, stroll or dance the equivalent of four times around the earth. Every day we ask our feet to take some 10,000 steps. We slap them down on hard surfaces as we walk, and pound them into the ground when we run. We torture them with ill-fitting shoes, and walk barefoot on floors that aren't free from fungus. No wonder many of us happen to have feet that hurt.

"The foot is a beautifully functioning structure which is absolutely not appreciated," says an eminent orthopaedic surgeon. "It can be flexible as a hand and yet its strength is awesome".

The human foot is indeed a marvel of biomechanics, with its 28 bones, 35 joints, 19 muscles, and more than a hundred ligaments. It is able to withstand pressures equal to four times our weight as we run. Since Homo sapiens stood erect, the human foot has undergone drastic changes: in the shape of its arch, in the strength of the ball as it became the major contact area in walking, and the diminished size and importance of toes coupled with the robustness of the big toe.

Still, if we are not careful, we can damage what nature has so carefully constructed. Neglect can cause crippling foot conditions, and these can also lead to knee, hip, and lower back problems

Here is a brief rundown of the common ailments afflicting the feet.

Calluses. As we get older, the fat padding on the bottoms of our feet, crucial for protecting important bones, thins out. This often results in calluses developing where the shoes and hard surfaces exert pressure against the feet. Though the outer skin on the sole of the foot is about 40 times thicker than it is elsewhere on the body, calluses come up, especially on the balls of the feet. When calluses get big or too hard, they pull the underlying skin, which can tear. And this torn skin can become painful.

In tropical countries like ours, most people go about in slippers or similar loose footwear with thin soles and not much a heel. This does save their toes from being squeezed as in tight shoes but the practice operates quite hard on their heels. The ball of the foot, derived of the cushion, grip and protection yielded by a good closed shoe, comes in frequent contact with the hard ground, even with sharp objects like small stones.

To prevent calluses, make certain your shoe has adequate cushioning, particularly at the heel. If a callus does develop, orthopaedic surgeons recommend using a pumice stone after bathing to sand down calluses. Soft cushions placed in the heel of your shoes, or under the ball of the foot, can also help.

Corns. If your toes are rubbed wrongly by too-tight footwear, hard knobs sprout on the tops around the joints. Soft corns grow between the toes too in response to the friction of one toe rubbing against the other. Once corns form, they can end up hitting each other—painfully.

To fight corns, make sure your shoes are not too tight so as to pinch toes. If corns are already formed, specially designed pads can be placed between the foot and the shoe.

However if corns, and calluses, are causing a good deal of pain or discomfort, you may need to visit a foot-care specialist. Professional trimming of corns and calluses—better avoid doing it yourself—can help, and so also specially fitted shoe inserts.

Ingrown Toenails. This is more an affliction of colder regions where closed shoes are worn most of the time. Ingrown toenails can afflict anyone even great runners. An ingrown toenail usually occurs when pressure from a tight shoe forces the nail of the big toe to dig into the nailbed. This results in swelling, pain, and infection, since the foot—the body part nearest to the ground—is a bacteria-rich environment.

Poor nail trimming can also cause ingrown toenails. If the big toenail is cut too short or left curved sharply at edges, the corners of the nail can act like a knife on the nailbed. Better train your nail to grow properly by cutting it straight across.

For immediate relief of pain, orthopaedic surgeons advise taking pressure off an ingrown toenail by wearing sandals or open-toed shoes. Soaking feet in warm water helps.

Hammertoes. That's another disturbing condition when you crunch your toes into shoes that are too narrow in the front—more common with the narrowly-pointed ladies shoes. The second toe, on getting crowded out, has no choice but to bend up and come down to rest on the tip of the big toe. Other toes can undergo similar contortions for lack of space. And your problem worsens when the contorted toes develop corns from rubbing against the shoe.

Athlete's Foot. This is a common foot disorder with people who go about a good deal barefoot. Fungi lurk everywhere: in your lawn, in the house compound, in the surfaces outside, even in your rooms. Millions in our country catch fungal infections in their feet through little cuts and abrasions.

Luckily these infections are not so dangerous. Good hygiene can take care of these, like regular bathing of the feet and periodic application of a sulfonamide.

Admittedly, the most important element in the care of your feet is the selection of proper shoes. Here are some tips when you go shopping for shoes.

Choose a style that bears some relationship to the shape of your feet. Comfortable shoes tend to be on the squarish side, with wide toe areas and room for your feet to spread out—shoes in C to E widths, instead of A and B. Your feet may look a bit bigger in them, but they'll feel better. Between comfort and image, opt for the former.

Remember that no two feet are the same, and that includes yours. Buy length to fit the longer foot, width to fit the wider one. And allow no less than half an inch of space between your longest toe and the front of the shoe.

Don't assume that your shoe size is forever. As we age, our feet get bigger.

Buy shoes at the end of the day when your feet are a bit swollen.

For added arch support, buy a shoe with a raised heel. A shoe without a heel, or a "negative" heel (soles lower in the back than front) is not good for the feet. Again avoid heels that exceed 2½ inches.

Select shoes made of soft leather, though they tend to be more expensive. Avoid synthetic leather which is stiffer.

Make certain that your shoes have adequate cushioning. While trying shoes in a shop, walk on some hard surface; the carpeted are of the store may give a false sense of padding. Better go in for shoes in which the heel and ball areas have extra cushions. It's the lack of adequate cushioning that often makes the bottoms of your feet like they're on fire.

Lastly, for your feet's sake, get rid of all those old shoes in your closet which no longer fit you. Give away these instruments of torture. If a shoe doesn't fit, just don't wear it.

The Care of Teeth

Dental decay and gum disease are among the most common disease afflicting mankind. And, ironically, the higher the standard of living, the more likely is their occurrence.

Both these diseases, which cause so much pain and suffering, are the result of bacterial action I the mouth, in the plaque which collects on teeth and gums. If it were possible to cleanse the mouth completely of the bacterial plaque and keep it that way, there would be no dental decay. Thus we know what should be done—the difficulty is carrying it out.

It is in this context that preventive dental care assumes crucial importance.

The Role of Diet

Within seconds of eating any sugary substance, acid forms on teeth and takes more than twenty minutes to disappear. Thus, small sugary snacks every two or three hours throughout the day will keep the mouth bathed in a dangerous acid state. For the teeth, the frequency of sugar intake is more harmful than the total consumption of sugar.

To many people sugar only means sweets. But the tooth-harming sugar is contained in many foods. In all sugars (including honey), even in tea and coffee, and in soft drinks such as colas and lemonades. Even strong fruit juices act upon the enamel of the teeth. In cakes, biscuits and desserts. In jams and marmalades. In chocolates and toffees. And in all lozenges and sugared medicinal preparations.

When we cut down sugar in our diet, we deprive the bacteria of the food from which they form the acid. Best is to shift over to sugar-free snacks, such as fruits: apples, organges, bananas. Or things like carrots, cucumber, nuts, milk, yoghurt.

Brushing the Teeth

A lot of people aren't brushing their teeth effectively; they don't brush correctly or spend too little time over it. Some tips from your dentist can be very useful.

Brush the top and bottom teeth separately. And do concentrate on the gum margins (which many people miss). The bristles to be moved back and forth with a gentle circular scrubbing motion and short strokes. Do not forget the teeth right at the back of the mouth and also the insides of the teeth. Finally brush all biting surfaces.

Do not put too much toothpaste on the brush, it will foam up and make you want to spit and rinse too soon. Once people get to the spit and rinse stage they stop brushing though some teeth have not been brushed.

Do not wet your brush before applying the paste or before starting to brush. It alters the action of the bristles and prevents them from removing plaque effectively.

People usually select a toothbrush at random, one that looks nice in its wrapper. The idea that brushes with natural bristles like hog bristles are better than nylon bristles is not correct. Nylon bristles are in fact superior, being made to exact specifications.

Brush heads should be small enough to reach all parts of the mouth and should have a flat brushing surface with a straight handle. The medium or medium soft (never hard) bristles should be set close together.

A toothbrush is due for a discard as soon as its bristles splay out. The average adult should probably buy about four brushes per year; presently this average hovers around one a year. Children need their brushes renewed more often as they tend to mishandle them.

At one time automatic brushes had become quite popular, but they aren't so common now. The main advantage of the automatic brush lies in the speed of its brushing. People who can brush effectively with the usual brush will not need an automatic brush.

As to the toothpaste, it's better to buy a well-known brand, if it otherwise has an acceptable taste. And a periodic change in the brand helps. Preferably buy one which contains a small amount of fluoride—this has been shown to reduce dental decay significantly. On the whole it is better to buy small tubes than the large "economy family size". In this way the tendency for some pastes to harden in the tube will be avoided because the contents will be used quicker.

Water spray irrigation units (such as Waterpik) aren't that attractive, considering the initial cost and the time and effort involved in their use. The money and time would be better spent on more effective brushing.

The same applies to mouthwashes and gargles used as a daily routine. Unless specified by your dentist for a specific condition, there is nothing better or safer than warm water or warm water in which a little table salt has been dissolved.

Dental Floss

Many dental experts assert that even the most careful brushing does not remove all the harmful substances from the crevices between the teeth, parts where the bristles cannot reach. They recommend the use of dental floss, a special silk or nylon thread, available wound in a spool. The floss is either waxed or unwaxed; the vogue today is for unwaxed floss, but the waxed one is easier to handle.

Competent flossing has the ability to remove plaque between teeth and on tooth surface below the gum line. But manipulating the floss correctly and safely is a ticklish operation, and can do with some expert advice. Adults and children over 10 are advised to floss at least once daily, preferably after the evening meal, when there's time to do it properly.

What's the right way to floss? Some tips from the American Dental Association are summed below.

Break off about 18 inches of floss and wind most of it around one of your middle fingers. Wind the rest of the floss around the same finger of your other hand. Hold the floss tightly between your thumbs and forefingers, with about an inch of floss between them.

Gently, use a sawing or a "shoeshine" motion to guide the floss between your teeth. When the floss reaches the gum line, curve it into a C-shape against one tooth. Don't jab or snap floss between teeth—it can cut into the gum, leaving an opening for the bacterial invasion.

Carefully slide the floss into the space between the gum and tooth until you feel resistance. Gently scrape the side of the tooth while moving the floss away from the gum. Be sure to follow these steps on the both sides of all your teeth—even the ones at the back.

Try to keep your fingers at the same level as the tooth you're going to floss, that's perpendicular to the tooth. Don't pull it up too high or down too low.

Toothpicks

Sad as it may sound, toothpicks like reading glasses, symbolize the onset of age. The older you grow, the more the fleshy gum tissues of your teeth recede, Fragments of food, particularly tenacious fragments of meat, get lodged between the exposed necks of the teeth. And it comes as a relief when one got rid of the offending matter with the help of a toothpick or piece of floss.

Dentists frown on toothpicks as these are known to injure gums. And what worries dentists more is the wide variety of implements people press into service to pick their teeth. A standard toothpick of wood or plastic is understandable. But people use paper-pins, points of knives, edges of visiting cards, even hair pins or bus tickets.

Whatever be the views of dentists, toothpicks continue in common use. People find them much easier to handle than floss. And you can't expect eating places to supply dental floss the way they stack toothpicks on tables or airlines pack one in the cutlery pouch.

Perhaps the best we can hope for are better quality toothpicks in the coming years, whether of wood or plastic. Our wooden ones presently are too fragile. They tend to break, sometimes creating their own obstruction.

Much scientific work is taking place to develop an anti-decay vaccine for the teeth—to bring immunity to the organism which causes dental decay. The research has shown promising results with monkeys. And it is hoped that, in the not too distant future, refinements in the vaccination materials, may enable humans to be made immune from dental decay. Till then the emphasis remains strongly on preventive everyday care.

3

Gender-related Health Issues

Gender and Health

Being a man can be damaging to your health. And damaging to your country, too, in terms of costs. Take the money wasted in locking men up, for example—men make over 90 per cent of the prison population. Or, take the havoc they wreak on roads with drunken driving.

Under the age of 50, men are more at risk of heart disease than women; the latter partially protected by the estrogen they produce until they reach the menopause. Women have more durable hearts. With men heart-related mortality rates soar after thirty-five, while women's heart problems don't usually crop up till forty-five.

Men's testosterone causes increased levels of bad cholesterol in their blood and suppresses the good kind, whereas in women, estrogen has precisely the opposite effect.

Throughout their lives, women have stronger immune systems than men, thanks to a higher number of T-cells.

Women have slower metabolism than men, which may mean that men's cells are placed under greater stress throughout life, or, put simply, that their life cycle completes itself sooner. No wonder, in societies where females suffer no discrimination in food or health care vis-à-vis males, women on average live longer by 4-5 years.

Women are less prone to cancers of the lung, bladder and the stomach, but more susceptible to such chronic conditions as arthritis and osteoporosis.

Women have better hearing and sense of smell. And their memory functions better and longer into old age as compared to men.

And because women have less of testosterone that contributes to baldness, they are less likely to lose their hair.

Men have a higher incidence of myopia, hernia, acne, and flatulence than women. And are heir to more genetic disorders such as colour blindness or left-handedness.

On top, men are natural exuberant risk takers: loving dangerous sports, binge drinking, and being sexually more predatory.

Men tend to take more chances with their health. And when things go wrong, are less inclined to do anything about it, much less consult a doctor. On average, men go to doctors half as many times as women. Indeed many men visit doctors only when their wives make them do so.

Even when it becomes imperative to see a doctor, men often don't do it properly. It could mean skipping on the case history or otherwise belittling the problem—both male patients and male doctors have absorbed lessons in being strong and silent. One survey of UK's National Health Service revealed that a consultation between a woman GP and a woman patient will last four times as long as one between a male doctor and a male patient.

If women risk cancer of the breast and ovaries, men equally risk prostate cancer, let alone problems with urination from an enlarged prostate.

Happily, in recent years, an increasing awareness of men's health problems is emerging. It is also being realized that improving men's health will improve women's health, too. After all, women suffer looking after their sick men.

Men's Health

With the health stakes so stacked against men, it is amazing that so much gets written and talked about women's health problems, while men's specific ailments attract so little attention. In that sense, men may well be victims of discrimination health-wise.

Of all the male health hazards, the prostate poses the biggest. It's an obscure, walnut-sized gland, located beneath the bladder. This gland surrounding the urethra—the duct carrying urine—contributes another 15-30 percent to semen coming forth from the testes. Nobody understands what precisely the added components do, but these are assumed to be crucial in reproduction.

Trouble from the prostate comes in three forms: prostatitis, benign prostatic hyperplasia (BPH) and prostate cancer.

Prostatitis is the inflammation of the gland, mostly caused by infection. It generally affects younger men in their twenties, thirties and forties. The usual symptoms are burning sensation when passing urine, along with an urge to pass urine frequently.

The standard treatment is antibiotics. Chronic prostatitis, however, calls for prolonged medication, even surgery.

BPH occurs when the inner portion of the prostate enlarges. Such a swelling can obstruct the flow of urine by pressing upon the urethra.

Obstructive symptoms of BPH include hesitancy (difficulty in actually getting started every time you try to urinate), a weak stream, an intermittent flow even with a full bladder (starting and stopping), straining to urinate, and dribbling urine after you have ostensibly finished urinating. Others complain of nocturia (needing to pass urine repeatedly at night), urgency (wanting to pass water immediately), even reduced sexual activity.

Urination by older men with an enlarged prostate presents quite a few problems, both physical and psychological. Having to wait for the urine steam to come on is certainly an embarrassment in men's room. You're like a creature from a world of slow motion marooned in a world of the speeded-up. You wait and wait, while younger men arrive, un-adjust their clothing, discharge themselves noisily (sometimes humming cheekily), zip themselves respectable again, and vanish, to be succeeded by others, while you're still at your unfinished business.

It often means getting up at all hours to urinate, taking forever to start, taking forever to finish, and never feeling like you've finished. Then the misery of holding out when it's most inconvenient (a long bus trip, for instance), or getting rid of the last urine drops before you zip up your fly, leaving an embarrassing dark spot on your trousers.

Presumably everyone with an enlarged prostate works out a strategy to save himself from embarrassments in public toilets. There are occasions when you stand before a urinal like your companion and make a motion of winding up at the same time he finishes but actually coming out unemptied. This could mean a surreptitious visit to the toilet soon after.

Wherever possible, some people make for an enclosed toilet; this affords more time in comparative privacy than an exposed urinal. Anyway a stream that has grown hesitant and intermittent is easier to operate standing over a toilet bowl than aiming at a cupped urinal.

The most annoying part is to manage a proper stop. Often you imagine you've finished. Even give yourself a few extra seconds to be on the safe side, and a few shakes, what's called "the shaking of the tree". And then suffer the mortification of a trickle down your leg or awkward spots appearing on the trousers. One is compelled to take a seat or cover one's front with something till those spots dry up. Maybe, such people should equip themselves with more absorbent underpants or even wear Depends (the Adult Incontinence Pants).

In youth it's no great deal to hold out urine for hours. With older men with enlarged prostate, it often comes with near uncontrollable urgency.

When urination problems become acute and medicines don't help (quite a few medicines are now in the market to shrink the enlarged prostrate), doctors have been recommending surgery. In a surgical procedure called TURP, a tube is passed through the urethra (penis) and bits of prostate tissue are snipped off by a tiny blade and sucked away. Repeated clippings eventually free up the passage, for some years at least.

By age sixty-five, about three-quarters of all men will experience BPH. What causes the enlargement of the prostate is still a mystery. It just seems to happen, like wrinkles on the face or hair on the shoulders, and the other signs of male ageing.

The worst is the cancer of the prostate. This is agonizingly common, the second major cause of death in males by cancer, next only to lung cancer. Among its victims are a whole lot of high-profile figures: Colin Powell, former US army commander; New York mayor Rudolh Giuliani; Rupert Murdoch, the media king; actor Charles Heston; Tiger Wood's father. If all men lived up to 90, almost everyone would have prostate cancer.

Yet prostate cancer is the cancer science knows least about. No one has a clue as to what causes it. While lung cancer is often attributed to smoking, esophagus cancer to alcohol, nothing in one's lifestyle has been identified to prostate cancer. Sex hormones may well be involved, as castrates don't get prostate cancer.

Prostate cancer is now diagnosed through the PSA test. In case of high PSA levels, further tests like a biopsy are undertaken. It can then mean radiation therapy or an operation called radical prostatectomy. The latter can successfully cope with prostate cancer if by that time the carcinoma has not spread beyond the prostate into bones or other surrounding organs. Of course, this operation entails profuse bleeding, and can have serious side effects such as impotence and incontinence.

The prostate is like a railway carriage sitting on tracks. These tracks are the nerves that promote an erection. The surgeon has to lift the prostate off these nerves without traumatizing them—a procedure calling for high precision and skill. Once damaged, these nerves take years to regenerate, if at all.

To some, the prospect of incontinence is worse than impotence. This is a possible ramification, because the upper sphincter, which helps retain urine, is lost during surgery. There is another valve below the prostate but does nothing much of its life. Now this lower valve has to be strengthened through prolonged physical therapy to stop the annoying urine leak. Many sufferers have to wear some sort of a sanitary pad under their underwear to take care of leaked urine. It's critical that the lower valve is not damaged during prostate removal surgical procedure.

Luckily prostate tumours are usually small, and they grow very slowly. Often their hosts die for other reasons before the cancer causes trouble. That has given rise to a peculiar medical dilemma these days: to operate on prostate cancer or to leave it alone? Which prostrate cancer will advance fast and which will advance slow is very hard to tell. That poses for both patients and doctors a cruel dilemma.

It is felt in many quarters that far fewer funds and research effort has been put into the study of prostate cancer, than say, of breast cancer.

Testicular cancer used to be relatively rare, about one in every 100 cancers in men, but the rate has doubled in the last 20 years. It's commoner in men in the 30-40-year age group.

And then all those problems of male sexual dysfunctioning. Some surveys show that the incidence of erectile dysfunction is quite widespread; something like one in 10 for men below 50, going progressively higher as men age. And the incidence is reported be rising rapidly. Maybe, men are now more forthcoming in talking about this problem.

Of late there is the growing trend to look up health web sites on the Internet for advice. But this can be no substitute for communicating with real persons, the very reason men don't go to their family doctors in the first place. That way, an over-reliance on the Internet alone can end up doing more harm than good.

Ins and Outs of Impotence

Impotence is defined as the inability to achieve erection satisfactory for an intercourse. At one time or another, almost all men experience the embarrassment and anguish of being unable to get or keep an erection. While this problem most frequently occurs in men in their sixties and seventies, it also occurs in thirties and forties.

An isolated experience—often from fatigue or mental preoccupation or alcohol—is soon rectified. Unfortunately, for many, the failure to get an erection is not a transient phenomenon but well-nigh a part of life. To Masters and Johnson, if the failure rate approaches 25 per cent of the sexual attempts, impotence is established.

"Erectile dysfunction" is of several types. Some men never have erection, others only in masturbation, others capable of erection with one partner but not with another. Others have only soft erections under all circumstances.

Generally the first reaction of the wife to episodic impotence of her mate is sympathetic and supportive. With repeated failures, however, this may give way to feelings of no longer being attractive or no longer being loved. She may even believe her husband has another woman. The man, on his part, starts avoiding behaviour which could possibly lead to sexual relations. Even hugs and pets are avoided. The physical loss of communication could well progress to periods of sustained silence between the couple.

Most men will not seek help for a problem with impotence until some deterioration of their marriage has occurred. And then they usually consult their physician. Unfortunately, few physicians are trained to deal with the problem, and frequently the answer they give is, "Relax and don't worry about it". An impotent man can neither relax nor stop worrying about it.

Over the past decade great strides have been made in understanding the causes of impotence. The most important finding to come out; around fifty percent of impotence appears to be the result of some underlying physical, rather than psychological, disorder. It could be an obvious cause such as prostate cancer surgery or an obscure one such as damage to blood vessels or nerves, a hormone imbalance, or adverse effects of medication. Much of this is amenable to medical treatment. That way it's become abundantly clear that loss of erection is not normal, natural, or inevitable. What's essential to treatment is achieving as accurate a diagnosis as possible.

At the outset, it's important to recognize that an erection is a normal physiological response that is involuntary, and not a response that can be willed. A man who does not understand this, or who cannot accept this, is not able to concentrate on anything other than his soft penis.

The penile shaft is all composed of tiny chambers. In a simplified manner, each chamber has two blood vessels. One is an artery that brings blood pumped from the heart. The other is a vein that drains blood back from the chamber into the general body circulation. At the point where an artery enters a chamber, there is a valve. These valves normally remain closed, preventing blood to flow into penile chambers, thus giving the penis its flaccid state.

With sexual stimulation, the valves open up, and blood rushes into chambers. As the rate of inflow is much faster than the outflow, the chambers expand, resulting in erection. Once the chambers are filled, the rate of inflow equals the rate of outflow, and the erection is maintained. Closure of the valves, as occurs following ejaculation, prevents further inflow while the blood already there drains out through the veins. The penis resumes its normal, flaccid state. And remains that way until the valves open again.

Each penile valve is controlled by two different types of nerves. The two respond to two different kinds of stimuli: one to direct gentle stroking of the penis or scrotum; the other to erotic thoughts, porno pictures or other sexually-exciting images. Generally both act together as during sexual stimulation. But they can function independently, too. This is important. For example, a person with severed spinal cord would still retain the ability to have an erection through the reflexogenic pathway.

And neither of these nerves are under the voluntary control of the brain. A man can voluntarily lift an arm or bend a leg, but he cannot voluntarily open the valves in his penis to produce an erection. No matter how hard he tries, the valves remain closed.

"Performance anxiety" or "fear of failure" is at the root of most cases of psychological impotence, say Masters and Johnson. And at no time this demand for performance been greater than it is today. Women, these days, want and expect sexual satisfaction. The result has been an increasing demand on men for more and better sex—which in turn has also given rise to an increase in "performance anxiety".

Where a man can accept an occasional failure as an isolated incident, he is unlikely to suffer any serious consequences. But if he believes there is something wrong with him, the stage is set for potential repeated failures. The fearful prospect of a recurrent failure becomes a preoccupation. A sexual encounter is no longer a relaxed and enjoyable affair, but instead a test of performance. His actions are no longer spontaneous but carefully planned to test his ability. The result is failure. And each failure only serves to reinforce the idea that something really is wrong.

Psychological impotence can develop at any age, beginning with the first attempt at sexual intercourse. However certain precipitating causes are common in one age group than another. And so could for convenience be broken down into three broad age groups: from adolescence to age forty, from age forty to age sixty, and beyond sixty.

Psychological impotence in the 40-60 age group generally has a slow, insidious onset in contrast to the sudden, acute situational onset prior to age 40. And the causes can be grouped into three categories: marital discord, the physical and psychological effects of ageing, and loss of interest in sex.

By forty, an overwhelming majority of men are married. If a husband and wife are not getting on well, their sexual relationship is almost certain to suffer. In some cases the wife develops a passionate aversion to sex and constantly rejects her husband's advances. Or a husband may be repulsed by a wife grown obese.

The physical and psychological effects of ageing are another significant cause for impotence, particularly as related to certain personality types such as hypochondriacs.

Loss of interest in sex is also important with regard to impotence in this age group. At times, there is only a loss of interest and this is misinterpreted as impotence. At other times the two co-exist. Loss of interest in sex occurs in some men without apparent cause. At other times, it can be a result of depression.

What about impotence in the age group 60 and beyond! The time has come to recognize and accept that sexual interest and activities continue throughout life. Regardless of age, people enjoy sexual sensations.
And sexual activity in the elderly frequently continues to include enjoyable sexual intercourse.

The false idea that it is natural for a man to lose his erection is one of the most significant causes for impotence in the over-sixty group. Some men stop having sex because they believe it is inevitable that sooner or later they are going to lose their erection. Others stop because they think they are "too old" for such things.

Another false notion is that we are born with a definite number of erections and once they are "used up" we are through.

Admittedly it's true that as men age, they respond more slowly to sexual stimulation. It takes longer to get an erection. This does not mean they are on the verge of losing their ability to get an erection.

Another effect of ageing is that it takes longer to reach orgasm. On some occasions, a man may not ejaculate at all. This is not harmful in any way; each episode of intercourse need not end with ejaculation. And this is important for women to understand. Even though an older man may not feel the urge to ejaculate, he can still desire and enjoy sex. A woman who does not understand this may feel she has not fulfilled her sexual obligation if her mate has not had an orgasm. She may put pressure on him to ejaculate, but he may be unable. This pressure can produce its own anxiety, even lead to impotence.

Perfecting the Male Pill

A male contraceptive Pill has been talked about for decades. Yet such a one has still to be marketed and gain popular acceptance.

The absence of a male Pill isn't as much a failure of science; it has a few other inhibiting factors to contend with. For one, the physical and social burden of unplanned pregnancy primarily falls on women. Willy-nilly most research has stayed centred on female contraception.

Again a woman would be hard put to trust a man who claims, he's on the Pill, more so in temporary sexual relationships. Even a married woman may apprehend some loss of control over contraception if relying entirely on her husband taking the Pill with the needed regularity—unless she oversees him doing it at the breakfast table itself.

This well-entrenched female distrust is showing some signs of wearing out. Among younger contemporary couples, men tend to be more helpful in housekeeping, in child-caring, and otherwise more supportive of their partners in gender problems—all in all, inspiring more trust in their mates. In a recent survey at Scottish family planning clinics, an overwhelming majority of women indicated their willingness to trust their husbands with the Pill. In fact they welcomed any move that would shift the burden of contraception to men.

Condom, the primary male contraceptive, has never been popular with men. In fact the whole history of the sheath is a four-hundred-year-long struggle between pleasure and protection. James Boswell (1740-95) in his famed diary complains that "engagements in armour" provided dull satisfaction.

Since then, condoms have vastly improved: thinner, burst-proof, leak-proof. They come lubricated, ribbed, perfumed, even flavoured. Coloured ones, with a choice of colours to match the mood. Yet no one has ever sung praises of the condom. The very requirement of slipping one on at a crucial juncture robs lovemaking of some of its spontaneity. Of course, in the era of AIDS, a condom can be lifesaving.

Meantime, research is on to perfect a male Pill. The basic approach is to craft a male hormonal pill, on the same principles as for women. The female Pill works by giving the body an additional dose of the female hormone estrogen, which in turn has the curious effect of switching off the woman's own supply. Similarly the male Pill supplies testosterone, the main male hormone, which in turn tricks testes into suppressing their sperm production. When a man takes a extra shot of testosterone, his system monitoring levels of testosterone for the requisite balance, sounds an alert and cuts down sperm production.

The problem with this hormonal approach is that you require large doses of testosterone to suppress sperm production sufficiently. Meanwhile such heavy doses give rise to worrying changes in the prostate, liver, as well as problems with weight gain and mood swings.

So progesterone—the female hormone—is added to reduce the testosterone dose. It's the same way, progesterone is added to the female Pill to cut down on estrogen quantity. But then too much of progesterone in the male Pill has its own side effects, the most worrying of which is breast growth. Researchers have to do a tight-rope walk; design a contraceptive cocktail that's effective and has minimum side-effects. Significant progress towards perfecting a male Pill has been reported.

Of late, a novel approach is being pioneered at North Carolina State University. This involves "blinding" of the sperm, through use of a synthetic chemical. It was discovered that an enzyme exists only in sperm cells which gives them the ability to recognize and fertilize eggs—giving sperm their chemical "eyes". Dr Joseph Hall at the Carolina University has hit upon a sugar-based synthetic that has the effect of inhibiting the work of this enzyme, and thus "blinding" the sperm.

At Immucon, a Montreal-based biotechnology firm specializing in the avoidance of unplanned pregnancies, has now received a patent for what promises a breakthrough in reversible male contraception. "One shot delivered in the arm is all it would require to safely sterilize a man for an entire year," says the company's president. And no side effects to speak off are anticipated.

Immucon's approach doesn't use or effect hormones in any way; instead, it targets proteins that naturally bind to the heads of sperm cells during their production. It's these proteins that help the sperm to attach itself to the exterior of the female egg and then carve its way inside to fertilize. The new vaccine targets the release of antibodies specifically engineered to combat those proteins. The experiments have proved highly efficacious on rats. Whether the vaccine would be 100 percent effective with human males has yet to be proved. But if a vaccine can accomplish all this without any side effects, that would be an incredible achievement.

The company also plans an oral or nasal vaccine that would last, depending upon potency, from three months to a year, followed by four-to-six week recovery period.

Separately, Gary Klinefelter of America's Environmental Protection Agency found that when toxic compounds reduced the amount of SP22 in animals below a certain level they become infertile. Researchers are now on the lookout for similar compounds which could cause temporary sterility in men, without serious side-effects.

A factor sorely inhibiting the development of hormonal contraceptives; most major pharmaceutical companies are shying away from it, fearing too much litigation. Only a few companies, such as Organon of Holland (one of the world's largest manufactures of the female Pill) are keeping up research on the male Pill. It is reckoned that a male Pill should be on the market in another 5 to 7 years.

Human trials of the testosterone-progesterone male Pill have just started in China, South Africa and a few other countries.

Perfecting a male Pill would be of immense interest to us in India. The country can do well to accelerate research on the subject. The government could even finance its development with some selected world-level companies in the field. The hormonal route to contraception holds the greatest promise: non-invasive, accessible, and yet easily reversible.

The Story of the Abortion Pill

After a decade of debate and controversy, the Indian authorities have finally approved the marketing of RU-486, the abortion pill. And it is now available in various pharmacies.

Lately the pill also gained the approval of the FDA (Food & Drugs Administration of USA) after years of wrangling. While in India the pill was opposed in some quarters for health hazards from improper, non-medically supervised use, in USA it was the anti-abortion lobby that had kept the pill out. It took 10 years of vigorous advocacy by the Reproduction Health Technologies Project to bring the abortion pill to market in the United States.

France, the country of its origin, allowed the use of RU-486 (now named mifepristrone) in 1988, followed quickly by China and Sweden. UK approved the same in 1991. Today most countries allow the marketing of RU-486.

How was the pill developed? And how it gained acceptance against heavy opposition? That makes an interesting story.

"I saw a lot of botched abortions when I was an intern," says Etienne-Emile Baulieu, the French doctor, biochemist, and the discoverer of RU-486. A pioneer in research on hormone receptors, Baulieu struggled for 20 years to develop an abortion pill; a pill that would do away with complications of the traditional abortion procedures.

During these researches he discovered that progesterone deactivated its own receptor before the onset of menstruation. That made him confident that an antiprogesterone agent would be effective in blocking pregnancy. He was terribly keen on having a drug that induced menses as well as an abortifacient.

In 1970 Baulieu isolated the uterine progesterone receptor. Secreted by the outer lining of the ovulated egg, progesterone prepares the uterine wall for implantation, should an egg be fertilized. Without continued progesterone secretion, the uterus cannot carry a pregnancy to term. Once the progesterone receptor was discovered, the next step in fertility control was to engineer a substance that blocked the uterine response to progesterone.

In 1980 the needed element got synthesized by a chemist named Teutsch in the Roussel-Ulcalf laboratory—and called RU-486; Teutsch was actually looking for new ways to make analogs of cortisone. Beaulieu became alert to the abortifacient properties of the new compound. But then the manufacturers were too frightened to investigate the idea. Beaulieu used his position as a consultant with Roussel-Ulcaf to nurse promising leads. And later mounted a fierce campaign to get the drug into the market when the company under pressure from its major shareholder, the German Hoechst A.G., yanked the drug off the assembly line.

Baulieu got a petition signed by 1,000 doctors and denounced Roussel's decision as "morally scandalous". He even persuaded the noted actress Sophia Loren, his long-time friend and former mistress, to campaign for it. The French government which owned about a third of Roussel, ordered the company to put it back on the market; the French minister of health calling RU-486 "the moral property of women, not just the property of the drug company". Professor Carl Djerassi, the renowned Stanford chemist who synthesized the first oral contraceptive in the 1950s, called RU-486 the *only* new discovery in fertility research since the Pill.

Roussel's policy since then has been to release RU-486 to those countries whose ministries of health request it. Now a majority of early abortions in Europe are done chemically with RU-486, and not surgically.

Speaking of RU-486, Baulieu says," People ascribe to it too much good or too much evil. It's either the work of angels or the devil. In truth, science has finally developed a drug for ending pregnancy, something that women have yearned for thousands of years."

He explains that RU-486 is no miracle drug; it's merely an instance of medical progress. And the pill does not demedicalize abortion. A woman takes the RU-486 pill in her doctor's presence. Two day later, she returns for another pill, this one containing a synthetic hormone that aids abortion by inducing uterine contractions. A third visit to the doctor is needed to confirm that abortion is complete. The success rate is almost 100 per cent in the first seven weeks of pregnancy. Though the procedure is considered safe enough, a medical follow-up is mandatory, since many women bleed heavily.

To the query whether all abortions will ultimately be done with RU-486, he comments," I don't think so. Some women won't like it. With a surgical abortion, you close your eyes and put yourself in the hands of the doctor. RU-486 involves a more active approach. You take the pill yourself, and the process lasts longer, since you have to wait 48 hours before the bleeding starts."

RU-486 can also be used as a morning-after pill, causing less discomfort than the other present-day remedies. Whether it can shape up as a regular contraceptive has yet to be established. However, it has an advantage over the standard contraceptive pill because of being estrogen free, and it is estrogen that gives the current contraceptive pill its harmful side effects.

RU-486 is also showing promise of treating some other health problems. It is known to shrink uterine fibroids. And it aids difficult births, reducing the need for Caesareans.

Of course, it is essential that RU-486 is administered under proper medical supervision. The way it should be administered and its aftereffects are best explained by Baulieu himself. The pill can only be purchased against a doctor's prescription, and is to be used under proper medical supervision.

RU-486 can be a great boon to women in a country like ours where currently too many take recourse to crudely conducted abortions, endangering their health and life.

Search for Good Sperm

At thirty-three Rajiv Misra heads a leading computer software company. He's happily married. But the couple's life is dogged by a dilemma: his mother had been affected by Huntington' chorea (an inherited neurodegenerative disease). Rajiv currently shows no signs of it but should he run the risk of having a child with the mutant gene.

Seeking genetic counselling, he is told that the empiric risk of his having an affected child is 20 per cent. Now the couple has three options. (1) Accept the risk and take a chance that the future baby will be unaffected or, if affected, will be amenable to therapy. (2) Utilize sperm from a stranger for artificial insemination. (3) Decide against reproduction because the risk is unacceptable, possibly adopt a baby instead.

Rajiv and his wife, Rani have been agonizing over the issue for nearly two years. Finally they opt for artificial insemination from a stranger. It has been particularly hard for Rani to overcome her abhorrence of the idea, of being inseminated by someone other than her husband.

Their gynecologist arranges a meeting with the director of Cryo-Genie India Ltd, the pioneering Indian sperm bank. The couple have ruled out any known donor. In fact they intend to keep this a well-guarded secret, and that includes the child when he or she grows up.

The sperm bank is asked to find someone with the same blood group as Rajiv's, same fair complexion, same dark eyes, preferably taller (Rajiv is 5′7″, and a university graduate from a good family; they want to "trade-up" on height at least. And, eventually pick up one from the 50 odd donors whose semen samples are currently held with the bank. Rajiv wished they had a donor who was an intellectual, someone outstanding, but the sperm bank's donors are mainly medical students.

In the sperm bank business, you're always on the hunt. A good man is hard to find. The man has to be more than just healthy and able to produce a healthy baby. Prospective parents commonly want donors with good looks, brains, and personality. In countries like USA or UK where public acceptance of donor sperm has gained significantly, cryobanks gear themselves to meet the varied requirements of their clients. Sperm is now sold like other consumer goods—with online catalogues, personal shopping, and other modern marketing techniques. In the Western world, many single women and lesbian couples are asking for donor semen—this getting more popular than baby adoption. These groups have all sorts of exotic demands, making it particularly hard for sperm banks to find the "right man".

The sperm bank product may be unusual but challenges are similar to any other retail industry: analyzing the customer base, obtaining high-quality inventory tailored to market demands, protecting and packaging, selling the product, and delivering it in good condition.

Surely there have been notable advances in treatment of male reproductive malfunctioning. For example, for males with low sperm count or poor sperm motility or erectile problems, a technique called ICSI (an expensive technique) is employed. Physicians extract sperm directly from the testes with a fine needle and the sperm so obtained is injected into the woman's egg in a petri dish. After the embryo has incubated, it's placed into the womb.

Yet there are many males whose sperm isn't fertile enough or they are not a position to use their own sperm like Rajiv Misra. No wonder, the business of cryobanks is getting brisker. In USA, 10 per cent of males in the age group 18-55 are deemed infertile. Dr Narendra Malhotra of Agra Test Tube Baby Centre, a top infertility specialist, puts the corresponding Indian figure at over 25 percent.

While you may be imagining something spacious and grand, a sperm bank is actually a small establishment. Besides the reception and office, it's usually a donor room, a lab, and a place for storing coded vials of sperm samples in tanks filled with liquid nitrogen, maintaining a temperature of minus 196 degree Celsius. At this temperature sperm can be kept for decades and still remains fit for use when thawed.

Some sperm banks have nice donor rooms, with subdued lighting and a good supply of inspirational material like porn magazines, a few even sporting porn videos. But then some others just direct the donor to an ordinary toilet.

It takes more to become a sperm donor than a wish to help the childless and earn some money (our donors get RS 100 each time; in USA the ruling rate is $50) Leading sperm banks are terribly choosy in recruiting a few good men. The acceptance rate may be as low as 10 per cent of the donor applicants. Not more than 25 per cent of intending donors for Cryo-Genie get selected, tells its director, Dr Pai.

Most cryobanks require that donors be between 18 and 40, and meet height and weight specifications. They should at least be two years into graduation. They must pass a thorough physical exam in which they're screened for HIV and other infectious and genetic diseases. Their health histories going back three generations are scrutinized.

Once a candidate meets all these requirements, his semen must have the minimum volume (5 cc), sperm count (70 million), and motility or swimming ability (2+ out of 4). The general standard observed by cryobanks is 20 million sperm per 1 cc vial of semen after thawing a frozen sample. Sperm banks put specimens into the deep freeze for six months as a quarantine measure (ours observe a period of 3 months), while donors are repeatedly serum-tested for HIV, hepatitis, and other sexually transmitted diseases. All this is very important as semen is one of the main routes of transmission of HIV and STDs. In fact, in most developed countries, the law specifically forbids use of fresh untested semen for artificial insemination. It's pity, in India many doctors are still making use of fresh untested semen for assisted reproduction.

Once the sperm samples are established as disease-free, they are thawed and tested for potency.

Recruiting donors is a never ending process. Many donors leave on their own (for a married man it's quite a crimp on his love life as he has to abstain 48 hours before a donation, with some cryobanks paying a bonus for 72 hour abstention, and often such donations are weekly affairs). Others are retired to guard against too many children getting the same genes. For example, in UK, once a donor has been responsible for ten pregnancies in a geographical area, it's customary to retire him. Our cryobanks are not observing any such retirement rule because they still don't get the feedback about successful pregnancies from the ordering 50-60 IVF (In Vitro Fertility) centres, let alone thousands of gynecologists.

Incidentally there are no banks for female eggs yet. These eggs are far more difficult to get at (it's almost a minor operation, with a mild anesthesia and special medical skills). And the technology of storing eggs is just developing.

Our cryobanks usually make 3 vials out of a single semen donation and sell at RS 300 a vial to IVF centres, who in turn sell at Rs 600 a vial. But then costs are incurred in keeping vials in liquid nitrogen both in storage and in transit. According to Dr Pai, the sperm count in Indian males has dropped significantly in the last 30 years. Whereas in 1960s a sperm count of 90 million was common, now they are lucky to get 60 million. He blames it on air pollution and chemicals in foods. That way it may not be a bad idea to open a collection centre in the hills near some institute of higher education. Why not one in Mussorie where the IAS Training Academy is located? Hopefully someday more donors from the elite would be forthcoming.

Currently the country's requirement of donor semen is put at a few hundred vials a month. According to Dr Pai, the two cryobanks operating today can easily meet the demand for some years. The two banks don't have any commercial or technical tie-up with any foreign cryobanks. However Dr Bhashini Rao who founded Cryo-Genie in 1993, was trained in USA.

As yet there is no licensing for sperm banks, though there are moves to draw up guidelines for such operations. "Sperm sorting"—such as "washing" and enriching it with Y chromosome which significantly increases the likelihood of getting a boy—is said to be practiced rather widely in the country. Our law, which otherwise forbids gender-biased techniques after the fetus is formed, is silent on "sperm sorting".

Presently quite often a couple approaching an IVF centre or a gynecologist for male infertility brings along a donor, usually a brother of the husband or even his father or father-in-law, with the idea that family genes would be preferable to outside ones. But a donor with such proximity to the couple can create many psychological and other complications in course of time. "I keep on persuading couples to go in for an anonymous donor, not a close relative," says Dr Narendra Malhotra.

And he's critical of some hakims or sadhus who claim to confer conception to women with infertile husbands. At times the woman is just drugged and raped by these people or their accomplices. Let alone the unethical and criminal approach, there is no guaranteed protection against HIV and other diseases.

Demand for disease-free donor sperm is set to grow in the country. And with greater sophistication among the intending users, our cryobanks will be called upon to offer a far greater range of choice, along with providing clients with detailed profiles of donors, including their lifestyle and achievements. Some cryobanks in USA and UK let the clients hear the recorded voice of the donor, even see his photograph. In quite a few cases, field enquiries are made to corroborate what the donor has said about his family's health history.

All in all, good sperm is hard to find.

IVF: Twins and Triplets

Infertile couples long for children, spend lot of money on IVF (*in vitro fertilization*), and are gladdened when their efforts bear fruit. But then, many a couple in want of one child gets saddled with twins or triplets; something the couple simply hadn't bargained for.

Currently one in three IVF births produce multiple babies. Cases of women giving birth to triplets are not uncommon. "The incidence of multiple pregnancy after IVF in Britain is about 25 percent. That is a real concern," says fertility expert Robert Winston of Imperial College, London. The epidemic of multiple births arising from fertility treatments is escalating. Between 1980 and 1997, the twin birth rate in the USA increased by 42 per cent, and triplet births increased by 370 per cent. Similar development is slated for India with the growing IVF births.

Women's bodies aren't designed to give birth to a litter. And imagine the impact on the fetuses themselves from sharing those tight quarters.

Now it's isn't all God or even the expensive fertility drugs but something more akin to medical malpractice. In most cases, multiple IVF births are avoidable.

Doctors generally implant more than one embryo in the woman, expecting that not all will develop into pregnancy. IVF procedures being costly, the incentive is to ensure a baby in minimum attempts. "If the couples have failed at an IVF attempt, they have a gambler's mentality where they ask for even more embryos the next time," says an IVF doctor.

Multiple embryos also inflate a clinic's pregnancy rates. If a clinic has 200 patients, it can report the creation of 150 babies, without mentioning that 30 patients had three babies each, while many others failed to have any.

A woman pregnant with more than two fetuses is at risk. She may require bed rest, hospitalization and medications.

And during development in the womb, fetuses in a multiple pregnancy are at a higher risk for lung problems and cranial haemorrhaging. While only 8-10 per cent of singletons are premature, the percentage rises to over 50 percent for twins and nearly 90 per cent for triplets. Multiples have a far higher mortality rate than singletons within the first month after birth. Multiples may also suffer long-term medical problems, including lung diseases and learning disabilities. And are prone to fiercer sibling rivalry than that between spaced siblings.

The parents of multiples are more apt to be exhausted, depressed and anxious. Imagine trying to teach three children toilet training at once or taking them out for a walk. Having multiples is also a tremendous financial strain that only grows as the years pass.

One way to minimize multiple births is to limit by law the number of IVF embryos that can be implanted in the woman at one time. Singapore has a law allowing only two embryos to be put in at one time. Netherlands has gone a step forward; now only one embryo allowed to be implanted. UK, Sweden, and several other countries operate a limit of three. We have yet to legislate on the subject.

Some IVF clinics abroad have started offering a concessional rate for the second trial. This helps reduce pressure from intending couples to have more than one embryo implanted.

Doctors say they implant numerous embryos to increase the woman's odds of becoming pregnant. But a study reported in August 1998 in the *New England Journal of Medicine* showed that implantation of two embryos is optimal—the chances of pregnancy do not increase beyond that.

Some infertility doctors—evidently untroubled by the superpregnancies they create through technology—are offering another technology: the termination of some of the foetuses. The physician injects potassium chloride into the heart of one or more of them. Usually the other foetuses survive, although the chance exists that the entire pregnancy will be miscarried. Doctors avoid the term *abortion*. They call the procedure *selective reduction*. In UK, if triplets, one can be culled. But if twins, no culling allowed.

Quite a few parents unwilling to go along with the option of culling. An infertile woman can find it emotionally wrenching to terminate lives she and her husband worked so hard to create.

Of late some scientists have put forward the idea that if we could culture the IVF embryo till Day 5, that is up to the blastocyst level and somehow prepare the uterus for favourable implantation (currently embryos are put back inside on Day 2 or Day 3), even a single transfer can yield a success rate of 50 percent. And the same has been achieved in a few IVF centres around the world.

At the leading Malhotra IVF centre at Agra, Ayurvedic medicines have been scientifically tried to help implantation. A slight improvement has been documented.

IVF practitioners are increasingly concerned with the phenomenon of multiple pregnancy. But they evidently await technical advances that could give a good rate of success with a single embryo, instead of gambling with multiples. The current success rate hovers around 30 per cent.

Postmenopausal Pregnancy

In November 1996, a sixty-three-year-old woman named Arceli Keh gave birth after lying about her age to a California infertility specialist and obtaining eggs from a younger donor.

Another woman, sixty-two, chose IVF with donor eggs after her nineteen-year-old son was killed in a car accident.

An Italian pioneer in infertility, Dr Severino Antinori, has helped seventy postmenopausal women become pregnant.

Researchers at the University of Southern California recently studied the outcomes for 77 postmenopausal women beyond the age of 50. Forty-two of the women had babies through assisted reproduction programmmes.

Yet there does operate a worldwide sentiment against postmenopausal pregnancy. It possibly flows from the idea that at some stage women should make peace with their biological clocks; be reconciled to have no more children once they reach menopause—the nature's halt to motherhood. In India, sentiment against older women bearing children is possibly stronger. For example, it's deemed somewhat embarrassing even for a menopausal woman to become pregnant when she already has a daughter with children.

With the technique of egg donation now available, women past menopause can question that closure. And there is talk of a technological breakthrough in freezing eggs. Once eggs can be frozen for storage the way semen is, a woman can have her own eggs frozen at youth, to be used for impregnation later in life.

Dr. Zev Rosenwaks, director of the Centre for Reproductive Medicine at New York Hospital, is opposed to pregnancy of postmenopausal women. He argues that the situation is not comparable to actor Anthony Quin creating the eleventh child at age seventy-eight. "Since men do not undergo pregnancy, there is no chance their baby's health will be compromised," says he. Since so few babies have been born of postmenopausal women, we don't really know what the risks will be for the baby or the mother, says he. To him, taking to trendy new techniques without an equal concern for the unknown risks is apparently inadvisable.

The American Society of Reproductive Medicine (ASRM) discourages egg donation to postmenopausal women. One reason is the scarcity of eggs—as compared to sperm. It also wants to protect older women against risks to their health by preventing them from getting pregnant: "the limit is not age; the limit is physical". Even healthy post-menopausal women have to resort to Caesarean births and face high rates of pregnancy-induced diabetes and high blood pressure, though these conditions are temporary.

But then there are dissenting voices that decry any rationing of medical services by age; it's like setting an age maximum on who can receive a kidney. They favour a policy born out of informed social debate, not left to individual physicians to decide in an ad hoc fashion. Many women delay having children, because of the exacting demands of their professional careers.

With advances in IVF techniques, there is likelihood of more and more postmenopausal women going in for pregnancy. The general health and longevity of women is improving, and so also their economic status. There would be the temptation to seek the satisfactions of pregnancy and the joys of child rearing, even when the baby comes of borrowed eggs. To some this would seem a more preferable option than adopting a child.

Dr Narendra Malhotra of Agra, a leading IVF specialist in the country, admits that the pressure and demand of post-menopausal pregnancy is "too much on the IVF clinics". In India the oldest woman who has achieved pregnancy by IVF is reported to have been 53 at a Mumbai clinic, while Jaipur and Agra have reported pregnancy at 47 and 48 years respectively. This was because the women gave their age wrongly, say the doctors.

According to Dr Malhotra, post-menopausal pregnancy should only be attempted in physically healthy women, and definitely of not more than 50 years of age.

What about men fathering children later and later in life? Be warned, say some doctors—men have biological clocks, too.

Men, like Murdoch, demonstrating their maleness by fathering children at advanced age. But, frankly, science doesn't recommend it. The older the father, the greater the chance of mental illness and disorders and diseases including some cancers.

It's a sperm thing. The older the sperm-carrier, the more chance there is of all kinds of mutations, deleterious as well as neutral. Researchers in Columbia University, New York have recently established a clear link between paternal age and mental illness. The American College of Medical Genetics puts the risk of producing a genetic defect as "four to five times greater for fathers aged 45 and above than for their 20-25-year-old counterparts".

All but one of a woman's eggs are produced before her own birth—-and they usually divide just 24 times. Men produce sperm throughout their life—at the rate of 176 × 10 (to the power 6) a day. Also the cells keep dividing—every 16 days. In a 20-year-old man, each cell will have divided 200 times. By the time he's 40, it'll be 660 times.

Each new replication means both that mistakes have more chance of occurring and that those mistakes are then perpetuated by constant replication. Also as men age, their testicles age with them. Blood supply reduces and testosterone levels drop—both important in the proofreading and repair of DNA. So mistakes are not as likely to be fixed. Finally there is the greater possibility of environmental damage from gene-damaging chemicals to older men.

With the mutation rate per cell division increasing with age, older men are heir to more problematic mutations and other genetic abnormalities. And so older fathers could mean more schizophrenics.

When asked what could be done, when there is a worldwide trend for men to bear children in later and later years, the leading geneticist J.F.Crow of the University of Wisconsin replies, "Well, there is of course a solution: collect sperm at puberty and freeze it till needed."

The Complication of Unclaimed Embryos

A peculiar problem is pestering many IVF (*in vitro* fertilization) centres; they are left holding unclaimed embryos in the freezer, some for years. And such storage doesn't come cheap.

Often the couples whose embryos are being held at an IVF centre, can't be contacted or don't respond. And, of course, they pay no rent for the keep. Yet the IVF doctors can't give the embryos away to other couples in a prenatal adoption without the consent of the owners, or even terminate embryos without consent.

On one hand, a human embryo is the most valuable and revered entity on earth. An entire movement is dedicated to protect its right to be born. Infertile couples are willing to spend a lakh of rupees per attempt to create embryos. Researchers see embryos as rich with medical possibilities, such as a source of cells that can be used to treat Parkinson's disease or Alzheimer's. The British Parliament has now passed a controversial law, allowing limited use of embryos for medical research.

And yet, abandoned embryos can be found in every IVF clinic. For instance, there are now more than 1,00,00 such souls on ice in the United States, and increasing at the rate of nearly 20,000 per year. Why are couples "forgetting" they have frozen embryos?

Female eggs, stimulated with drugs, are harvested and singly an egg is mixed with sperm to create an embryo. Generally up to three embryos are deposited in the uterus. Many clinics store and freeze unused embryos for later use, though the implantation rate for such frozen embryos is somewhat lower.

If the initial attempt doesn't work, the couple can have the surplus ones defrosted and implanted more cheaply—and less painfully—than if they began the whole cycle all over again (expensive fertility drugs, gg retrieval procedures, and so on). But once couples get the babies they want, they lose interest in the embryos held in the IVF freezer.

Clinics differ in how to handle the disposition of frozen embryos? One American clinic only allows embryos to be frozen for two years. But that doesn't make sense. If a woman gets pregnant with fresh embryos in her initial IVF attempt and gives birth nine months later, she may not be ready for a second child when her first one is just one year and three months old.

In another clinic the doctor is dead set against destroying embryos. So when one couple who thought their family was complete wrote about termination of its embryos, the doctor angrily responded that the clinic would give them the embryos in an envelope to take home and terminate themselves.

The fate of frozen embryos has now assumed the shape of a major social debate, with UK taking the lead on the vexed subject. The British Human Fertilisation and Embryology Act lays down that frozen embryos should not be stored for longer than five years— nless both parents specifically consent to longer storage. Physicians who fail to destroy the embryos on schedule face jail or fines or both. And the Human Embryology and Fertilisation Authority has been sending letters to sixty-one clinics, reminding them of this obligation.

Clinics in Britain annually send parents a letter asking if they want continued storage of their embryos, or donating them for medical research or to be used by another couple, or to have them destroyed. And if they receive no response, the embryos are destroyed within the stipulated period.

The Vatican condemned this destruction of frozen embryos, calling it "prenatal massacre". Some Italian women even volunteered to "adopt" embryos, similar to taking in an orphaned child. But the British authorities rejected such offers. The then Prime Minister John Major denied a last-minute appeal by anti-abortionist groups to delay disposal, merely saying, the destruction was the "will of Parliament". Over 3,000 embryos across England were accordingly removed from storage; some were simply allowed to defrost, while others were placed in a solution of vinegar and alcohol and then incinerated.

Such a law has little chance of getting passed in USA, with its strong anti-abortion lobby. Already, a Louisiana law prohibits termination of in vitro embryos. The law declares such embryos to be "juridical persons" and requires that each embryo be registered through something akin to a mini-birth certificate. If a couple believes that they have enough children and do not want to use the extra embryos themselves, the state can swoop in and give the embryos to other couples. This is somewhat ironical: a woman has a right to abort an eight-week-old fetus but her eight-cell embryo stays protected.

How many unclaimed embryos are held in India's IVF clinics is not exactly known. The numbers can't be large, but in due course we would be facing a similar problem of unclaimed embryos. We don't have strong anti-abortion sentiments and so should be in a position to legislate about the disposal of unclaimed embryos.

Seeking Prime Sperm

Robert Klark Graham had launched a plan to create human beings at their best. At his ten-acre Escondido farm, California, Graham established the Repository for Germinal Choice. There he collected the sperm of Nobel prize-winning scientists and, later, other geniuses.

Graham, a wealthy optometrist and inventor, did not provide this valuable sperm to just any interested or intelligent female; he believed that only one out of every fifty women was qualified to bear the children of his Nobelists. The women had to be members of Mensa, an international society of people who are in the brightest 2 percent of the population, according to certain IQ tests.

Women began calling or writing to him from all over the world. Scientists who believed they were geniuses were vying for opportunity to donate sperm, to help produce superkids.

The Repository (which had earned the epithet "notorious") closed its doors two years back. But then Virginia's Fairfax Cryobank stepped into the breach with its "Fairfax Doctorate Donors". Since 1999 the firm has been offering, at a third more than usual prices, sperm from Ph.Ds in law, medicine, and other disciplines. Cryos offers three grades of sperm, including an "extra" version that contains twice the number of highly motile sperm as its "regular" brand.

Sperm banking is now global, like any other consumer product or service. The Internet has added a new dimension to artificial insemination: the possibility of viewing a photo of the donor and, in some instances, listening to a tape of his voice. The digital dads seem more like part of a dating service than a medical clinic.

Consumers are no longer limited to the small donor pools locally. The Denmark-based Cryo, for example, is aggressively marketing its product over many countries; it has the avowed goal of becoming the McDonald's of sperm banking.

As recently as 15 years back, a one-line description of the donor was the industry standard. Now, a dozen-page medical and family history is typical. Today's sperm shoppers want to know more than the cause of the donor's maternal grandfather's death or the shape of his nose. For instance, over 100 sperm banks operating in the United States offer catalogues with varying amounts of background information on available donors, and thousands of profiles are available on-line. Some even offer baby pictures of donors, current photographs, and 10-minute videotape bio, even a donor essay about his interests and hobbies.

The Egg Donors

A sperm donor spends a few minutes in a room that looks like a college boy fantasy. It has soft-and-hard-core magazines and a comfortable couch under subdued lighting. And he gets paid for an activity that's associated with pleasure.

In contrast, an egg donor faces a gruelling medical regime. She gets fertility drugs injected daily for two weeks. The painful shots cause the woman's moods to swing widely. She may experience headaches, cramps, and nausea. She bloats up and risks kidney trouble.

The monitoring of egg donors involves daily visits to the clinic for blood tests and ultrasound screening. When the ovaries are ripe, as many as several dozen eggs are removed with a fifteen-inch-long needle inserted through the vagina. A general or local anesthesia has to be used for the procedure. According to some studies, she also has a greater chance of getting ovarian cancer later in life.

Because of the risks presented to women who are recruited to be egg donors, some clinics prefer to use their own IVF patients as egg donors. Since these women are already taking fertility drugs, they seem to face fewer additional physical risks by donating. Some clinics even offer their IVF facilities to women at a reduced cost if they are willing to give some of their eggs to other women (a temptation for the doctor to pump her up even further with hormones to ensure that she produces dozens of eggs for donation). Some clinics even do nothing to prevent patients from being solicited by other patients. At times, an infertile woman who cannot produce eggs will show up on an egg retrieval day and ask an IVF patient to share some of hers.

Egg donors, of course, get good money. As compared to something like $50 per sample for sperm donors (ours banks pay as little as Rs 500), egg donors can rake up $2,000 or more for one harvesting. Sperm is plenty, eggs are scarce.

Again, while frozen sperm and frozen embryos have routinely produced pregnancies, freezing eggs poses its hazards. These get damaged when thawed, and so donor eggs are commonly fertilized within twenty-four hours of harvesting. Lately a special technique has made it possible to freeze eggs. In October, 2002, the first baby is born in UK of a frozen egg. Once the technique gets refined, women could store eggs in their 20s when they are highly fertile, and use the frozen egg for impregnation, if needed, in later years.

Egg donors have started advertising directly through papers and the Internet. One such ad reads, "Hungarian Egg Donor. . . . age 25, weight 100 lbs. Very attractive, in perfect health." (the way height is important for sperm donors, weight is a crucial factor for egg donors).

And there are Web sites that list out particulars of egg donors with them. For instance, at the Web site of the Centre for Surrogate Parenting and Egg Donation in Beverly Hills, there are three hundred egg donors available. Each fills forms listing her favourite books and movies, her weight, her own and her parents' health history, and her "philosophy" of life. The biodata, along with photos, determines how couples choose a potential donor. A top-class donor can cost $5,000, and on top, all the medical expense of the egg transfer. Incidentally the rejection rate for egg donors is high; four out of five get rejected on health and other grounds.

Majority of egg donors in America and Europe are young women from Russia and other East European countries who are looking for much needed cash. Young British university students are known to be selling their eggs for thousand of pounds in the American market as a way of paying off their student debts. Although it is illegal in Britain to pay women any more than unspecified "expenses", American clinics are allowed to reward donors handsomely for the unpleasant and potentially risky procedure. They pay these foreign girls travel/hotel expenses, and a hefty fee.

All in all, donated eggs from women volunteers are scarce, with prices escalating. So a search is on for alternative sources of genetic material to produce babies.

Researchers are focussing on the biological fact that all of a woman's eggs are created prenatally. A woman actually has her maximum number of eggs—about 7 million—when she is twenty-week-old foetus in her mother's womb. By puberty, only around 300,000 remain.

With millions of abortions each year, some scientists have begun to think the unthinkable—using female foetuses as a source of eggs for infertile women.

But other scientists believe that bypassing natural selection can have disturbing results, including a serious risk of abnormalities. Anyway the idea itself has raised a public outcry. "I don't believe that, like rag dolls, babies should be made up of discarded bits of humanity," said Baroness Strange in the British Parliament. In 1994, Britain passed a law making it a criminal offence to use foetal eggs or ovarian tissue for fertility treatment. Some other countries are considering a similar ban.

Egg donation for infertile women is still in its infancy in India. However, with the spread and advancement of IVF in the country, egg donation is set to figure significantly. We have to tackle the spectre of substandard labs undertaking such work. And a movement towards better ethical practices through self-regulation by its practitioners, backed by legislation and enforcement.

4
Healthy Travel

The most carefully planned holiday, business trip or expedition may be ruined by illness, much of it preventable. It is therefore logical to put nearly as much effort in protecting your health while abroad as you have in planning your itinerary.

Unfortunately, it is not in the best commercial interests of travel companies to emphasize the possible health hazards of destinations that are being sold to potential customers: most holiday brochures limit health warnings to the minimum legal requirements.

According to Dr Richmond Dawood, a physician in London who specializes in travel medicine, as many as a third of travellers suffer short-lived episodes of gastro-intestinal problems when they are abroad. We, living in India, do develop greater immunity to food infections, yet it isn't uncommon for us, too, to suffer from stomach upsets during foreign trips.

Dawood, an inveterate traveller himself, is the editor of *Traveler's Health—How to Stay Healthy Abroad* (OUP, 1986); the fourth edition coming out in 1999. The book assembles 45 specialists, top in their fields, from several countries, who provide practical advice on prevention and treatment of various health problems. And it makes mention of a host of minor upsets that can ruin a journey, such as trouble with contact lenses, insect bites and sunburn.

The message is simple. There are teeming health hazards for the unwary traveller, especially outside North America and Northern Europe. But they are easily avoided if you take a few simple precautions.

According to the experts, serious diseases can be missed or mis-diagnosed when you get back home. Malaria, for example, can mimic the symptoms of other diseases—high fever, lassitude, headache and joint pains. And the malaria menace is growing in many places. Similarly tuberculosis is a re-emerging scourge. Any suspicious fever should be checked.

And you are advised to adopt a pro-active approach to vaccinations; getting the basic shots in plenty of time, coupled with "fine-tuning" of specific shots at short notice, dependent on your destination. And carrying a mini medical kit: your favoured painkiller, Band-Aid for cuts, and a tube of anti-septic cream, plus a supply of your prescription medicines.

"With food and water hygiene, you have to learn what to look for," Dawood says. "You have to accept that a fly in a five-star hotel hasn't suddenly become clean." This means choosing food that has been freshly and thoroughly cooked and served hot. Avoid salads that may have been washed in polluted water, so also prepared buffets (mayonnaise and Russian salad, for example, are notorious sources of food poisoning). What looks appetizing can be a poor guide to food safety. In fact, curries served hot are often safer than Western food.

Fruit should always be peeled. "Wash it, peel it or forget about it," remains excellent advice. Above all, never drink unbottled water (make sure the bottle is opened in front of you). Even avoid ice in drinks, particularly in non-alcoholic drinks (only a few hotels make ice from bottled water). Don't assume tap water is safe outside USA, Canada, North and West Europe, Japan, and Australasia.

Expose minimum skin area to insect bites. If you're outdoors in the evenings, wear long-sleeved shirts and use a good insect repellent. Avoid wearing scent.

A crucial matter is health insurance. Make sure it covers all your needs and is there when you need. Current health insurance policies issued by Indian companies are based on reimbursement principle—the insurer meeting the cost in the first instance. Now this is clearly an unsatisfactory arrangement. You may not get home if you are refused treatment or not allowed to leave until bills have been settled. In many other countries they have health insurance policies wherein you get a card that ensures all costs of treatment in the first instance. Some policies even cover the cost of a business colleague to replace you if you're sick or injured during a trip.

Hopefully, with the opening up of the health insurance sector, we should look forward to increasingly user-friendly health insurance policies, particularly for travel abroad.

Most airlines serve elaborate meals to Business and First Class. And it's hard to say no to a glass of Chardonnay, grilled swordfish with nuts, followed by chocolate tart and a glass of port. Nevertheless the overwhelming advice from doctors and experienced business travellers is to eat lightly on board. And to avoid alcohol, including wine—at 30,000ft alcohol deemed doubly potent. But then you can afford to be indulgent at meals and drinks served just before deplaning.

Of late doctors have been highlighting the risk of blood clots from sitting long hours in very cramped conditions, such as obtain in crowded economy class with narrowed seats and restricted legroom. Blood clots formed in the legs can move up right to the heart. WHO has now undertaken a comprehensive research programme to investigate the unresolved issues regarding travellers' thrombosis. Airlines can no longer disregard the problem, notwithstanding their obvious anxiety to squeeze in maxim possible passengers.

Meanwhile it's important, you do some leg exercises while sitting long hours in a cramped plane seat. Airlines are now suggesting some special leg exercises while staying seated. And you should also avail of every opportunity to stretch them out standing or walking.

Hazards Facing Frequent Business Travellers

These days many business travellers average 25 business trips a year. And business travel seems set to stay at high levels, notwithstanding advances in communication technology. Businesses find no substitute for face-to-face contacts with their far-off customers and clients.

Frequent flying poses its own risks; not so much the risk of a hijack but physical and psychological hazards that affect regular travellers.

Medical researchers are generally agreed that the risks to the health of frequent travellers are real and varied. These include a potentially greater risk of deep vein thrombosis, or blood clots in the legs, especially for those taking flights lasting over three hours.

And the somewhat controversial issue of exposure to ionizing radiation; the same attracting increasing attention lately. Cosmic radiation increases with altitude (exposure doubles every 6,000ft) and can pass through the structure of an aeroplane. On a rough comparison, you get the equivalent of a chest X-ray every four hours of flight. Those doing more than 1,50,000 flying miles per year may well receive twice the safe limit.

Along with the physical toll to which frequent flyers are subject, their psyches may be taking a beating. A 1997 clinical study compared the health claims of 4,700 managers and professional workers of the World Bank who engaged in international travel to 6,000 of the bank's employees who did not travel. The findings showed that travellers accounted for three times more claims for treatment of anxiety, stress and other psychological issues that their stationary counterparts.

Women business travellers undergo the added concern for personal safety and greater risk of sexual harassment. They often opt for flights and hotels more with an eye to safety than convenience.

Since September 2001, the requirement to report early and the elaborate security drill at airports have given a new dimension to the stress of air travel. No wonder, incidents of "air rage" are on the rise.

Work-wise, the impact of interrupted sleep cycles and jet lag can be profound. Stressed-out travellers whose sleep patterns are interrupted can actually have significantly impaired decision-making capabilities. "I've seen a lot of bad decisions made by jet-laggged employees who weren't alert," warns Smolensky, a professor of environmental physiology at the University of Texas.

Quite a few employing companies are giving increasing attention to the risks, physical and psychological, affecting their frequent business travellers. They are putting in place policies that would ameliorate the position.

To help make the trips easier, allowing employees to choose their own airlines and enroll in airline clubs to give them a more pleasant place to spend layover time. Employees to keep their frequent-flier miles they acquire during business travel and to use them towards personal vacations and other rewards. Encouraging employees to factor a Saturday-night stay into their plans.

All in all, the time seems ripe for employers to adopt strategies to deal with the health issues and anxiety surrounding frequent business travel.

Business Travel: Staying Connected to Family

Telecommunications, it was assumed, will reduce the need for business travel. But business travel hasn't decreased with new technologies. Indeed it has been registering a noticeable rise.

According to the statistics compiled by the Travel Industry Association of America, average business trips per year went up from 4.7 in 1988 to 6.3 in 1994. And the duration of such trips went up from 3.2 nights in 1991 to 3.6 in 1994. Nights spent out by frequent flyers grew up from 72.4 in 1989 to 88.7 in 1994. And a new class of super-frequent flyers has emerged who do over fifty airplane flights a year.

More likely the travel schedule of most business travellers makes them spend between three weeks and three months away from their family. Now this quantum of travel by working fathers can strain family relationships.

What makes it particularly tricky is the fact that everyone at home assumes business travel is fun, exciting, even glamorous. Sometimes it is. But such travel can get stale pretty fast. And it can be both exhausting and lonely.

How you handle your goings and comings—and your time of absence from home—has a big impact on your family's reactions to your travels. Here are a few strategies that could help you stay connected to your wife and kids during all three phases of a trip: before you go, while you're away, and when you return.

Obviously, before you commit to a trip, you have to weigh carefully the necessity for it. Business travel consumes not just the time while you are away, but all the time it takes to get ready to leave and all the reentry time.

Instead of travelling the night before, consider departing very early the morning of the meeting. If you're a frequent flier, this could save you quite a few evenings for your family over a year. For example, a Delhi-Mumbai early morning flight could perhaps do as well, obviating the need of flying the night before.

Announcing your trip to your family as far in advance as you can, helps them absorb the fact of your absence. Especially with small children, mention your trip repeatedly. What these children most need to know is when you are coming back in concrete terms that fit their sense of time. For example, it may not mean anything if you tell your four-year-old, "I'll be back by Saturday morning," if he doesn't know his days of the week. Better connect your return to one of the week's regular events: "I'll be back to take you to the chocolate store."

Children under three, in particular, may not understand that you are coming back at all. Start a project with them to be finished when you return. Remind him of it when you talk on telephone.

For children ten and older, show them a map of your route—the cities, countries, continents or oceans over which you will be flying. With a good atlas or a home computer with access to the World Wide Web, you may show your family what locations you are going to and what it looks like. Web sites, such as HYPERLINK http://www.travelcity.com http://www.travelcity.com or HYPERLINK http://www.travelcom.es/ http://www.travelcom.es/ let you zoom in on many major cities and global landmarks. Incidentally, don't romanticize your trip; you're going for work, not vacationing.

Psychologists suggest that by helping with packing, children become used to the idea of your departure—and of your eventual return. Young children can "help" you pack by figuring out ways to squeeze socks into your suitcase. The family can have a special meal or a special dish at home to signal your departure. Or you can drive to the airport to "wish daddy good luck".

Phase two of travel is staying connected while you are away. Besides the usual telephone and mail, new technologies have created more options, including fax, e-mail, and videotape. If you use them in ways that fit your child's stage of development and the rhythms of your family's life, the are all excellent ways to keep in touch. Taking along a small family album—kept duly updated—is deemed a help against homesickness.

On telephone if you ask a child, "What did you do today?" you're likely to hear, "Nothing." If you simply ask, "How was your day? you'll probably hear, "OK." For better connectedness, ask specific questions about what he ate that day or what game he played at school.

Try to establish a "best time" to call that will work for everybody in the family. That will also help establish your telephone call as a daily ritual for connection while you are away. It's the act of calling that is important, talking about things that would perhaps not in themselves justify a phone call.

And if on calling home your wife complains or describes the problems she is having, do not—repeat, do not—offer immediate solutions. What she probably needs much more is your empathy and appreciation. After that, if she wants your advice, you can give it.

In a sense, the telephone is as confessional as a psychiatrist's couch, because it allows you to talk to someone without distractions. People often find it easier to deal with intimate or difficult topics. In fact, people often do more serious talking on the phone than they would have done face-to-face because they are more focussed when talking on phone and actually forced to listen to what the other was saying.

Then the final thing is that when people are apart and talk on the phone, they actually have to make some things explicit which face-to-face they may let go. That they miss each other, for example, which may never be said otherwise. What the phone does is allow people to get things sorted out and to build up, a set of explicit understandings, which they may never have talked about together at home.

The third phase of business travel is returning to your family. Don't expect to be able to pick up with things as they were before you left, especially if you've been away for the better part of a week. Reunions have their own rhythms.

Give everybody a chance to readjust, without expecting a dramatic welcome. Reestablish contact with each of your kids separately, such as sitting on your child's bed for a few minutes to reconnect. After you have established contact with everybody separately, reunite with the whole family by doing something together—going out for a treat or an interesting visit.

Buying your child a big gift every time you travel overemphasizes objects as signs of your love. Small inexpensive items can be fun if chosen imaginatively. In a rush you can even do with those hotel or plane trinkets: miniature soaps or lotions, tiny jars of jam or ketchup.

And lastly, on occasions (after accumulating sufficient frequent flyer miles) you can take your family along on a business trip. Planned properly, it could be a mini-vacation for them without interfering with your business commitments.

Tips for Women Business Travellers

Women travelling on business faced particular problems: harassment, humiliation, loneliness, discomfort, danger. And things haven't improved significantly, despite promises by the travel trade to change attitudes and practices—a lot of lip service but little real change.

This is borne out in a survey conducted recently by Total Research Corporation of Princeton, New Jersey, reflecting the views of 217 frequent women travellers in the United States and 136 in the United Kingdom. Even though women account for a growing proportion of business travellers—40 per cent in USA and over 20 per cent in UK—they say they are still not getting a fair deal. They continue to face indifference and disdain, if not rampant sexism, by airline, hotel and car-rental staff. Women believe they receive inferior service because of their gender.

Many choose room service in hotels because they feel intimidated. If a woman is brave enough to come down to the restaurant, she often gets shoved behind a pillar.

No wonder, a move is afoot to set up special hotels exclusively for women. Zurich, for example, now has one; "Hotel Lady's First", a hotel for female guests only. The Hotel has been specially planned for business women who want a relaxing stay in Zurich. And now, even some Indian hotels, are into keeping a particular floor, deemed the safest and most convenient, for unaccompanied lady guests.

Personal safety being an overriding concern, a majority of respondents laid emphasis on airlines to make more secure arrangements for women travellers when planes are delayed or arrive very late at night.

And hotels to pay more attention to giving women more secure rooms away from stair-wells and elevators. And they want airports to provide a security presence at taxi stands late at night.

In hotels, room design should be more woman-friendly. For example, there should be a socket within hairdryer's reach of a mirror and proper ironing facilities.

For more information on hotels for women travellers, refer to HYPERLINK http://www.redcarnation www.redcarnation hotels.com)

In choosing a hotel, smaller is better; you want the staff to be familiar with guests and with you. The smaller the lobby, the more noticeable the loiterers.

Ask for a room near the elevators and away from any renovation work. Anyway ask for a room as far as possible from emergency exits.

The Please Make Up the Room sign tells everyone you're not there. Better call housekeeping instead.

Have your room key ready when you leave the lift, instead of fumbling for it in your purse at the door.

Stand near the elevator buttons with your back to the wall.

Make sure your room door has double locks. For extra security, better bring along a rubber doorstop.

Put expensive clothing on hangars under other garments. Thieves usually take what they see.

Lock valuables in the front-desk safe.

In public lavatories, use the corner cubicle.

On overnight flights, take your purse with you when you go to the lavatory.

Don't exit a taxi until you're sure you've arrived at your destination. Pay while still in the vehicle so that you can be sure you've received the proper change.

Stay close to your valuables when passing through airport security.

If you place your carry-on bag on the floor when sitting in a restaurant or other public area, put your foot through the strap; don't leave it loose.

Rent a mobile phone or bring your own.

Be cautious of hatchbacks, as they leave your luggage in plain view.

When possible, park so you won't have to back out. It makes for a speedier departure.

On flights to new places, talk to female attendants and passengers on the plane about the safety of your destination.

On the pavement, keep you handbag away from the street side, and on escalators, away from the opposite ramp.

Study your map before going out. Once on the street, use a pocket-sized guidebook to avoid looking like a tourist. Ask the concierge to mark any dangerous areas on your map.

Dress down. And avoid jewellery. Even a chain that's fake gold can be ripped off your neck.

Be wary when getting off a bus, a train, or an escalator; that's when pickpockets tend to strike.

Carry photocopies of important documents.

Divide money for small and larger purchases so you don't have to expose a wad of money. Become familiar with foreign currency before you have to use it.

Have tips ready for porters and doormen.

Should a car start to follow you, turn immediately and walk the other way.

Cross over the road to avoid anyone threatening or suspicious.

Ask directions from families or women with children.

To make an outside restaurant reservation, better ask your concierge to do so, and have him say "Please take care of our guest, she's coming alone and will need a taxi home."

Here are a few general safety tips for women who happen to travel alone:

Trust your instincts. If you have any doubts about getting into a car with someone or meeting him somewhere, don't do it. And don't feel bad about not turning up to a prearranged meeting if you've had second thoughts.

You may find it useful to wear a wedding ring, even if you're not married. Or carry photos of a scary-looking "boyfriend".

Avoid eye contact with strangers. Wearing sunglasses should do the trick.

Plan any journey in terms of daylight hours.

Be careful about disclosing where you are staying.

If groped on public transport, you may wish to draw attention of other passengers to the fact—loudly.

"The art of travelling is learning to behave like a chameleon," said a noted woman traveller. "Blending into the background is not only a prerequisite to understanding and observing a different culture, it also keeps you out of trouble."

For women, dress is the first line of defence and the most immediate symbol of respect. How you dress can be construed as camouflage or an invitation; it can make you one of the crowd or a moving target.

The Air in Aeroplanes

Anytime you stuff over three hundred people in a metal can, stick them some thirty thousand feet up in the sky, and give them a fairly limited supply of outside air to breathe, they can't be comfortable with it.

The cabin air in flight is low in pressure, ordinarily equal to that obtainable at an altitude of 6000-7000ft (this cabin pressure, produced by concentrating the oxygen in outside air, is a compromise between the requirements of human health and the economics of pressurization). At sea level air presses on us at 14.7 pounds per square inch. At six thousand feet this pressure is down to 11.78 psi. The 20 per cent drop in squeeze also implies 20 per cent drop in air density, and consequently 20 per cent fewer oxygen molecules per cubic feet. Your lungs and heart have to work harder to get the requisite supply of oxygen. Admittedly most of us adjust to the reduced amount of available oxygen in planes.

At sea level the body tissues are saturated with approximately 21 per cent oxygen and 79 percent nitrogen, in the same proportion as the air itself. This situation however undergoes a rapid change as the jet climbs; rising in under 20 minutes from takeoff to the cruising altitude of over 30,000ft. Your body now contains 20 per cent more nitrogen than the air around you. Unlike oxygen, nitrogen is inert and can't burn. You get rid of it by breathing it out—the blood picking up the excess nitrogen molecules to be exhaled. But nitrogen isn't easily soluble in blood; it can't escape fast. So your tissues swell up with the trapped nitrogen. That's why your shoes feel tight and so also rings on your fingers. And the reason why wearing of loose clothes and taking off one's shoes is recommended on long flights.

The change in pressure also poses a problem for our ears. Usually they respond to the change by "popping", making the pressure inside the ears the same as the pressure of the cabin. But if one has a cold or sinus trouble, popping isn't easy because the tiny channels between the nasal passages and the middle ear are likely to be blocked by the swollen membranes of the nose. This is particularly a problem during descent. The air pressure in the cabin increases while the pressure inside your ears remains low. You end up with a vacuum-like effect in your middle ears that sucks your eardrums inward. It hurts, plus it muffles your hearing.

A well-known way to clear your ears is to try sucking on something (why airlines distributed sweets when planes weren't pressurized) or just yawning. This activates the muscle that opens your Eustachian tubes. Taking a decongestant an hour before the landing also helps.

The cabin air gets very dry; its humidity dropping down to about 10 percent against the average of 25 per cent to which we are usually accustomed. The reason is simple; at cruising altitude humidity outside a jet airliner is practically zero as it flies above the cloud level. And aircraft ventilators remove what little moisture comes in. In fact much of the moisture inside a plane comes from the breath and sweat of passengers.

In the dry cabin air your body cells start drying up. Thirsty cells pull water from the blood. Not that a normal person can't cope with the contingency but 3-4 hours of continued exposure to it does produce a definite degree of dehydration. That's why it's recommended that you drink plenty of water or juice—preferably 8 ounces every hour. Alcohol dehydrates by speeding the passage of fluids through the system. Again coffee and tea are diuretic—produce more urine and so drain the body of fluids. The best fluid to combat dehydration is plain water; no other drink is hundred percent water. Even sugar in it retards water's action to some extent.

Another disturbing aspect of flying is the high of level air pollutants you encounter in the cabin of a crowded commercial airliner. Most of the modern jets deliver only between 40 per cent to 60 per cent of fresh air in the passenger cabin; the balance is recirculated air. Newer jets are coming up with greater capacity to recirculate cabin air; all because fresh air is expensive. The thin, cold air outside a plane at high altitude isn't fit to breathe. Jets use up fuel as they turn that air into something breathable.

The recirculated air is no doubt passed through particle filters. These can remove pollen, dust and mould but they are usually ineffective against viruses, cigarette smoke and carbon monoxide. Researchers have found bacterial-colony counts as high as 256 per petri dish on commercial airliners, compared to 15-20 in restaurants. Again carbon dioxide levels in cabins of commercial airliners average about 1800 parts per million when outdoor air contains only 400 parts. First-class and business class passengers also get the same recirculated air but they enjoy a better quality because of less crowding.

If you find your cabin air too stale, you could complain to a flight attendant and ask that the pilot turn up the ventilation system. Sometimes pilots run it at two-thirds or half capacity because they're under orders to save fuel. Pilots don't know how stuffy cabin air may be because they have just the opposite. The cockpit is virtually windswept, with up to 20 times more fresh air than passenger get. More ventilation keeps flight equipment cool, and the pilots awake and alert.

An even simpler way to get better air is to give the overhead vent a twist. On planes that have these vents—many modern ones no longer sport these—the air that comes out is usually fresh. By opening the vent you create a pocket of better air around yourself.

To Overcome Jet Lag

The fuzzy, queasy sensation of jet lag has sometimes been likened to having your brain gently squeezed. And now a researcher in UK claims the feeling has scientific backing. Kwangwook Cho, of the University of Bristol Medical School, who carried out brain scan of scores of Bristol Medical School, who carried out brain scan of scores of flight attendants found that chronic jet lag appeared to shrink a frontal part of the brain, inflicting a temporary loss of memory and coqnitive skills.

Ads luring travellers to distant lands stress the comfort and excitement of it all, the new places, people and life-style, and the sense of romance and adventure. The possible fatigue, indigestion, headache, irregular bowels, difficulty with sleeping and concentration—in fact, generally feeling 'below par'—finds no mention. These are the symptoms of jet lag, and they are being experienced by more and more people as flights spanning the globe become more common.

Why do we get jet lag? And what can we do about it?

The world stands divided into 24 one-hour (15 degree longitude) time zones—apart by about 1,000 miles at equator, and between 600 to 800 miles in temperate regions.

When we jet across time zones, our body clock is out of synch with the time environment of our destination. And the body clock takes its own time to adjust. During this period of adjustment we experience the discomfort and debilitation of jet lag.

A few other explanations of jet lag have been advanced. One is that it's "in the mind". This may be partially true—expecting you'll suffer jet lag hardly helps—yet the abnormal timing of bowels and sleep, and the feeling of fatigue can't be all explained in psychosomatic terms.

Some others attribute jet-lag largely to the anxieties and inconveniences of today's intercontinental flights, such as crowded cabins, limited legroom, airport tension, and dry air in aeroplanes, often coupled with in-flight indulgence in alcohol and heavy food. These can surely exacerbate fatigue, but even those travelling in comfortable conditions don't escape jet lag, either.

It has also been argued that, with practice, the body becomes more able to adjust to a time zone transition, a kind of 'learning' effect. Some travellers maintain they get used to jet lag—in the sense they learn to live with it. Yet others find the problem becoming worse.

Here are some estimates of how long jet lag will last.

West Ward	Up to 3 time zones	4-6 time zones	7-12 time zones
	- nil-	2 days	3-4 days
East Ward :	Up to 2 time zones	3-5 time zones	6-12 time zones
	- nil-	3-4 days	5-6 days

Older people tend to be nearer the upper limit of any range than do younger people.

What is this body clock that's causing trouble on transmeridian flights? Scientists have come to understand that an elegantly engineered clock deep in the hypothalamus governs natural body rhythms. Evolved over thousands of years, this tiny cluster of nerves, smaller than a pinhead, called SCN, regulates our cycles of sleep and wakefulness. It not only receives information about light and dark from the eyes, but also from its own dedicated pathways of nerves.

In the predawn still of the night, much before we finally awake, hormone levels start surging in the bloodstream. Pulse beats faster and blood pressure rises (possibly one explanation why heart attacks mostly occur at that hour). By the time our brain awakes, the body's functions are automatically reaching daytime levels of activity. And when night falls, the biological clock adjusts the system downward to sleep; the body temperature lowers and the brain activity slows down.

The advantage of the body clock is that it prepares us and other mammals to be ready for the coming environmental condition, such as a new dawn. A tree is different; its leaves only move in response to the sun, and not before in anticipation. And so the response of the leaves to change direction for getting maximum sunlight is necessarily slow, and always behind the ideal with respect to the changing positions of the sun.

Under normal conditions, the 25-hour cycle of the human biological clock—why it's 25-hours instead of 24 is still a mystery—is automatically, without our knowing, reset each morning by the light of the dawn so to conform to the 24-hour schedule of day and night.

Having an intrinsic 25-hour period means we are biologically programmed with a steady westward drift of time cues. That's what makes westward bound jet travel across time zones less disorienting for the body clock than eastbound.

What practical steps can you take flying across 4 or more time zones (3 or more in case of eastward flights) to reduce the rigour of jet lag?

As far as practicable, begin to adjust your life-style to the new time zone a day or two before the departure date. One possibility is to go to bed one or two hours later than normal and to get up one or two hours later, if you're journeying west. And to do the reverse if you're going eastward.

Immediately on taking off, set your watch to agree with the local time at your destination. And during the flight try to sleep if it's nighttime at your destination and, if it's daytime there, try to stay awake. Of course, you'd often encounter the problem that the in-flight schedule of meals and other activities is sometimes arranged to accord with time in your departure zone.

Suppose you're taking a midnight flight from Delhi to London, 5½ time zones away to the west. It would still be evening in London. On this 10-hour flight, eat a light supper in the beginning, and sleep (at least nap) for the next 7 hours or so, preferably with an eye mask. Exposure to bright light during sleeping time interferes with the anti—jet-lag effort. And then you get up for a breakfast and deplaning.

At your local destination where it would be just morning, avoid the temptation to take a nap during the day. You could sleep a little early on your first night there.

Light exercise and brisk walk taken at your accustomed time by the new local time will help you adjust quicker to the new time zone. Again try to make meals of the correct type (breakfast, lunch, etc,) at your adjusted time.

Recent researches claim that properly timed light and darkness could reset the body clock much quicker. Books and charts have come out which guide the air traveller as to when to seek bright light and when to wear an eye mask. *How to Beat Jet Lag: a practical guide for air travellers* by Dan A. Oren and others (Holt Co, 1993) is one. Tom Houpt at the Harvard Medical School and the Institute of Circadian Physiology have prepared a similar guide chart, called "MidnightSun". Portable light visors are also being designed to focus strong light into the wearer's eyes whether in flight or elsewhere in the absence of bright sun.

There is as yet no magic pill to counteract jet lag. Tablets containing melatonin—the hormone produced by the pineal gland at night—have, however, shown promising results. A melatonin pill can be taken a few hours before sleep is required in the new time zone; this helps bring on sleep. A nightcap in the form of alcohol may well induce sleepiness but it can often result in disturbed sleep.

In short, the best advice for combating jet lag is to adopt a new routine in accord with your new time zone, to strengthen all possible time-cues, and to reset the body clock as quickly as possible.

Food in Flight

Few passengers ever realize how highly complex is the task of providing them food and drinks on a flight. Many others often confuse inflight catering with foodservices found in airports.

Whenever a commercial flight takes off anywhere in the world, it is provisioned by inflight foodservices. Over 9,000 commercial aircraft fly everyday from some 1,000 airports. And carry over 755 million people in a year. Inflight catering is currently a four-billion-dollar industry (at wholesale rates: the retail equivalent would be double that amount).

In the beginning, airport foodservice consisted of simple luncheon counters adjacent to single runway airfields. The emphasis was on simplicity and quick service. It was not until 1936, with the development of DC-3, that the first airplane galley was introduced. With no electric power available to heat food, all hot foods and liquids were boarded at ready-to-serve temperatures and held hot in thermoses. Only after World War II, came the aircraft which generated electric power during flight and it was possible to divert power to the galleys to brew coffee on board and to keep food hot.

Meal service trays used to be set on pillows on passengers' laps, till the lap pillow was replaced by alternative supports. The pillow was still used to support the meal trays of passengers seated in bulkhead rows as late as the 1970s.

One means of meeting the hunger needs of passengers would be for them to bring their own food onto the aircraft, just as many bus and train passengers do. In China, it's still an accepted practice. But almost everywhere else the same stands abandoned on grounds of health and security; many a passenger may be unaware of the time and temperature parameters for potentially hazardous foods. Yet alternative means of meeting passengers' food needs have not been completely given up. For example, in places passengers pick out cold items from a complimentary food cart set up in the boarding area. This is more common in USA for short commuter flights.

Serving of food and beverage has become an expected part of airline services today. And food is no longer only a means of assuaging passengers' hunger but often the component of a competitive strategy of the commercial airline. Indeed, satisfaction of passenger hunger may be the least important reason motivating airlines to offer food and beverage services.

At some stage airlines also began to realize that foodservices were an important distraction helping the passengers control their fears of flying as well as helping the flight crews manage the behaviour of their passengers.

On flights, feeding passengers increases their blood circulation in the stomach. This slows down blood circulation in other parts of the body, resulting in a reduction of tension; drawing the blood away from the tensed muscles leads to their relaxation. No wonder, one of the best ways to calm irate passenger is to first feed them, and after they have finished dessert, come to talk about their grievances—a common tactic among flight attendants who have to deal with difficult passengers in very confined work areas.

Liquor, of course, plays a similar role to that of food. But then its excessive consumption can not only contribute to passenger dehydration but also at times lead to passenger behaviour problems. The inflight alcohol intake by individual passengers and signs of inebriation are monitored by flight attendants.

In addition to the physiological value of food and beverage services helping to relieve the tensions and fears of passengers, they also are of psychological value. They provide a diversion for the passengers, helping to keep them from becoming bored—something to do to pass the time, particularly on long flights.

While inflight foodservices have many things in common with other food outlets, these are unique in some ways. For one, people who prepare, package and deliver foods and beverages to airlines have little opportunity for direct contact with consumers of their products, unlike keepers of food stalls and restaurants. They only learn about passenger likes and dislikes indirectly through the airline and flight attendants.

Another unique feature is that the preparation site or inflight kitchen is far removed from where the food is served. The food products must be able to withstand holding conditions in the kitchen, the transport conditions, and the extended hot or cold holding period that occurs between the time these are loaded on an aircraft and are actually served. Hot foods are generally prepared one day ahead of the day they are going to be served, and rapidly chilled to a temperature of 40 egree F. And at this temperature they are kept right till heated in the plane galley ovens just before serving.

For inflight foodservices there is no margin for error. The whole thing calls for great care, control and inspection. The right products in the right amount must reach the right plane at the right time. Any error can delay a flight, with the caterer incurring heavy fines. The caterer has to keep track of flight changes, parking gate changes, and changes in the configuration of various types of aircraft. And there's simply no time to go back to the kitchen for shortages. The unloading of food waste and the loading of fresh provisions has to be done with maximum efficiency and speed; the caterer's men are usually the first to enter an arriving plane through its rear service door.

Airlines lay all possible emphasis on the wholesomeness and quality of food. Firstly, food served on flights undergoes more handling and transport than is typical of most foodservices. Therefore, there are more opportunities for spoilage or contamination to occur. But more important: any incidence of food-borne illness on a flight can have a very adverse effect on the concerned airline's ticket sales. And nowadays legal liabilities from public suits can be crippling to the airline's finances. No wonder there have been so few cases of food poisoning on planes.

The travelling public possibly doesn't know of another food safety precaution that airlines take. They provide the flight deck crew with individual meals containing different foods. They want to avoid a possible situation where both the pilots might become ill from a contaminated food product and both be potentially unable to fly. Even crew members on long flights are provided with quality food—approximating to the one served to the first class or business class—to help them keep fit and alert for their exhausting work.

Latest trends in airline food are heralding a few significant changes. There is greater use of branded items, individually pre-packed, bearing names of famous firms in food industry. These products—even items such as sandwiches, cold cuts, cereals, desserts—are popular with passengers, as people fancy eating familiar foods, not the traditional airline fare. More and more of branded items are being pressed into use as airlines are moving towards more cold meals and fewer hot meals.

Airlines are concerned with quality for all classes. And insist on their caterers to prepare products in accord with very rigid specifications—the Continental's instructions for preparing a turkey sandwich run into a full page. However maximum attention is currently being levied on meals in the business class. Here are customers who are commonly frequent flyers. And being mostly from the business community, their goodwill can bring the airline higher business from their companies. Anyway airlines make much more money from a business-class flyer than from the one riding in the economy class.

Despite all this, inflight food has still to outlive its image of being rather boring and unappetizing. This calls for even greater attention on the part of airlines, and there are indications that this would be forthcoming in good measure.

Special Inflight Meals for Health

Most air travellers assume the only choice they can exercise over inflight food is to specify a vegetarian meal. Actually many airlines now offer a variety of special meals for health, medical or religious reasons.

Take passengers suffering from diabetes mellitus. There is the special Diabetic Meal (DBML). Here are the guidelines of that meal as drawn up by the Inflight Food Services Association. IFSA came into existence in 1972 and represents major airlines and inflight caterers.

DBML Diabetic Meal

Use lean meats; do not fry foods.
Use low fat dairy products.
Use high fibre foods wherever possible—fresh fruits and vegetables and whole grain breads and cereals.
Canned fruits must be water packed or in their own juices. Use unsweetened fruit juices.
Use polyunsaturated fats.
Omit any items with high fructose, sorbitol, mannitol, zylitol, and sugar.
Specialized, commercially available diabetic products and sugar substitutes are acceptable.
Omit cakes, pastries, sweet biscuits, sweetened breakfast cereals, ice cream, and sweet sauces.
Low fat: (30 per cent or less of energy intake).
Protein: approximately 10 to 12 per cent energy intake.
Calories: approximately 2,000-2,400 in 24-hour period.

There is an ever-increasing number of requests for special meals. This trend is the result of passengers' increased concern with healthful foods, a rising percentage of elderly passengers, and the public image of airline food as "unhealthy".

At one time various airlines were serving different type of special meals and a good deal of confusion prevailed among passengers over those meals. Until major airlines got together and standardized Special Meals. Meal codes were then agreed upon so that a passenger ordering a particular type of meal on any airline anywhere in the world could be assured of getting the type of meal desired, if the airline offered it.

Medical guidance for special meals was based on the latest information from the American Dietetic Association. Each airline still has the latitude to individualize the special meals served to fit ethnic, regional, or cultural needs by creating its own menus while staying within the parameters of the special meal guidelines.

Currently the coded list consists of 22 Special Meals.

BLML	Bland Meal
DBML	Diabetic Meal
GFML	Gluten Free Meal
HFML	High Fibre Meal
LCML	Low Calorie Meal
LFML	Low Cholesterol, Low Fat Meal
LPML	Low Protein Meal
LSML	Low Sodium, No Salt Added Meal
NLML	Non Lactose Meal
PRML	Low Purine Meal
VLML	Western Vegetarian Meal
VGML	Western Vegan Vegetarian Meal (no dairy, no eggs)
AVML	Indian Vegetarian Meal
RVML	Raw Fruit Vegetable Meal
SFML	Seafood Meal
SPML	Special Meal
KSML	Kosher Meal
ORML	Oriental Meal
HNML	Hindu Meal
MOML	Moslem Meal
CHML	Children's Meal
BBML	Baby Meal

When passengers request special meals (done in advance, often through travel agents), the airlines ask their inflight caterers to prepare these meals individually. Since all special meals require individualized food products preparations and handling, they are labour-intensive, costly meals for the caterer to prepare. Thus, the increasing demand for them is adding to airlines' operating costs.

Yet this facility, which is now available on most international flights and even domestic flights in America and Europe, can prove particularly beneficial to passengers with diabetes or other health problems. What is needed is a more widespread awareness among air travellers of this added facility.

Passengers, even otherwise, are getting more health conscious. You see a trend towards lighter foods, such as for salads, and for fat-free pretzels as an alternative to peanuts for snacks with beverages. And a marked preference for wines, even bottled water vis-à-vis hard liquor.

Suffering Motion Sickness

Passengers helplessly vomiting out of cars and buses on hill journeys are a frequent sight.

Motion sickness is a normal reaction of humans, in common with animals, while exposed to certain motion stimuli that occur during passive transportation. The term itself was first used in 1888 by J.A. Irwin to denote sea sickness and train sickness. Added since then are road sickness, air sickness and space sickness.

And, despite this diversity in environments, there is a commonality of symptoms, notably nausea (the word nausea comes from the Greek word *naus*, meaning ship), vomiting, pallour and cold sweating. An attack of motion sickness is always uncomfortable and frustrating, often embarrassing, occasionally as debilitating as to cause prostration.

What exactly causes motion sickness? Thinkers and scientists have pondered over it for centuries. And, even with all the intensive research in the last few decades especially with reference to space sickness, many questions still remain unanswered.

Various theories about motion sickness have been advanced from time to time. "Sailing on the seas proves that motion disorients the body," wrote Hippocrates. As sea sickness was characterised by vomiting, the focus of inquiries has been the stomach. But stomach is not the seat of motion sickness; only an upset stomach makes matters worse. Incidentally, summer heat has nothing to do with this nausea. And, contrary to the popular impression, the roots of motion sickness are not psychological; it's a real physiological ailment.

The pivotal role of vestibular sensory system in motion sickness has been recognized for more than a century following the observation that deaf mutes were immune. The vestibulary system in the inner ear comprises the paired otolith organs and the three semicircular canals. While the fluid-filled canals are stimulated by head movements, the otolith apparatus is stimulated continually by gravity and also by sudden linear acceleration. It was believed that overstimulation of these organs from provocative movement caused motion sickness. But this hardly explains absence of motion sickness in horse riding.

The most widely held explanation today is that motion sickness is "sensory conflict". The circuits in the brain that control body orientation, balance, and movement receive an overload of inconsistent signals. When there is a sustained mismatch of sufficient intensity it builds up excitement in neural centres, resulting in motion sickness.

The relatively slow development of motion sickness and the persistence of symptoms after withdrawal of provocative motion suggest that the act of vomiting is achieved by the accumulation of a chemical agent released by the brain that had been burdened by conflicting signals.

On the basis of a lifetime of experience in a stable environment, our central nervous system develops the ability to predict sensory signals it should receive when certain body movements are made. Our brain appears to compute the difference between the actual and anticipated sensory signals as a way of detecting external disturbances. Otherwise, the world would seem to move whenever we moved our head, for instance.

In normal activities such as running, jumping or dancing, conflict signals are small, since the body's behaviour is almost completely predictable. On a rolling boat or a winding hilly road or a plane caught in air turbulence, however, the body movements a person undergoes are unpredictable, so there is an overload of error signals to the brain.

People vary widely in their susceptibility to motion sickness. In general, women, especially when pregnant or menstruating, are more likely to suffer from motion sickness than men. Infants less than two years are usually immune. Children from two to twelve are most susceptible. From twelve years onward, susceptibility declines with age. Illness may raise susceptibility greatly; indeed, an experience of provocative motion may bring out the symptoms of the disease before they would otherwise have appeared.

What can be done to prevent motion sickness, or at least to reduce its rigour?

As motion sickness is due to a neural mismatch induced by motion stimuli, any procedure which reduces sensory conflict or the physical intensity of the motion will be a palliative. Visual-vestibular conflict can be minimized if you keep in sight an earth-stable visual reference. Thus it is better to be on deck when aboard a ship with a view of the horizon or in the front seat of a car and able to see the road ahead. A pilot, for example, free of symptoms in the cockpit, may experience motion sickness in a viewless cabin.

If below deck in a ship or with scant outside view in a vehicle, conflict is less with the eyes closed than with open. A restricted head movement and provision of body restraint like a seat belt is beneficial, as is the assumption of a recumbent position.

Reduction in the intensity of the motion is a help. If the bus driver can take bends more slowly and avoid powerful acceleration and braking, or the pilot can seek less turbulent air and avoid making steeply banked turns, that's a gain for motion sufferers. Anyway, one could try for a seat where the motion is least, usually in the middle of a vehicle or plane or in the middle of a train carriage.

Adaptation or habituation to the provocative motion is "Nature's own cure", although there are some people to whom such adaptation comes dismayingly slow. Again adaptation to one type of motion does not necessarily confer protection on transfer to another; a bus driver adapted to hill driving may well experience sea sickness for the first few days of a sea journey.

Many medical remedies have been claimed to be beneficial in preventing motion sickness, but relatively few are effective and none affords complete protection. Nevertheless, there are a number of drugs of proven value which increase tolerance to provocative motion and allay the development of symptoms.

The effective drugs are in two pharmacologically distinct classes: the anti-muscarine and the anti-histamine. The former, like Scopderm or Dramamine act quicker but give short term protection; the latter, like Avomine or Avil are more persistent in their action but slower to take effect. Both are sedative to some extent, and there could be side effects such as dry mouth. And one problem is always there; the drug taken orally may get regurgitated.

Science has yet to find a perfect preventive for motion sickness. Yet some understanding of the sickness itself helps the unfortunate sufferer against undue anxiety and panic.

Vacationing with Allergies

If you have allergies or asthma, you know they're always with you, even when you travel. So, to ensure that your vacation is relaxing and enjoyable, you should take special steps about your allergies or asthma.

Incidentally, the word "asthma" of Greek derivation (known since the time of Hippocrates) refers to the act of "panting", a condition of people with widespread narrowing of bronchial airways.

Travel by Car, Bus or Train. When travelling by car, bus or train, potential allergens or irritants can include dust mites, indoor moulds, and pollens. Mites and moulds can lurk in the carpeting, upholstery and ventilation systems of vehicles. In case of a lengthy auto trip, better turn the air conditioner on while keeping the doors open for at least ten minutes prior to entering the car. This should help in removing dust mites and moulds.

Air pollution can worsen allergy and asthma symptoms. To avoid excess air pollution when travelling by automobile, travel in early morning, when the air quality is better and you can avoid heavy traffic.

Travel by Airplane. Air quality on planes can greatly affect the allergic or asthmatic person. Airliner cabin air is a unique environment, providing something different from what people breathe on the street, at home, or in office.

Cabin air is 50 per cent re-circulated and about 50 per cent "fresh"— meaning drawn through the jet-engine air intakes, compressed, and diverted to the cabin. In addition, the fresh and re-circulated air is routed through filters through filters which can trap various particles. The air flows into the cabin from ducts in the ceiling and is sucked out through vents along the floor at the cabinet wall.

That way, window seats on airplanes have better ventilation flow than the aisle seats. They're a good place to sit if you're a sufferer of allergies or asthma.

The main controversy over cabin air surrounds the decision by airlines to save money on fuel by reducing the amount of fresh air available. Drawing in and distributing fresh air requires compressors, and compressors need power. That means more jet fuel per flight. The compromise arrangement often results in airliner cabins having a high level of pollutants.

Other Allergen Sources. Hotel rooms often contain large concentrations of dust mites and moulds in carpeting, mattresses and upholstered furniture. Ask while making hotel reservations if there are allergy-proof rooms available. If you are sensitive to moulds, request a sunny, dry room away from areas near indoor pools or basements.

If you have food allergies, be cautious in eating outside. It calls for particular care when eating airline food. And better carry your portable epinephrine in case you have a severe reaction while in flight.

Almost any food can cause allergy. But milk, eggs, wheat, chocolates, nuts, and fish are known to cause most troubles. It may all sound funny, but the symptoms are no joke to the person experiencing the allergy.

Why are a few people sensitive to some foods while the rest of us can consume them with pleasure? Physicians are not certain about the process of allergy, but make out that some people possess an overabundance of the antibody immunoglobin E. An allergy is essentially an overreaction of the antibodies in repelling a foreign invasion of the body. Allergists believe heredity is involved.

Persons suffering from sinusitis or ear infection can experience significant ear pain in flight. Sipping liquids, swallowing often and chewing gum, can help alleviate the discomfort.

Back-care in Travel

After an enjoyable 5-day trip to Singapore, Kapurs were homeward bound. As the plane came to a halt at the IGIA, Ravi leaped out of his seat to retrieve the heavy hand-luggage stowed overhead. A sudden twinge in the back; he ignored it. Next morning Ravi woke up in excruciating back pain.

Sitting long in plane, train, bus or car, and heavy lifting of luggage can hurt your back. If you never had back problems before, you could develop some. And if you already have them, you can make them worse.

Back experts have been coming up with a few spine-saving travel tips.

If you're on a plane or train, get up and walk around for a few minutes every hour. On long car trips, stop every hour and walk around. Sitting increases pressure in the vertebral discs and this makes it all the more painful for people with lower-back problems.

If there is no room to walk in a plane or train, better stand up periodically. Standing upright reduces the strain on the lower back.

There is even an art of sitting for long hours. A small pillow (the sort provided in planes) tucked in the gap between your lower back and the seat counteracts the tendency to slump.

Sitting slumped over an extended period plays havoc with the back. While standing, the lower portion of your back—the lumbar section—normally curves inward (towards your abdomen). But when sitting, it tends to slump outward. That squeezes the ends of the vertebra discs, cutting off their supply of nutritious fluids.

It is useful to empty your back pockets when sitting for hours. Sitting on a thick wallet or a bunch of keys gives an unnatural twist to the spine.

Sitting long with legs crossed (more common with women wearing skirts) is bad for the back and for the legs, too. Crossing the legs shortens leg muscles, reduces circulation to the legs, pushes out the lower back, creates uneven weight on hips and pelvis, and irritates the sciatic nerve.

When you can't even stand in a plane or train, fidget frequently. Stretch your arms overhead; lean to one side, then the other. Shift around in your seat. Changing position assures that the discs' supply of fluids isn't cut off.

Again, in a plane or train, it helps if you rest your feet on a briefcase or carry-on bag on the floor. This elevates your knees above your hips, taking the pressure off the back of the legs and keeps the lumbar spine curving more inward than outward.

For automobile drivers, an anti-slumping strategy is to tilt their rearview mirror a little bit upward. This keeps them sitting up straighter, in order to watch what's coming behind.

Another important element in back-care is to lighten luggage loads.

Backpacks are good; they take the load off your back and put it on your abdominal muscles. Just remember to wear the backpack over both shoulders.

Even a heavy purse hung all the time on one shoulder drags it down.

Better limit your travelling bags to less than 15 kilos in weight if you suffer from back problems. It's preferable to distribute the weight evenly by carrying one small suitcase in each hand. A large suitcase carried in one hand is particularly hazardous to your back. The idea is to avoid a situation where all the weight is on one side, resulting in asymmetrical loading on the spine.

With two smaller suitcases, position them close to your sides, bend both knees, grasp the handles and slowly straighten the knees. And maintain an upright posture.

Lifting heavy packages to overhead racks or bins is dangerous, particularly if you already have a bad back. Better stow such items under the seat. And there's no shame in securing some friendly help if a heavy package has to be hauled up or down.

Preferably travel with suitcases that have attached wheels and retractable handles. Or, in the alternative, you carry a light collapsible luggage carrier with wheels. And, wherever possible, push rather than pull.

Lifting heavy bags is riskier in the early morning hours. Fluids pool in your spinal discs while you sleep, making your lower back extra sensitive to irritation on waking up. If you're leaving early in the morning, better load your car the night before. In case this isn't feasible, make sure you do some gentle stretching movements before commencing the loading.

Some make out that backache is the result of poor anatomical design; human spine not yet fully adapted to the upright posture. Yet our spine is a miracle of design and a wonder of engineering—and incredibly complex—which researchers are just beginning to unravel.

Keeping this complexity in mind, experts advocate prevention strategies than cure, especially in modern-day travel. The track record of existing therapies for chronic back pain is rather poor.

5
Medicines, Doctors and Hospitals

Evolutionary Approach to Medicine

In "Why We Get Sick" (Times Books, 1995), Randolph M. Nesse and George C. Williams propound an evolutionary theory of medicine. Their thesis is that our bodies have been genetically programmed for life as hunters and gatherers over a hundred thousand years. And though our way of life has changed dramatically since then, our genetics have not.

In the light of the same, the two authors come up with some fascinating findings. Their lively explanations of certain health problems, however, would be hard to prove or disprove. One reason why medical scientists don't seem greatly excited about it.

Why do babies cry so often? The authors' explanation: infants cry to be picked up, since thousands of years of evolution has taught them that the safest place to be is in their mothers' arms.

And why do children loathe dark green vegetables that adults know are good for them? This childhood aversion is a defence mechanism inherited from Stone Age days. Prior to the advent of agriculture, most plants were full of toxins designed to discourage browsers. Children can't easily deal with these toxins and developed the wisdom to avoid them.

Indeed the authors connect the origin of morning sickness to the same. It was a reflex to keep women from eating foods that might harm the foetus.

And they are somewhat critical of doctors who routinely try to bring down a fever. Fever, they say, is the defence mechanism of the body for putting the invading bacteria at a disadvantage. Suppression of fever may bring comfort to the sufferer, but it could prolong the illness.

They even theorize how pathogens have developed survival strategies through millenniums of evolution. For example, cold viruses which spread by human contact are better off when their hosts move about and infect others. No wonder, these viruses are kind enough to let us walk about. On the other hand, malaria makes us immobile; thus making us an easy prey to more mosquitoes.

What about decrease in appetite during fever? Invading bacteria need iron. One of the body's counterstrategies, they say, is to deny them iron. In a genetically programmed reflex, the appetite centres of the brain respond with nausea to meats and other iron-rich foods.

And in health, we have a desire to gorge on sweets and fatty foods. This was a good strategy of stocking in nutrition during the Stone Age when rich foods were so scarce. The same no longer holds true but it isn't easy to suppress the ancient reflex.

And why one of our commonest complaints is back pain? To the authors, our lower backs are still not fully fit for upright posture; the evolutionary process yet incomplete in this respect. It all results in a good deal of backache.

The book's main message: treating sickness symptoms routinely is probably counterproductive. A better bet is to gain insight into the body's evolved wisdom and as far as possible to come to terms with it.

Mind Your Medicines

Why did the dusk fall so fast on the golden age of antibiotics? One miscalculation was to assume that a steady stream of new drugs would always be available. Another lay in supposing that bacterial resistance would evolve glacially slow the way it happens with other evolutionary changes.

Bacteria have responded in an astonishingly short time with packages of genes that counteract each of the five major classes of antibiotic.

For most diseases there are still one or more antibiotics that work. But the antibiotics of last resort are often far more expensive, beyond financial reach in poor countries.

The ritual of prescription has lost some of its value. Much of the time people don't take the prescribed drugs. At times, a drug is even given to someone for whom it wasn't prescribed. Quite a few people, it seems, don't follow the schedule. And a lot don't follow the take-with-food, finish-all-this-medicine kind of directions.

Another area of medicine misuse is self-prescription. Most of us are not doctors, so why do we all feel qualified to prescribe medicines for ourselves and our dependents? The hazards of playing doctor are obvious. But then, we are all, to a varying degree, hypochondriacs.

Under continuing push from pharmaceutical companies for higher sales, more and more drugs are being taken off the list of prescription medicines and sold over the counter as home remedies—converting them from Poms (Prescription-Only Medicine) into Pees (Pharmacy drugs). One argument advanced is that it would relieve physical pressure on overworked doctors. The other; it saves people consultation fee for everyday ailments.

Regulations on the advertising of drugs are there. But ad campaigns are busy enticing consumers into using drugs whose number and complexity is ever on the rise. In the big league of consumer spending are pain relievers, remedies for colds and coughs, vitamins and minerals, laxatives, and skin treatments. There is simply too much to swallow. Someone has yet to come with an effective scheme that would guide and protect consumers in the field of self-prescription medicine.

Safety becomes paramount as stronger and stronger drugs are coming off prescription. For example, the ubiquitous workhorse of headache business is paracetamol. Yet an overdose of paracetamol can be lethal.

In Britain, since January 1995, it places upon the counter-staff of every pharmacy a duty to satisfy themselves that a medicine can be safely supplied to a person who asks for it, and to make sensible judgements about when to involve the pharmacist (the latter have had four years' training).

Many of us here also seek advice from shop chemists. At times shop chemists volunteer advice on their own. How good is the quality of that advice is a grey area. Indeed there is a worrying element of laxity in observing regulations about drugs that can be only be prescribed by doctors.

Pack details and leaflets which are supplied with each pharmacy product are supposed to echo warnings against improper use. There is currently a Plain English Campaign in UK to make instructions on the pack and the leaflet understandable "at a reading age of nine". We need something similar here. And so also a campaign advising consumers to read carefully and without fail what's written on the pack and the accompanying leaflet.

Another area of concern: where drugs don't mix.

There are now thousands of drug compounds on the market to treat all manners of maladies that went untreated a generation ago. Some of these potent drugs can interact with each other in unpredictable ways.

"Drug cocktails" have acquired a legitimacy from several lifesaving applications. For certain strains of tuberculosis you need a cocktail of four antibiotics to kill the bacterium. You need a cocktail of four to six antiviral drugs to quell AIDS.

Now it's for your doctor to decide about the safety of various drugs he prescribes. But these days, people can have more than one doctor. Make sure that each one of them knows what the others are prescribing. And don't forget to tell even of vitamins or herbal remedies you may be taking on your own.

The consequences of adverse interaction are far more serious with the elderly, who are often taking several medicines at one time. The amount of fat and water in the body changes with age and with it comes a tendency to respond to treatment differently from their younger counterparts.

Doctors Now and Then

How differently doctors work now from the way they worked fifty years back! Possibly no other established profession has changed so much in recent times.

The modern medical man largely functions as if medicine was invented after the Second World War. In fact doctors are almost embarrassed about the past. Not so long ago allopathy had hardly anything to offer except opium and bromides, bloodletting and purges.

When as children we reported sick, the first thing a doctor would ask was to stick out our tongue. Proper bowel motions enjoyed top priority then. And your general condition was mostly gauged through an examination of your nails and pupils, temperature and pulse. Now straightway before you even finish narrating your woes, your blood and urine and possibly stool, have to be sent for laboratory tests. And it often entails a few shots of X-rays. Irregularity of bowel motion, howsoever it may rattle you, doesn't really bother doctors anymore.

The most significant change has taken place in what the doctors tell now and what they told then. In a 1961 study of cancer I patients, only 1 in 10 doctors told patients they had cancer; by end of 1970s, 1 in 4 doctors said cancer diagnoses was shared with patients; towards the end of 1980s, almost all the doctors said they preferred to disclose cancer diagnoses. In fact the pendulum may have swung so far that patients are inundated with information about their illnesses. Some loose-lipped doctors have even got into the habit of thinking out loudly in front of patients about all conceivable complications of a case. They are possibly worried that they won't figure out the diagnosis until it's too late. Of course, they are doing it from the best of intentions but in the process they sometimes scare their patients needlessly.

It's good that doctors are spending more time explaining illnesses to their 'patients. Only some doctors remain unskilled in exactly what to say to patients or their near-ones. Understandably a few medical colleges have started emphasizing the importance of bedside manners. Perhaps the best strategy would be reveal a moderate amount of information and then assess the patients desire to know more. The issue is to tailor communication to the needs of the patient.

However in many quarters-especially in our conditions, a common complaint persists that doctors aren't telling enough. One area where doctors sometimes don't tell enough is the possible side effects of a medicine. Some doctors feel that the patient made aware of it may suffer magnified side effects through auto-suggestion. Yet a few recent studies have revealed that people who were adequately briefed about the side effects were better able to discriminate inconsequential effects from more dangerous reactions.

Contrary to the earlier pattern, patients are now encouraged to ask more questions and supply more details of their illnesses. Being too shy to specify one's condition or too nervous to do the asking could well mean the doctor missing some salient points of the ailment. In most cases the suspicion that something is seriously amiss can be deduced from the patient's account of his symptoms. The distinction, for example, between the many types of headache can be made solely by differentiating its site, type, periodicity, and exacerbating or mitigating factors. Simply saying: "I've a headache" is useless, as the busy doctor working on the basis of probabilities would just check your blood pressure and issue a prescription for pain-killers.

By contrast: "I don't usually get headaches, but for the last month I wake every morning with a crashing headache which mostly gets better during the day but is made worse by coughing," will, unless the general practitioner you consult is a complete ignoramus, ring sufficient bells to take it seriously.

So, you are now advised to be self-confident, to reflect on the precise nature of your symptoms, and to tell the lot to your doctor.

That brings us to the question of "your doctor". Nowadays you are repeatedly being exhorted to "consult your doctor" before taking up a particular exercise or a special diet or a drug. But then I've no "doctor", and I imagine there must be many like me. All the ones I go to are now specialists, whether it's for eyes or ears or teeth or heart or prostate or bone troubles. In fact no doctor of my acquaintance proclaims himself as a mere general practitioner. Where has the good old tribe of GPs vanished?

At one time you used to look for a specialist, now you have to be on the look-out for a general-purpose doctor.

Medical Mistakes

Some time back there was this case in Sawai Man Singh Hospital, Jaipur, the premier hospital of Rajasthan. Vimla Regar, a 25-year-old woman, was admitted for the removal of kidney stones, but in a patient mix-up her uterus was removed. The latter operation was meant for another Vimla in the same ward, a 45-year-old. And there was an attempt to hush up the matter, to tamper with the papers. The state authorities suspended the surgeon and the supporting staff members, while ordering an inquiry.

Occasionally we hear of outrageous mistakes in hospitals: the wrong leg amputated, the wrong kidney removed, or surgical swabs left in the abdomen. Though much publicised, such blunders are relatively rare. Far more common are sundry medical mistakes and lapses in patient care: a harried doctor misdiagnosing someone's illness, a ward nurse making an error in dispensing medicines, or a chemist misreading a doctor's handwriting on the prescription.

The phenomenon of medical mistakes in USA has been studied at some length by the Institute of Medicine (National Academy of Sciences). A recent report claims that between 44,000 to 98,000 Americans die every year as a result of medical errors. And the report outlined a series of recommendations aimed at reducing these errors by 50 per cent in five years. The basic approach is to model remedial action similar to that adopted by the aviation industry, with focus on collecting information on errors and using this knowledge to devise safer systems and procedures.

The report also recommended the creation of a nationwide reporting system and a new federal agency, the Centre for Patient Safety, to coordinate the collection and analysis of the data.

An influential section of medical opinion in the country has, however, challenged the report's estimate of deaths from medical errors. Doctors make out that it is often impossible to determine whether a patient died from a an error in healthcare or from the disease itself.

There is also the difficulty to decide what is or is not an error; a common definition of medical error has yet to be evolved. Charles Bosk in his book *Forgive and Remember* has developed a classification scheme for errors. Some errors, he states, are clearly "technical"—an artery nicked or a knot tied too loosely in a surgical operation. Others are what he calls errors of "judgement"—misdiagnosing an ailment. And errors are more difficult to pinpoint in medicine than in surgery.

A move is afoot in USA that would require hospitals to report all errors that result in serious injury or death; less harmful errors to be reported on voluntary basis. Of course, how many errors will actually get reported is another matter; there's the normal human tendency to cover up one's mistakes.

That brings us to the general question of medical ethics. Should doctors voluntarily confess to their mistakes, instead of the odd chance of being found out? And, going a step farther, should patients be informed of doctor's errors?

Senior surgeons are known to confess their errors among colleagues in informal settings. This method of acknowledging errors without disclosing it outside the profession somewhat solidifies the power of senior surgeons, who are seen as strong enough to confess their errors to their colleagues. Other surveys, however, indicate that most doctors remembered their major mistakes, but few talked about these to colleagues, friends, or even family members.

David Hilfiker is one of the few doctors who has broken the silence and taboo on disclosure. In his memoir *Healing the Wounds*, dealing with his life as a family practitioner in rural Minnesota, he catalogues the sort of mistakes he made: misreading an X-ray, mistakenly aborting a fetus that he thought had died, not adequately assessing the emergent nature of a patient's complaint.

Hilfiker reasons that telling patients of our mistakes is good because the burdens of physicianhood are too heavy; we should tell for the good of our souls. His rationale is that physicians need forgiveness for their mistakes in order to maintain their spiritual health, and this forgiveness can only come from patients.

And there is some evidence that patients do come to know about their doctors' mistakes. Many a patient can recount a series of misdiagnoses and the resulting complications.

But then any admission of medical mistakes to patients could give rise these days to a malpractice suit. Clearly the current surge in malpractice suits has changed doctors' behaviour. Disclosure in a world where medical errors are expected to be compensated has its costs; doctors clam up on their mistakes.

Doctors are supposed to be honest. Lawsuits and departmental punishments are supposed to help them that way. But lawsuits and other punishments represent a system that doesn't trust doctors to be honest on their own. Excellence is no longer internal to the profession. Instead, it resides in the regulators, who are seen as morally superior.

What's the incidence of medical errors in India? The phenomenon, it seems, has not been the subject of any detailed study or research. Again no major hospital is known to be collecting statistics of its medical errors in any systematic manner.

The health ministry, however, recently commissioned a study of how hospitals were dealing with complaints. The Delhi-based consumer association, Voice, conducted a sample survey of 81 hospitals in Delhi, Lucknow and Hyderabad. The study revealed that only 21 per cent of hospitals kept accessible complaint boxes. And these again weren't being opened on a regular daily or weekly basis.

Yet what came out as a surprise was the fact that the great majority of complaints related to sanitation, utilities or billing. The fact that the complaints relating to the quality of clinical services did not figure prominently reflects upon the poor awareness and low expectations of consumers regarding healthcare services.

Dr N.S. Dixit, a noted heart specialist, is particularly critical of the manner in which medicines are dispensed. Any error there can have more serious consequences for the infants and the elderly. Errors, he says, occur with prescriptions that can't be read clearly: "Incidal" the anti-allergy drug, for example, read as "Indiral" a beta blocker. The latter can produce a strong reaction in an asthmatic patient. An error check becomes all the more difficult to trace as many a chemist here avoids giving a bill, listing out the medicines. And our pharmacies commonly dispense medicines in the physical absence of a trained pharmacist. Again prescription drugs are being routinely dispensed without insisting on a prescription.

Dr K.P. Mathur, with a lifetime experience of managing government hospitals, traces most medical errors to the pressure of numbers in public hospitals. Doctors dealing with outdoor patients (the outdoor was really outdoor, E.M. Forster once commented, seeing patients lined under a tree). Doctors can't spare more than a few minutes for each patient, whereas they need time to make a diagnosis. The result; they often fail to go into a patient's medical history. In their hurry, doctors can miss all sorts of clues.

And Dr Mathur blames lack of facilities and adequate trained staff for many errors in public hospitals. Of course, there is a sort of medical audit in most hospitals, where cases of death and prolonged hospitalisation are reviewed by a senior-doctor team, in consultation with the concerned doctor. But that's about all. No hospital operates a system of looking for and documenting medical errors, not even a prestigious institute like the AIIMS, Delhi.

"Just telling doctors and nurses to be more careful won't do very much," says Dr Mathur. "We need to change the system that allows errors to happen." And the first thing to do in this direction is to reduce patient pressure on hospitals, something not at all easy to manage.

Yet both the doctors concede that there is need of a greater awareness about medical errors, big and small. Possibly an NGO or a semi-government organization could specialize in surveying, researching, and documenting the phenomenon.

Hospital Visiting

> Whether to ignore my host of disquieting symptoms and have to spend my days visiting friends who have surrendered to theirs, or to surrender to my own and spend my days being visited by friends who are thereby being punished for being well.
>
> —Ogden Nash in his poem *Hospital Doors Haven't Got Locks Anyhow*

As a people we stand second to none in demonstrating our warmth when it comes to visiting hospitalized relatives and friends. Indeed hospital authorities have a hard time limiting the number of visitors and restricting them to visiting hours. Here they are counting on two emerging trends to ease the pressure: hospital stay progressively getting shorter, and the distances visitors have to travel getting longer, and that also in the trying conditions of urban traffic.

One of the burdens of the hospitalized is that he or she has, in a sense, to play host to the healthy. Howsoever uncomfortable you may be feeling, you've to display by word or deed due appreciation for the trouble someone has taken to visit you.

Lying in a London hospital for a retinal eye operation, I found no one ever visiting the other patient in the room. My wife, who was good enough to stay most of her day with me, couldn't help asking this middle-aged Englishman about it. "I've told my wife not to visit. What's the point of her coming when I can't see her; both my eyes are bandaged," was the reply.

On the other side, is there an appropriate visiting etiquette?

Small children, for one, shouldn't be taken along. They are in no position to sympathize with the sick. And it's a job keeping them entertained or even still. With their busy fingers, children are again highly vulnerable to hospital infections. Fruits and flowers are the only permissible offerings. Flowers are particularly welcome with women patients. Women love getting flowers. Women are moved when they get flowers. All women. Every woman.

The sick should only be visited during visiting hours unless specifically asked otherwise. Anyway no visiting before breakfast when the patients are being prepared for the day. I once had the mortification of being visited by a senior service colleague when sitting on a bedpan in a Jaipur hospital. He said, he had just looked in while on his morning walk. With a sheet wrapped around me, he couldn't conceivably figure out as to what exactly was I doing. But to me it was no fun prolonging the proceedings with the bedpan edges biting into the buttocks. Mercifully, an angel of a nurse arrived, and made a questioning sign whether I was done with? Getting my nod, she asked the gentleman to step out for a minute. "Oh, I'm leaving anyway," he said, and walked out briskly after giving me a hearty handshake.

Some visitors claim too much expertise with regard to a patient's illness. "Oh no, you can't assume it as a one-time affair. These kidney stones form again and again. My brother was operated twice for it, and that made me read a lot on the subject. The trouble lies with some of the new foods: even too many cola drinks can leave a fine sediment that eventually hardens into stones."

Or, they may be too innocent: "Where exactly is the prostrate? Amazing how surgeons can get at it without cutting open the stomach."

Others could bore the visited by telling some obvious jokes about the illness, such as the punctuation jokes to a colon patient or farting jokes to someone with a distended stomach.

If you've a mind to entertain through humour, anecdotes about doctors, nurses or interns go rather well.

Difficult Patients

Naresh, 40, a sales-tax inspector, lies in a general medical ward of the Delhi Safdarjung Hospital. He had swallowed some 40 sleeping pills in a suicide bid. After emergency measures such as stomach pumping, he's now being treated for liver damage.

In the beginning Naresh lay passive, refusing food. And needed much coaxing for medicines. With the life-threatening phase over, he has started complaining about lack of hospital facilities and nursing attention. He keeps on calling nurses for sundry little things: tidying up his bed, getting him water, or sending a message. He was particularly nasty to one night nurse who delayed giving him the urine bottle. Indeed he has come to harbour the grievance that the nursing staff has started avoiding him purposely, and ventilates this view quite often.

Is Naresh a difficult patient—the way he has been dubbed by the nursing staff?

The term "difficult patient" is not new to nursing. Difficult patients are the ones who make nurses feel frustrated, uncomfortable or ineffective. By and large, nurses like to be liked and to feel useful; in nursing, job satisfaction is important.

A difficult patient is described as demanding, uncooperative, unappreciative, and generally unlikeable. This includes patients who grumbled, complained, or were over-dependent or overly questioning. And others who displayed behaviours expressing withdrawal (refusing to interact), passivity (non-compliance), manipulation (practicing devious means), aggression (confrontation, anger), or even violence.

Difficult patients are actually difficult people. So dealing with difficult people means dealing with difficult behaviour: noisy, complaining, cringy, grumpy, or generally dissatisfied. Their attention-needing displays could include feigning discomfort, making seemingly unsubstantiated complaints, or seeking constant attention that does not reflect their actual level of need.

The need of attention from staff is important in its own right for some patients, and the resulting possession of such attention from nurses has a value all of its own. Actually every patient presents his or her own set of individual needs and problems. So what is it particularly that dubs him or her as more demanding than another? And how do nurses decide that a certain level of being demanding is too much, and therefore "attention seeking" as opposed to an acceptable need of nursing attention? This is by no means an easy issue.

Nurses tend to avoid patients who, they think, make excessive demands; they are afraid that when they encounter the patient again, a new or additional demand will be made. And this view may be passed on from one nurse to another during handovers or at team meetings. As a result there is often an increase in "detachment" or gradual withdrawal. This, in turn, makes the patient more needy and more demanding. A vicious circle emerges.

The health care sector can be a minefield of anxieties, complaints, fears and frustrations. And hospitals by the nature of their environment and patients by the nature of their necessity provide a highly emotive atmosphere.

Today, patients (and their attendants) are far more assertive and aware of their rights than ever before. They ask questions regarding prognosis and seek additional information about treatment. Many nurses find themselves still struggling to cope with the new scenario.

Aggression and violence from patients, or more particularly from patients' relatives and attendants, is on the increase in healthcare. All nurses face confrontations on a daily basis but the areas more prone to aggression are Accident and Emergency departments.

Admittedly nurses have a hard task, especially when dealing with what they perceive as "difficult patients". Here are some ways that can help them cope better with the problems.

The ward environment is filled with alien sights, smells, and behaviours, which generally generate feelings of fear, anxiety and uncertainty in patients. Nurses have a duty, therefore, to make the first move in alleviating a patient's misgivings.

It is increasingly recognized in healthcare work that compliance and cooperation is best achieved by involving patients in their care and adopting regimens to suit their individual needs and lifestyle as opposed to forcing patients to suit hospital-based routines. Nurses would do well to share control with patients. "Difficult patients" are commonly the product of a rigid regimen and frequently labelled when reluctant to comply.

Guidance and advice is commonly required but the nursing role is not to coerce, force or insist, even when choices made cannot be condoned. There are situations when a patient's views may be overridden, but in the main, it is the duty of the nurse to respect the wishes of patients who are fully informed.

In patient-nurse relationship, little things are, in fact, big things. For the patient, when vulnerable or afraid, minor worries and irritations can become major anxieties. The well-liked nurses not only possess sunny disposition, they also take care of "little things": a welcomed smile, a hand on the shoulder at the right moment, giving a few minutes when a patient is upset, changing water of his flower pot, and so on. These little things can have a lasting impact on patients, and give amazing satisfaction to the nurse, too.

It's important to keep your commitments. Nurses are commonly heard to say, "I'll just be back in a minute". Minutes can easily turn into hours and even longer. Such breaking of a commitment can be very destructive of patient-nurse relationship. The golden rule: aim to make promises, formal or informal, that can be kept amidst your busy schedule.

There are many situations in nursing when an apology coupled with an adequate explanation could avoid escalation of patient anxiety, dissatisfaction and resulting anger. There are undoubtedly numerous situations that are out of immediate control of nurses: busy routines, cancelled appointments, difficulties contacting doctors, increasing paperwork, unrealistic patients; the list is endless. Yet what is controllable is the nurse's ability to communicate with the patient, to offer acceptable explanations.

Some patients will always be easier to handle than others. But this does not mean that the difficult ones (many a patient isn't patient) can be avoided for their genuine needs. Patients, too, must recognize and take some responsibility for their actions.

How Good are Placebos?

Webster Dictionary defines a medicinal placebo as a preparation of little or no therapeutic value given merely to please the patient. The word comes from the Latin "placebo," meaning "to please". Originally, a placebo was the pejorative word for professional mourners. By extension it came to mean doing something to please someone. Around a hundred years back it acquired its modern, medical meaning—something given more to please than benefit the patient.

Yet the placebo effect is real. In studies of new drugs, between 30 to 60 per cent of patients are known to benefit from taking a dummy pill, generally a sugared pill. Some recent experiments have shown that surgery produces still a higher placebo effect—the bigger and more dramatic the patient perceives the medical intervention, the bigger the placebo effect. Big pills have more effect than small pills, injections more than pills, and surgery most of all.

J. Bruce Moseley, an American surgeon had grown sceptical about the specific benefit of the standard arthroscopic surgery for arthritis of the knee. He persuaded 10 middle-aged male patients to volunteer for the study, and got clearance for the experiment from the Houston medical authorities.

In the summer of 1994, all the 10 were wheeled into the operating theatre, draped, and anaesthetized. All of them then dispatched to the recovery room and sent home next morning equipped with crutches and a painkiller. But in reality only two had undergone the surgery of scraping and rinsing of the knee, three had rinsing alone, and the rest no recognized medical procedure at all, except for the incisions to make the fakery look real.

The placebo worked. Six months after surgery, the 10 patients still didn't know whether they had been faked out or not. But all of them reported much less pain. None were unhappy with the outcome of the operation. Later the experiment was repeated with another 180 patients, and the results were the same. Apparently the symbolism of surgery—the shedding of blood, the prestige of surgeons, even the scars—proves a powerful force in recovery.

As an offshoot of these and similar experiments, the taboo on placebo surgery is fading. In fact some surgeons are arguing that new surgical procedures, like new medicines, ought to be tested with placebo controls.

For years, scientists have tried to come up with a plausible explanation for the placebo effect. A common explanation is that people who have experienced relief in medical settings or from ingesting a pill are primed, like Pavlov's dogs, to expect relief. Another explanation is the release of endorphins: the placebo pain relievers stimulating the brain's own analgesics—the natural pain relievers. A third makes out that taking a placebo in an atmosphere of hope gives the patient the authorized licence to cease playing the part of the patient.

All these explanations rely on the same element of expectations. Here we have to make a distinction between illness and disease. Hope can often soften the experience of illness—illness is what the patient perceives, though hope cannot cure the underlying disease—disease is what the doctor finds.

Numerous surveys support the notion that the emotional alliance between the doctor and the patient is itself a therapeutic forc—the sick are often frightened and, in their fear, a little childlike. A compassionate and optimistic physician can be, as one writer puts it, "a walking placebo". Indeed one of the great classical doctors, Gelen, wrote in AD 300: "He cures most in whom most are confident." A physician who can marshal a placebo response with his or her words and manner (without actually dispensing a placebo pill) probably comes closest to what may be the professional ideal.

For centuries, allopathic medicine consisted of almost nothing but the placebo effect. The patient who got better after a bleeding or a purge got better in spite of it, or because of its symbolic value. Except for a few tried remedies, such as quinine for malaria or vaccine for smallpox, most other drugs were essentially placebos.

Things changed dramatically during the second half of the 20th century with the coming of all those drugs and techniques that fought many diseases successfully. This perhaps made doctors neglect the part of medicine that is not science at all—the placebo effect. Modern medical training again lays emphasis on full disclosure to the patients. And there is the growing concept of informed consent—the patient made to understand the line of his treatment and obtaining his general consent for it.

Today's patients themselves are often far from pleased to hear how well their placebos have worked. Some people feel insulted, or silly, as if they were being told, their illness was all in their mind. To others placebos smacked of deception and quackery, and what's worse, upended the logic of modern medicine.

Yet the placebo phenomenon is real. If placebos are lies, these are "lies that heal". Repeated studies have shown placebos working well for certain conditions—pain, depression, blood pressure, gastric ulcers, insomnia, colds, coughs, fevers, and some stomach complaints, even warts. Yes, warts. Doctors are known to have got rid of warts by painting them with an inert dye and telling the patients that when the colour wore out, the warts would be gone. Actually it's not unheard of for placebo effect to exceed those attributed to the active drug itself.

Some doctors have therefore started suggesting that if placebos accomplish as much in research setting, why not let doctors deliberately prescribe them. Such a strategy, they feel, would be appropriate for conditions like mild to moderate depression, pain, asthma and hypertension.

In support they reason out that the multibillion-dollar success of Prozac and similar pills may be attributed largely to the placebo effect. The expectation of improvement, not adjustments in brain chemistry, is said to account for 75 per cent of the drug's effectiveness. Or for that matter, antibiotics to treat a viral infection like common cold (in fact antibiotics are a dangerous placebo as it contributes to the problems of bacterial resistance—cough drops, vitamins, and tonics are at least not harmful). Such preparations, however, assuage the common longing to leave a doctor's place with something in hand.

The placebo effect can occur when conditions are optimal for hope, faith, and trust. It might sound sentimental, but then sentiment, working hand in hand with science, can make medical practice so much more powerful. Surely, there is something to be said for a little benign deception. Placebos aren't real medicine, but if they help in healing, why not exploit their power?

The Marvel of Melatonin

You want to stay young. You want better sex, better sleep, better health and longer life. Well, Dr Steven J. Brock and Michael Boyette claim to have the answer in their book *Stay Young the Melatonin Way* (Vermillion, London, 1995)."If there is indeed a Fountain of Youth, it's probably located between your ears: a tiny conical gland at the centre of your brain known as *pineal gland.* It releases almost undetectably minute quantities of a substance known as *melatonin* into the bloodstream."

In a similar vein, Drs Walter Pierpaoli and William Regelston in *The Melatonin Miracle* (Fourth Estate) make out that the "master hormone" could boost the immune system, relieve stress, prolong sexual vitality, even extend the human lifespan to 120. In tests they had found that mice fed with melatonin thrived far beyond their normal lifespan.

A spate of other publications have come up extolling the virtues of melatonin; a notable one is Josephine Arendt's *Melatonin and the Mammalian Pineal Gland* (Chapman & Hall, 1996). No wonder the sales of melatonin have soared, more so in USA. Last year, it sold more than aspirin in California.

The pineal gland is connected by a direct pathway to the eyes, and so is directly affected by light and darkness. Melatonin production steps up with the coming of the night—it's often called the hormone of the night—and almost ceases with the start of daylight.

When you feel sleepy in the evening, it's because the pineal gland has started pumping melatonin into your bloodstream, where it begins the physiological changes that prepare us for sleep, such as lowered body temperature and lowered blood pressure. In the morning, bright sunlight hitting the retinas of the eyes shuts down melatonin production almost completely. It is these chemical changes that promote sleep at night and keep us alert in daytime.

The pineal gland's propensity to darkness and light, evolved through millions of years of man's sync with the sun, is not easily fooled by artificial light. To affect pineal production of melatonin, you need light with intensities of more than 1,000 to 2,000 lux. Indoor lighting is generally in the range of 200 to 500 lux, while bright daylight approximates 100,000 lux. Even on a cloudy day brightness is in the region of 10,000 lux.

This mysterious hormone, researchers are discovering, has far-reaching effects on some of our basic bodily processes such as sleep, immunity against diseases including cancer, even ageing. Indeed the discovery of melatonin is regarded as a big breakthrough in medicine.

Researchers were hampered in their efforts because of the scarcity of melatonin produced by humans or even that obtainable from animals. Eventually they have learned to make synthetic melatonin. It's a white powdery stuff made from beans, chemically identical to natural melatonin. The supplements typically come in capsule or tablet form; each capsule of 1 to 5 milligrams. The actual amount of melatonin in each pill is very small, the rest inert fillers. Of course the best melatonin is the homegrown variety—the one manufactured in your own body.

The implications of melatonin were first studied with respect to sleep. In old days life was a lot simpler. Day in and day out, human bodies followed the natural rhythms of the sun. Now these rhythms stand topsy-turvy for many of us. Some nights we go to bed early; on others we stay up beyond midnight. Many work night shifts or travel through night.

To make the best of body melatonin, a lifestyle is advocated that duplicates as much as possible the daily rhythms of darkness and light. Once you look at lifestyle from this new perspective, you'll quickly find simple strategies that help you keep up with your body's rhythms.

If you're sleep deprived, you're probably also melatonin deprived. And this can lead to a host of health problems.

A capsule of melatonin taken an hour before sleeping time can be more helpful against insomnia or other sleep disorders as compared to the usual run of sedatives or sleeping pills. The latter not only disturb the natural sleep patterns, they bring on the morning-after drowsiness.

As the role of melatonin in regulating circadian rhythms became clearer, the idea of employing it to counter jet lag has come up. This is done in combination with light therapy. Detailed charts have been drawn up, indicating when to expose oneself to sunlight and when to stay in dark, with reference to the time zones crossed, westward or eastward. Broadly speaking, flying westward, you should avoid exposure to morning sunlight at your destination. Travelling eastward, avoid sunlight in the afternoon. And this is supplemented with synthetic melatonin, to be taken at prescribed times.

Along with vitamins, melatonin is now known as an eminent free-radical scavenger. An antioxidant, it fights the damage caused by the oxidation of free radicals—the renegade compounds that can upset the delicate and complex structures of living cells. For example, the wrinkled skin is really the result of skin collagen breaking down under assault of free radicals contained in the sun's ultraviolet rays.

There is really no escape from free radicals. All day long we breathe them, more so when the air is polluted with carbon monoxide or tobacco smoke, or our food and water with pesticides. So these have just to be neutralized for healthier living. To melatonin's advocates, the best strategy is to keep one's production of this hormone at optimum levels through adopting a favourable lifestyle, aided by a diet and regime of exercise that help fight off free radicals.

Old age is now being regarded not as a collection of unrelated problems but as a progressive deterioration of basic body functions. And some researchers attribute it largely to the declining levels of melatonin production as we age.

New discoveries indicate that it is in fact the pineal gland, the body's biological clock, that controls ageing, and that this gland's daily production of melatonin establishes the basic rhythm of life for every organ, every tissue, every cell within the body. Someday, scientists hope, this clock can be reset, thus increasing human longevity.

No wonder, using melatonin supplements as medicine is growing in appeal. It's non-toxic, cheap, easy to administer, and sold in health food stores. It's become the world's most fashionable hormone.

But critics are not wanting of this "Melatonin Madness". They feel that there is no data on the long-term effects or what it does, for instance, to pregnant women or unborn babies. Dr Michael Hastings, a neuro-biologist at Cambridge University terms it a simplistic nonsense that we age with decrease in levels of melatonin. "The pineal gland stays the same size throughout our lives and there is a gradual decrease in melatonin during adulthood, not a sharp drop crying out to be remedied".

Some are even sceptical of it being a wonder drug as a sleeping aid. They deem its sleep-inducing effects as rather mild. All they concede is that melatonin supplements are useful in fighting jet lag and can treat cyclical sleep disturbance, such as that experienced by blind people who lose their sense of day and night.

So the debate goes on. On one side are ranged the melatonin enthusiasts who extoll its miracles. Ranged on the other side are those to whom believing in the melatonin miracle calls for a leap of faith.

Is the Sun Setting on Pax Antibiotica?

In the 1960s the surgeon-general of the United States announced that infectious disease was conquered. Now we know how mistaken the assessment was. Who will have the last laugh: man or bacteria?

For billions of years bacteria colonized the planet, learning to cope with every environmental threat. Human beings appeared much later; just a few hundred thousand years ago.

Once people didn't know anything of bacteria, and were always intrigued when someone died of wounds. Only a hundred years back scientists were able to see microbes in their millions through microscopes. And then one smart Frenchman, Louis Pasteur, came up with the idea that these tiny creatures were responsible for deaths.

Pasteur's discovery persuaded people to pay attention to personal hygiene, build sewage systems and filter water supply. Hospitals laid great stress on sanitary practices: scrubbing, antiseptic drill, patient isolation. This did help in reducing infections and deaths, but the bugs stayed active whenever given a chance.

Till, in 1928, Sir Alexander Fleming discovered a chemical (he named penicillin) that killed bugs—the antibiotic, literally "anti-life". It was a miracle drug, successfully fighting all sorts of infections. In due course, many more antibiotics were found. Human beings thought they had beaten these tiny little things. People were lulled into a false sense of security.

Bugs knew otherwise. They invented systems that made it impossible for the antibiotics to get inside their cells. As fast as human beings discovered new chemicals—today, more than 8,000 antibiotics are known and about 100 are widely used—the bugs created new ways of surviving them. Bacteria anyway have a much longer track record at adapting and surviving than human beings. "Although man can build a better mousetrap, nature always seems to build a better mouse," says one exasperated researcher.

It is evolution at work through natural selection. When you kill billions of bacteria, a few survive. These few happen to have a system for defeating the antibiotic. Then they reproduce fast—under optimal conditions, bacteria double every twenty minutes—which gives them a decided advantage in evolving new mechanisms to evade a host's defences. And bugs have a nasty habit of passing their resistant genes across other species. The careless and rampant use of antibiotics has left us with some highly resistant bacteria.

Take the most common bug, *Staphylococcus aureaus* (SA), which infects wounds and cuts. Penicillin killed SA promptly. But by late 1950s, 90 per cent of SA became penicillin-resistant. Methicillin was introduced but within two years, strains resistant to methicillin appeared. Then came vancomycin, the powerful antibiotic. Now there are reports of vancomycin-resistant strains of SA in USA and Japan. Currently the main hope is centred around a new family of compounds, Synercid and Linezolid.

The most likely places where you get infection are hospitals. "The irony is," says the doctor of a famous hospital, "that you could roll around in the gutter outside this hospital and you might never get an infection that would cause you any problems. You come inside this clean hospital and you're in much more danger of serious infection because hospitals are where patients infected with resistant organisms are gathered together." That way, every hospital needs a special infection-control team.

It is likely—certain, in fact—that within years, all new antibiotics will encounter newly resistant strains. So we must learn to use these precious drugs sparingly and well. This isn't simple as we have become accustomed to regular use of antibiotics. In animal husbandry, even in agriculture, animals and crops are routinely dosed with disease-preventing antibiotics. Resistant genes can move easily from animal bugs to human ones.

In medicine, doctors and patients have got to stop routinely using antibiotics. Doctors, especially under pressure of patients' rush, are among those who often over-prescribe antibiotics. Patients usually insist on antibiotics, or stay unsatisfied till they have secured a generous prescription for the same. And then many a patient taking to self-medication with antibiotics—our pharmacies commonly dispensing these drugs without insisting on a prescription. Adding to the confusion is the indiscriminate sharing of a prescription by members of a family for similar symptoms.

In many developing countries, including India, a lot of people are guilty of underdosing, which further promotes bacterial resistance. This has particularly happened in TB treatment, as the full course of treatment requires a combination of expensive antibiotics to be taken regularly over a prolonged period.

Indeed, if a virulent bacterium resistant to all known antibiotics appeared and spread, human beings could be in desperate trouble; it will be like living in the pre-antibiotic era prior to the 1940s.

The actual situation, however, is not so alarming. A vigorous hunt is on for new ways to overcome bacterial resistance. And computers have vastly speeded up the process of discovering new medicines and their formulations. Just when we need a break in the worsening war of drug-resistant microbes versus antibiotics, new technologies are galvanizing the pharmaceutical industry into action.

Researchers are working furiously to uncover the private lives of bacteria, probing what mechanisms the microbes use to survive antibiotics. Special attention is being focussed on drug-resistant bacteria that cause pneumonia, tuberculosis, sexually transmitted diseases, and wound infections.

One new way to attack antimicrobial resistance is to design drugs that disable the antibiotic-resistance mechanism in bacteria. For example, it has been discovered that the bacterium *Pseudomonas aeruginosa*, which causes a variety of diseases, including pneumonia and infections of urinary tract, uses hundreds of pumps to eject the antibiotic out of its cells. So a drug is being designed to target and disable these pumps, after understanding the pumps' molecular biology.

Researchers are also busily looking for simpler remedies, and so examining thousands of plants and herbs for their antibacterial properties.

Certain types of honey, for example, has been found a good anti-infection agent for wounds. Honey has outperformed conventional antibiotics in treating infected wounds and burns. And, unlike most other antibiotics, honey actively promotes wound healing.

Well, most of the medical profession is still not convinced, but honey as an antibiotic is now undergoing extensive trials. Worker bees regurgitate nectar from flowers into the mouths of waiting hive mates. And it is fanned till most of the water in the nectar has evaporated. At the same time, their enzyme-rich saliva turns the sucrose into glucose and fructose, which leave a desert in which bacteria cannot survive. Protection comes in the form of bees' enzyme, glucose oxidase, which makes the brew acidic and hostile to most bacteria. And then honey has hydrogen peroxide, a chemical once used to disinfect wounds in hospitals.

Of course, not all honeys possess equal levels of this antibacterial property. The most potent one comes from New Zealand when bees have picked nectar from tea trees.

Whether someday microbes will acquire immunity against honey has to be seen. Incidentally there's no proof that eating honey confers any immunity against bacteria; it's only local application that matters.

How Aspirin Works

Many of us nowadays take one baby aspirin (81 milligrams instead of the usual 325 of the regular aspirin) at breakfast, a sort of an insurance against heart attack and stroke. Do users have a clear idea how the drug works?

Aspirin, one of the most-used drugs in human history, had its 100th anniversary celebrations recently. As a part of festivities in the German town of Leverkusen, the headquarters of Bayer AG, the owning company's skyscraper was all draped with cloth strips to look like the largest package of aspirin in the world.

Interestingly, despite aspirin's widespread use for over a century, much remained unknown as to how the drug worked. Only in the last 20 years some important discoveries have been made. But a good deal still remains unknown about aspirin. Researchers are busy unravelling its mysteries.

About 2,400 years ago, Hipocrates prescribed bark from a white willow tree for such ailments as pain and ague. The active ingredient of willow bark is salicin, a bitter-tasting substance. From it, chemists made a chemically simpler version called salicyclic acid, prescribed as a fever reducer. The problem was that its side effects were ferocious—enough to begin eating away the lining of the stomach.

In the late 1880s, Bayer AG, a major dye manufacturer, diversified into the pharmaceutical field. One of its chemists, 29-year-old Felix Hoffmann, whose father was being administered heavy doses of salicycle acid for arthritic pain and had his stomach lining eaten away, hit on the notion of adding an acetyl group to it. The resultant acetysalicyclic acid (called ASA) proved highly effective against pain and fevers but with much milder side effects.

A wonder drug was born, and its name changed from ASA to ASPIRIN. Aspirin was originally sold as a powder, like many other medicines.

Spurred by its meteoric success, there cropped up in course of time a dizzying array of aspirin-containing products: Anacin, Ecotrin, Bufferin, Excedrin, Motrin, just to name a few. And several brands of just plain aspirin came into the market. Anacin (containing mostly aspirin, with some addition of caffeine, and originally meant for use by dentists) proved a particularly difficult rival, being touted as offering "fast relief".

Commercial exploitation of aspirin led to prolonged legal battles that lasted some twenty years. These are brilliantly captured by Charles Mann and Mark Plummer in their book *The Aspirin Wars*. Eventually the courts ruled that the word *aspirin* was by then generic in the public mind, and so no longer saved by a patent.

Aspirin has seen dramatic ups and downs. For instance, Sterling Co in USA, which took over Bayer AG in that country during the war, had once taken a bold-faced ad: "Does Not Affect The Heart". The government objected, there being no evidence either way. The ad was withdrawn. Fifty years later, Sterling is advertising that aspirin does affect the heart, but in a beneficial manner.

As a pain reliever, aspirin began encountering serious competition from drugs such as Advil and Tylenol. The latter had the advantage of producing less serious effects on the gastrointestinal tract.

At one time it seemed as if the heyday of aspirin was over. Till one Californian doctor named Lawrence Craven found that a daily dose of aspirin seemed to prevent coronary thrombosis (the building of blood clot in the vessels supplying the heart), a major cause of heart attacks. By the 1950s the anticoagulant effects of aspirin came to be widely perceived. Doctors began telling people at risk for heart attacks that an aspirin a day would keep the grim reaper at bay. Consumption of aspirin soared to unprecedented heights.

Epidemiological research during the 1980s also revealed that regular aspirin use could protect against the risk of colon cancer by as much as 50 percent.

On the downside, long-term use can cause gastrointestinal ulceration or bleeding. And wounds take longer to heal with aspirin in the system. No wonder, there are quite a few doubting voices about the perceived benefits of aspirin. This is doubly so for women. Most studies of aspirin effects have been done on men. Only now a giant study of aspirin's effects on women is underway in USA. The results are not due until 2004.

How exactly does aspirin work? The first major insight came from the British pharmacologist, Sir John Vane, who shared the Nobel Prize in Medicine in 1982. Vane found that aspirin blocks the formation of molecules called prostaglandins, which cause inflammation, pain and fever. And this aspirin does by stopping the enzyme (known as COX) that catalyzes the production of prostaglandins.

One of these prostaglandins, called thromboxane is produced in the tiny blood vessels called platelets. Aspirin halts thromboxane production, and without it the platelets are less sticky. They move more easily into the blood, and thus help against blood clotting and consequent heart attack.

The cardiovascular benefits of aspirin have now garnered scientific support. But then aspirin can produce gastrointestinal problems. Researchers are busy figuring out whether they can have formulations that retain aspirin's benefits while reducing its side effects.

Talking of Temperature

According to a new American study, our average body temperature is 98.2°F, not 98.6°F as elders and doctors have always said.

The myth of 98.6°F dates as far back as 1868. A German physician Carl Wunderlich was investigating the cause of fevers. In this context he collected temperatures from 25,000 people to arrive at his average of 98.6°F.

Philip Mackowiak, an infectious disease specialist at the Veterans Affairs Medical Centre, Baltimore, recently gathered 700 temperatures during a vaccine study. On checking his records, he found that Wunderlich had been off by nearly half a degree-the average coming to 98.2°F.

A likely explanation for the discrepancy is that the thermometers used by Wunderlich were too crude to calibrate with the precision that is available to present-day researchers.

Mackowiak's findings highlight another fact that we are indeed warmer in the evening than in the morning. Again men's temperatures do tend to be lower than women's.

These variations have been largely ignored for the last century. People wanted one number, something easy to remember. Mackowiak now makes out that a healthy temperature can be as low as 97 or as high as 99.9.

But this doesn't mean that your thermometer can just be thrown away. A temperature of 99 or higher in the morning, and anything over 100 in the evening still qualifies as fever.

What Should Doctors Tell?

My father, aged eighty, had his chest X-rayed as a part of the preliminary fitness test before a prostate operation. The young radiologist-a golfing acquaintance of mine-took me aside and said, "He has fibrosis in the left lung. It looks like cancer. And surgical intervention for it is almost ruled out at his advanced age."

The old man was puzzled and upset over the postponement of his prostate operation. "Your friend, the radiologist, behaved as if I had only a few more days to live," he muttered. I mentioned fibrosis in the left lung. "But that's there for the last three years, since I had an attack of pneumonia during my Canada visit. And it had come out benign in the biopsy test."

We consulted a heart-lung specialist who found my father quite fit to undertake a prostate operation. Two years have gone by. The old man is staying sprightly.

Here was a radiologist who was somewhat loose-lipped, I mean in the habit of thinking out loudly. Nowadays you come across such horror stories where the doctors have spoken before the tests confirmed things like a cancer diagnosis.

Of course the doctors are doing it from the best of intentions but in the process they sometimes happen to terrorize their patients needlessly. The thinking-out-loud trend may actually be a nasty side effect of the much-heralded change extreme towards much sharing of information and decision-making between the two.

It's good that doctors are spending more time explaining illnesses to their patients. Only some doctors remain unskilled in exactly what to say to patients or their near-ones during the extra time. Perhaps some blame for the same has to be shared by medical colleges. These are now emphasising the importance of bedside manners as well as on the desirability of looking for the worst-case scenario when diagnosing and treating patients. "To miss the one-chance-in-ten possibility would carry with it a terrible burden;" say a medical professor. "Doctor worry these - days that they won't figure out the dignosis until it's too late." In this situation there are doctors who unload all sorts of anxiety on patients. Doctors, and patients too, have to realise that doctors aren't expected to perform miracles or deliver instant gratification-say, an immediate diagnosis with exact information on the seriousness and the duration of the illness.

Apparently the best strategy for doctors would be to reveal a moderate amount of information and then assess the patient's desire to know more. The issue is to tailor communications to the needs of the patient. In an ideal adult doctor-patient relationship, patients shouldn't force their doctors into guessing games, while doctors should satisfy all the information needs of a particular patient without causing undue alarm or anxiety.

Of course there is the other complaint-and a more common one in our conditions-that doctors aren't telling enough. Studies on the subject reveal that shielding patients from the truth is usually not in the patient's best interest. And it leads to mistrust just at the time that the doctor needs to be seen as an ally.

Another area where doctors sometimes don't tell enough are the possible side effects of a medicine or the pain involved in a medical procedure or test. Some doctors feel that the patient made aware of all this may suffer magnified side effects or pain through auto-suggestion. Yet a few recent studies have clearly found that people who are adequately briefed about the side effects were better able to discriminate inconsequential effects from more dangerous reactions. And greater knowledge did not lead to greater side effects or more anxiety about the treatment. Many people if they know pain is coming, can steel themselves against it.

The sharp decline in the acceptors of I.U.D. in the country advance warning of the loop's side effects. Presumably they didn't so as not to discourage the persuaded persons or there wasn't enough time for it in those crowded camps or hurried campaigns. A majority of Indian women are malnourished or anemic. I.U.Ds. do increase menstrual flow. The adverse effects came up-with the acceptors not properly briefed-and they broadcast their dissatisfaction to others. Thus a body blow was dealt to a promising breakthrough in our family planning programme, O!ai,.I.:1ly due to poor or faulty doctor-patient communication or follow-up.

Hospital staff make a practice of not telling patients about their illness and its treatment in the belief that it might confuse or worry patients, and so make the situation worse. Yes, there is that possibility. But there is also ample evidence that not V telling the patient about his illness may have even more disturbing effect. Mothers given a lot of information about the ailment of their children suffered less distress, say over a surgical event, than mothers not so well briefed.

The handling of recognized uncertainty, in diagnosis or therapy, is a particularly important feature of doctor-patient interaction. Despite all the advances of medical science, nearly half of what the medical profession does is of unverified effectiveness. Again there may be several methods of treating a disease, medicinal and surgical, and not yet clear which are most effective. In general there tends to be a bias in favour of operating surgically. In the charged atmosphere, with the patient and his family in a state of anxiety and tension, a decision to operate certainly "clears the air", and makes everybody feel better .

Many patients will be shocked if they came to know of doctor's uncertainties, particularly in areas of chronic ailments. The patient's problem: he has to distinguish between his doctor's personal ignorance or ineptitude, and the limitations of medical science.

Another tricky area of doctor-patient relationship is the role of placebos in treatment. A placebo, defined as an inert substance given for its psychological, not physiological, effect relies on the gullibility of patients. The usual placebo these days is an antibiotic, a tonic, a tranquillizer, vitamins, or some such compound (with backward patients an injection has a higher placebo effect than something takenorally). It has been estimated that 35-35 per cent of the modern day prescriptions are unlikely to have any specific effects on the disease for which they are ordered. Yet patients are readily persuaded that they are receiving appropriate treatment. And the process is aided by some element of self-deception on the part of doctors too. If a doctor admits to himself that the treatment he is giving is frankly inactive he will inspire little confidence in his patients-unless he happens to be a remarkably gifted actor.

Critics of placebos make out that all this is a huge waste of money; sugar drops come out cheaper than medicated pills. Those advocating the use of placebos argue that if the therapy is "beneficial" to the patient, besides being harmless, then why should it be abandoned because it is unscientific?

Doctors face a few other problems. Being uncomfortable (about expressing their ignorance, there is the temptation to "diagnose" something whether it is there or not. Patients are again pressing them for reassurance (it's only a sprain, no arthritis), or even wanting to be "certified" sick so that they can play the "sick role". In this demand for diagnosis, a doctor may well diagnose a non-disease (disease absent but diagnosed). This can in turn mean some unnecessary treatment and diminished perception of health by the patient. For instance, diagnosing hypertension and then "treating" it is not an infrequent failing. The "treated" hypertensives are often more *t* depressed and complain of more symptoms than the untreated: ones. That way the hypertension label can have quite an unsettling effect on the work and marital life of the one so labelled.

Recent surveys of doctor-patient communication have brought out some simple but interesting points. It has been observed that patients forget much of what the doctor tells them. Patients remember best what they are told first. Intelligent patients do not remember more than the less intelligent. Older patients remember just as much as younger ones. And moderately anxious patients recall more of what they are told than the highly anxious ones and those who are not anxious at all. Patients relax more when no desk is there between them and the doctor. And medical instructions are best understood and carried out where patients are made to write these out in their own hand.

The Marketing of Medicine

Over six hundred private nursing homes are said to be operating in Delhi. And new ones are coming up allover. Diagnostic laboratories and X-ray units have sprung up in every locality. And then all those private practioners with their consultation set ups and drug dispensing. The business of medicine is surely boomimg. Health care has become commercialized as never before, and professionalism seems to be giving way to entrepreneurial ism.

Eventually government-run hospitals will largely cater to government servants, especially influential officials and other public men who manage to get extra care or the indigent who have nowhere else to go, leave aside cases seeking some specialised treatment. Patients who can pay may well gravitate to private nursing homes and private doctors.

Even the not-for-profit institutions run by charities and voluntary organisations are coming under increasing pressure. Now, forced to compete with run-for-profit nursing homes and poly- clinics with respect to facilities and equipment, their altruistic approach is apt to get distorted.

Management decisions are now often based more on considerations of profit than on the health needs of the community. Many voluntary hospitals have begun avoiding or limiting services to the poor, while actively promoting services that can be charged.

Again attracted by profits in private hospitals and diagnostic labs, big money had started moving into the business of health care. This trend is set to accelerate in coming years. In cities like Bombay or Delhi, the commercialized private sector of health care may already be outmatching that of government and philanthropic bodies.

Admittedly private sector is making commendable contribution in supplementing public effort in the field of health care, yet its unbridled expansion poses a few pitfalls. If most of our physicians become entrepreneurs and most of our hospitals and health-care facilities become businesses, patients who can pay will get more care than they need and poor patients will get less and less. In a commercialized system the cost of health care will continue to escalate. And even government intervention may fail to control the rise in charges. Medical care is in many ways uniqely unsuited to private enterprise. It is an essential social service. Private sector is capable of making a notable contribution but it must remain alive to its social responsibilities; it just can't conduct health care like any other business.

Commercialization of health care raises another crucial question: are private practitioners businessmen? From its earliest origins the profession of medicine has steadfastly held that physicians' responsibilty to their patients takes precedence over their own economic interests. In modern times this theme has again figured prominently in many medical code of ethics. The International Code of the World Medical Organization, for example, says that "a doctor must practice his profession uninfluenced by motives of profit".

Such lofty pronouncements may be discounted but doctors still are not like any other businessmen. Their medical education remains heavily subsidised by society. Again hospitals provide physicians with many facilities, staff and specialised equipment, thus relieving doctors of many of the kinds of overhead costs that businessmen must pay. Physicians have also been enjoying a privileged position in society, virtually assured of high social status and a good living. These privileges have been accorded with the expectation that they will remain competent, trustworthy and will give precedence to the health care of their patients over their own profiteering.

The relationship between physicians and patients is quite different from that between businessmen and customers. It's another matter that patients are entitled to the protection available as consumers. Patients depend upon their physicians for advice. Most patients do not have the expertise to evaluate their own need for medical care. This relationship of dependency assumes that doctors will be acting in the best interests of patients rather than of themselves. It's nowhere like businesses persuading consumers to buy more of their products without being unduly bothered about the needs of particular consumers for such products.

The health care situation is quite different, where the provider of the services protects the patient's interests by acting as advocate and counsellor. Sick and worried patients cannot adequately look after their own interests, nor do they usually want to. Moreover, a sick patient often does not have the option of deferring his purchase of medical care or shopping around for the best buy. He may seek the opinion of another surgeon if the first one is not convincing, but he will very shortly have to trust someone to act as his beneficient counsellor.

Some skeptics question whether doctors paid on a fee-for- service basis can really give advice to patients that is free of economic self-interest. Others, on the opposite side, defend doctors by saying that there is no social contract between the doctor and his patients. Consequently physicians and private hospitals are free to sell their services in any lawful manner they choose. And it is for the patient to guard himself against overuse of services or unnecessary tests or against surgical operations that are not strictly called for-like the "Buyer Beware" in the marketplace. But would that be not asking too much of a seriously sick patient and his worried attendants?

One way in which medical practitioners are making more money is to refer their patients for tests or other services to enterprises in which the practioners have a share or some other financial interest. Thus they both are paid for their professional services and share in profits resulting from the referral of their patients to a particular facility. Some doctors make deals with wholesalers of prescription drugs and sell those drugs to patients at a profit. Or accept expensive gifts or elaborate hospitality from drug companies whose products they patronize. In entering into these and similar business arrangements, physicians are trading on their patients' trust—a clear violation of the traditional ethical rule for medical practice.

Advances in technology have also promoted the commercialization of medical practice. In an earlier and less technologically sophisticated era most physicians were generalists rather than specialists. They had mainly their time and counsel to offer, commodities that commanded only modest prices. Now a multitude of tests and procedures provide lucrative opportunities for extra income. This inevitably encourages a business approach to medicine and an overuse of services.

How best can a patient cope with this emerging scenario? The good advice: he has to heal himself. He has to be a "health- active" patient, demanding a greater role in his own health care, even if branded as uncooperative or too argumentative by his doctors. Consumers have to be the primary practitioners in the new health-care system.

Most of us grew under a medical system where the physician was all-powerful. Even now a majority of patients continue to be passive. They feel that there is little they can do to improve their health or to manage illness. They accept everything said by their physicians as "doctor's orders". There are others who may occasionally seek a second opinion but they will almost always go along with what their doctor recommends. They demonstrate childlike obedience, hanging on to their physician's every word and rarely questioning their doctor's decisions. Indeed, they sometimes act as if they were more interested in pleasing their doctor than in getting well.

But now a new breed of health-active, health-responsible consumers is coming up fast. These highly motivated men and women are determined to play an active role in their own health. They will not hesitate to disagree with their health advisors, even explore alternative therapies. They understand that medical treatment involves substantial costs and risks as well as potential benefits. If they aren't satisfied with a doctor's recommendation, they may seek a second, third, or even fourth opinion.

When faced with a health problem, they will search out additional information, through reading or asking their more- experienced friends. These are the most enthusiastic and tireless seekers of health information. They refuse to relinquish control of the key decisions pertaining to their health or of their dependents. They make a lot of querries and do not hesitate to question their physician's suggestions. But it would be a mistake to assume that these individuals are "anti-doctor", They question the doctor because they want to understand their treatment and participate in it.

This trend, beginning in the mid-1970s, is actually a product of the Information Age. The goal of the Information Age system is to empower the health-active, health-responsible people to do everything they possibly can to stay healthy and to manage their own health problems. With the help of the increasing information available on health -through books, magazines, papers, TV, radio, even through computerised information - people have taken to regulating their diet, cutting down on smoking or alcohol, and doing appropriate exercises. And they prefer to use their physician as consultant, not one calling all the shots. They want to discuss things out with their physicians and then reach agreement instead of hearing authoritarian pronouncements.

Sensitive doctors are encouraging this process. They make every effort to make the client feel trusted and responsible. In fact some were never comfortable playing God and they welcome the new more equal relationship with their patients. Some hospitals are also allowing, even encouraging, patients to see the related charts and X-rays and reports, and discuss these with their relatives and friends.

Possibly the best check against increasing commercialization of medicine is the health-active, well-informed patient who takes a good deal of responsibility about his own health.

6
Men and Women Ageing : An Explanation

The Puzzle of Ageing

Why do we decay as we grow older? Why do things go increasingly wrong with the elderly? Why does the body's capacity to heal itself diminish alarmingly with age?

Of course, each person's body ages in unique ways, but an average person can expect some of the following changes over time.

Ears: Ability to hear low frequency tones decreases in 60s. Between the ages of 30 and 80, men lose hearing more than twice as quickly as women.

Eyes: Difficulty focussing on close objects begins in 40s; ability to see fine detail decrease in 70s, from age 50 susceptibility to glare increases, and ability to see in dim light and to detect moving targets decreases.

Lungs: Maximum breathing capacity diminishes by 40 per cent between Ages 20 and 80.

Bones: Bone mineral loss begins to outstrip replacement around Age 35; loss speeds up in women at menopause.

Brain: Memory and reaction time may begin to decline around Age 70.

Gerontology, once a backwater science, is today a hotbed of research. Many a scientist is busy trying to unravel the puzzle of ageing. The idea is not so much to extend human life span, say to 150 years, but to make people's final decades of life more active.

Biologists, on a rough count, have advanced some 330 different theories of ageing, with a consensus nowhere in sight. An overall understanding of the why of ageing in humans as well as in other mammals remains elusive.

There's the widely held belief that all things deteriorate over time, worn out by use, whether it's cars or kitchen gadgets. But then living organisms are different from machines; the former composed of cells that can repair themselves through splitting and forming perfect copies. That brings on the unanswered question: why with age cells lose their capacity to replicate?

Another popular theory that life span is somehow tied to the metabolic rate. The quick nervous mice die within months while the lazy turtles can last as long as a century. But then the hummingbird has 1,200 heartbeats a minute and still lives for over ten years. Similarly birds have high metabolic rates, high body temperatures, and high glucose levels—all things that are supposed to be bad for you—and yet survive for remarkably long periods.

Steven N. Austad, an evolutionary biologist, has now come up with another explanation of animal longevity in a new book *Why We Age*. The basic idea is that the force of natural selection has great power to favour good genes and act against bad genes.

Austad's most exciting work on the ageing puzzle has been with opossums (also called possums), a rat-like New World mammal with an average length of 100 centimetres. He compared the rate of ageing between opossums in South Carolina with opossums in a specially selected offshore island.

The South Carolina opossums bred early, were incredibly prolific, and died within two-three years. To predators, the slow-moving, easy-to-spot opossums are an easy catch. In contrast, Sapelo island was opossum heaven: very few predators and plenty to eat. The opossums there bred late, had smaller litters, and were living 50 per cent longer than their mainland counterparts.

Austad's explanation: mainland opossums have an inherited trait that causes them to age rapidly at the age of 2. In the wild, an opossum would be lucky to dodge foxes or owls long enough to be affected by this trait. There is really no evolutionary pressure to remove the destructive trait from the genes pool.

The island opossums, with their far better chances of survival from predators, aren't investing all their energy in producing offspring quickly and copiously; they breed late and breed fewer, investing in better immune systems and other ways of keeping themselves healthy longer. And thus over millenniums delayed their collective rate of ageing. Austad is now working with tissue samples from the island and mainland opossums to prove that the difference in life span is, in fact, due to difference in the opossums' genes, rather than external factors. These genes could be a gold mine for biologists seeking genetic clues to mammalian ageing in general, and human beings in particular.

Austad cites a good deal of evidence that in many species late breeding and fewer births lead to longer life. And the same may hold good for humans. Life span is getting longer in populations with fewer children bred relatively late.

And he has an explanation why diseases like cancer are overwhelmingly the afflictions of the old. According to a basic principle of the evolutionary biology of ageing, if a gene has two effects—a helpful one early in life and a harmful one later—natural selection would actively favour it, despite the damage it does to older individuals. Prostate and breast cancers, he suspects, are by-products of inheritances that gave us an early advantage in siring and suckling infants, respectively.

Our best hope, Austad suggests, may lie in genetic engineering, by finding the mechanism of slow ageing that have evolved in other species. We may then be able to produce gene therapies that stave off some of the ill effects of time. However he concedes that ageing being a result of evolutionary adaptation, it isn't amenable to any easy or quick tinkering "I should see it becoming common for people to live to be 100, but I'd be surprised if we could extend human life much beyond that."

The reigning paradigm of ageing is the free-radical theory. According to it, over the years cells are damaged by toxic products of oxygen metabolism, a process otherwise necessary for life. Much ageing research is focussed on ways to destroy those free radicals. While the role of free radicals in ageing has gained widespread acceptance, it can't be the whole story. Birds, for example, burn oxygen much faster than mammals their size, yet they usually outlive them by a wide margin.

You can stop smoking. Avoid excess in alcohol. But there's one toxin you can't escape: oxygen. With every breath you take you gulp oxygen.

Oxygen is mostly good. It combines with fats and carbohydrates to churn out the energy that gets us through the day. And it nourishes the blood that courses through our veins. But during this interaction, a small amount of oxygen is regenerated in the form called a free radical or oxidant—the very critter that causes iron to rust. The oxidants careen about, binding to and disrupting cell membranes, proteins, DNA and other cell structures. Over years, this damage adds up, making you an older, frailer person.

Oxidants are said to bombard the DNA inside every one of our cells—an adult human body contains on average a hundred thousand billion cells, that's one followed by 14 zeroes—around 10,000 times a day. Luckily, most of the assailants are intercepted by the body's antioxidant chemicals. And proteins patch up the damage caused by the radicals that do get through. But eventually, as the theory goes, our tired cells get less efficient at repelling free radicals while repair work becomes sluggish. The damage accumulates, we begin to rust from inside out.

Some researchers think the key to ageing is to understand how oxidative damage works. Once that is known, it shouldn't take long to increase life expectancy.

Experiments on flies and rodents have shown some promising results with antioxidants such as lipoic acid. Fruit flies bred with a dose of SODI, an antioxidant enzyme that breaks down free radicals, lived 40 per cent longer than normal fruit flies did in a University of Guelph laboratory. Notably, the phase of life extended was youth, not old age.

If antioxidants work for flies and rats, what about human beings? Can you down a daily antioxidant supplement that would extend your years? "Don't count on it," say most researchers. Vitamins, especially C and E, are very good for those whose diets are deficient in them. Many older people have diets that could benefit from this kind of supplementation, let alone benefiting from the placebo effect. The fact that a deficiency is bad for you does not, however, mean that a surplus will do you good. For one, your body can absorb only so much of these vitamins; the rest goes the way of other wastes.

A more pleasant alternative is munching on fruits and vegetables that are high in antioxidants. With a supplement, you never get the benefit of a fruit or vegetable that contains hundreds of compounds. Right now researchers can't even identify all the compounds, much less to explain, how they might work together to fight free radicals.

Till something dramatic turns up, your best bet for fending off cellular damage from free radicals—and thus improving your odds for a longer, healthier life—is to eat lots of fruits and vegetables. This, of course, has been the conventional wisdom, but now it has the backing of science.

Here are some foods rich in antioxidants.

Fruits: oranges, plums, cherries, strawberries, red grapes, prunes, raisins, grapefruit

Vegetables: Onions, green chillies, spinach, beets, corn, eggplant, carrots, various sprouts.

One of the best-known ideas about ageing holds that animals that eat less live longer. Laboratory experiments have shown that if you reduce the daily feed of insects they live longer. For example, a spider who normally eats eight flies a day lives longer if fed only three. And diet restrictions work on lab mice, too. But there is no conclusive evidence the same happens with mammals. Admittedly gluttony is no good for longevity but whether fasting or dieting helps to prolong life is not proved. Mammals, it seems, do best when they consume what their bodies are adapted to handle.

Scientists see no reason why the same wouldn't work for us. Lighting the load of food is seen to reduce wear and tear on the body and may delay the slow descent towards death from free radicals and other aggressors such as the highly seductive but tissue-damaging sugar, that weigh down the eater of a normal diet.

In effect, it would mean restricting daily caloric intake to round about 1,500, instead of 2,000 calories the average-sized human consumes every day. And this again has to be four-five small meals a day, predominantly vegetables and fruits.

Now this is a prescription that could keep you painfully thin and perennially hungry, let alone you missing most of the fun in food. One is not sure whether many would bargain for decades of such living—eating broccoli, distilling water, gobbling garlic—just to add a few years to their life span.

Yet you can train yourself to fewer calories. There are all kinds of tricks you can play on yourself, some as basic as using smaller utensils so that a reduced portion does not look so small. Set realistic targets that gradually replace sugary and fat foodstuffs with fruits, vegetables, and fish. These measures are best adopted as early in adulthood as possible, but it is never too late to start. But researchers do caution against trying a radical change in eating habits at an advanced age.

One dieting tip that is often found effective is to eat slowly, so that your body has time to signal to the appetite centres of your brain that food has arrived. Then ask yourself at the appropriate time, "Do I really need this extra spoonful or morsel of food?" If the answer is no, stop eating. Simple, cheap, and it works if you can manage to slow down on eating.

If antioxidant supplements are mostly out, and the "famine diet" presents an unappetizing scenario, and gene engineering is still decades away, all that you can do to prolong life is to manage a balanced diet with plenty of fruits and vegetables, coupled with regular exercise. Walking is fine exercise if you do not have the amenities or inclination for other sports. Using stairs instead of lifts is a good idea, not only because the exercise is more taxing than walking, but also because the slight jolting you get as you walk downstairs stimulates your osteoblasts to build more bone.

Cultivating a sunny disposition, curbing bursts of anger that could trigger a stroke, and leading an active life can assuage the ageing process, yet there is little evidence these actually beat ageing.

The quest to beat ageing goes on. But far too many factors seem to be involved in ageing—at least several key processes are involved.

A few studies of the lives of certain individuals who managed to live up to a hundred or more have thrown up some common features. Everyone was given to taking a regular, substantial breakfast, and leading an active, moderate life lived mostly in fresh air.

How the Old Feel? Here are the Musings of one 70-Year-Old Man

I think about age all the time. I think about age the way younger people think about sex. I haven't stopped thinking about sex, but its mysteries no longer tease me. Ageing is still a mystery—not so much in the tangible signs sneaking gradually and irreversibly that I strive to stave off. The signs I watch more closely are the diminishments—little things I can no longer do or do as well.

Thinking about age is thinking about death (it's another matter, I was more afraid of death at 50 than I'm now). Will I come face to face with it in one year or ten years? And what exactly will be the form of greeting? Which indignities are in store? Once I thought I'd like to die than live with certain physical humiliations; now I'm more amenable.

People talk of the joys of contemplation in old age but the pleasure in such retrospection doesn't come unalloyed. One is often reminded of mistakes that can't be undone. It's a rare man who can review his career without some lingering regrets. Even Rupert Murdoch, the media baron, ruminates, "What have I done? How much time have I wasted in endless meetings with no decisions? Company conferences? Studying overlong reports? Yeah, I guess I've wasted at least half my life."

Kindly friends keep on greeting, "You're looking very well". But the telltale signs of age are obvious; there's nothing ambiguous about being seventy: advancing baldness, graying eyebrows, wrinkled neck, drooping furrows from mouth corners. The other day a fortyish-looking fruit-seller who used to address me as *uncle* called me *pitaji*.

I find it hard to follow what's being said when people talk in a crowded room—the embarrassment got over by smiling inanely.

Often I have to get out of bed in the dead of night with a non-negotiable need to go to the bathroom and then taking forever to finish the business—courtesy, enlarged prostrate. And I can no longer pare my toenails, as if the feet have receded or the arms got shorter.

I still manage 9 holes of golf twice a week but every time I end up with new aches and twitches I hadn't dreamed of even ten years back.

The whole business of body maintenance is getting increasingly complicated, expensive, and time-consuming. Frequent visits to dentists, ophthalmologists, ear specialists, orthopedics, urologists, test labs, let alone repeated trips to the family physician. More and more doctors are figuring in my address book and less and less of friends.

I'm aware what's happening to me is nothing novel or new. Some variation of it happens to all ageing human beings. Still it's a cause of some wonder to undergo changes that hadn't been willed.

Magazines and papers carry stories about sex for the elderly, Viagra adding another dimension. But in their heart, people approaching seventy-five well-nigh know they are staring into a sexual abyss. In fact a stage comes when you love women in general but lust for no one in particular. Over years my sexual perspective has undergone an unbelievable change. An excellent meal is now nearly as important, and so also a good night of rest.

Brain, they say, withstands ageing better than the body. Yet that hasn't stopped significant erosion in my memory for names. The other day at a get-together I couldn't recall the name of a former service colleague with whom we had shared many social evenings including rounds of bridge.

Recent researches indicate that a brain duly stimulated does compensate nicely for many losses in efficiency. No wonder there is this curious tendency, especially in the media, to shower praise on the eighty and over-eighty staying productive. People find it hard to hide their disappointment when in response to their query as to what I do, I admit to doing nothing. Of late I've taken to replying, "I'm killing time, till time comes to kill me."

Possibly what disturbs me most in going seventy is the growing isolation from the young; bulk of my social contacts are limited to people within an age differential of 10 years. One is desperate to be heard by the young, believing one has something interesting to say. The young, however, have little time or inclination for it—their concern may be more with the Spice Girls or Daler Mehndi, of whom I know next to nothing.

And there is the craving for love from one's children; the need for their love, not their money. With dead friends nearly outnumbering the living—on an average I now make one new friend in a year and lose two—

there's a greater fallback on one's children and grandchildren. But the young, at best, extend ritualistic deference. The nostalgic image of the extended family is a myth. Probably the generations have always found it difficult to live together.

Managing independently, what I and my wife strive for the most is to save each one for the other. My job is a little easier as she's six solid years younger. Anyway it is said: "If you want to live a long time, it helps to be a woman".

One of the many things young people don't know is that everyone no longer chronologically young is privately young, or at least younger; we all have an age, at which subjectively, we stopped ageing. I put mine at 55—the mental age at which I believe I've stayed since then. It makes for a kind of double life; one life in the actual world where the numbers accumulate, and the other in a dream world, a no-man's land.

Some of my friends read a meaning in their lives. They nurture the visions of a rebirth. I'm convinced there is no afterbirth. When we die, the world vanishes forever. We lose wives and children, brothers and sisters, houses and belongings, the fragrance of flowers, the warmth of the winter sun.

Knowing what one will lose makes living even more precious. I'm getting increasingly choosy about spending my time, and the books I read. To savour the dwindling hours and days, especially of daylight. To laze over morning cups of light tea. To stay more in the open.

It has taken me seven long decades to realize that I was no different from anyone else in my desires, ambitions, affections. I had taken it for granted, I do not when, how and why, that I was unique.

The realization that I was hardly different from those whom I thought were inferior—though tinged with a certain remorse—has been followed by a sense of peace. To be free from the obligation to appear special in one's speech and conduct!

And then the ultimate consolation of old age: "If you don't like growing old, consider the alternative."

"Growing old is great". That's a lie, propaganda, myth.

"You're not getting older, you're getting better." Better at what? Better than whom?

"Ageing gracefully." If anything, at seventy I'm ageing disgracefully.

Is seventy too young to be old these days? It could be different for each, some of us ageing faster than others. Yet there's nothing ambiguous about being seventy.

The poet Auden once said, seventy was a good age to die (he popped off at 66). Barring a misfortune, I could last another ten years, if there is anything in the doctrine of hereditary longevity. But already my dead friends outnumber my living friends.

Mercifully one good piece of news for those "over the hill": alcohol retards ossification of arteries, say some medical researchers. I can continue with my daily dose of a drink or two.

And the pervading feel of a mild depression. Perhaps it's a natural and even sensible state to be in when entering one's seventies. Well I wish my inability to sustain depression beyond a few hours doesn't desert me.

There is this curious tendency to view with approval those older persons who continue to work, and to deplore those elderly who just give up. Press is particularly fond of praising eighty and ninety-year-olds who work every day. People find it hard to hide their disappointment when in response to their query as to what I do, I admit to doing nothing. Of late I've taken to replying, "I'm killing time, till time comes to kill me."

Possibly what disturbs me most in going old is the increasing isolation from the young. There is this temptation to dispense vast quantities of advice. One is desperate to be heard, believing one has something interesting to say. The young, however, have little time or inclination for it—their concern may more be with the Spice Girls, of which I know next to nothing.

At times it astonishes me as to how I got so far; something of a feat to have reached seventy in a world of illnesses, germs, accidents and disasters. It makes me study the obituary page with more than passing interest—often relieved that someone died younger than older than me.

Growing Older More Slowly

A recent study found that when the majority of fifty-year-olds look into the mirror, they readjust their image and see themselves as about thirty-five. Gloria Steinem, the noted feminist writer, once remarked at being told she looked so young at fifty, "This is what fifty looks like."

And what about today's 35s? The age of thirty-five, formerly the threshold of middle age, is now merely the end of a protracted adolescence.

In my boyhood, there was no such thing as a teenager. You went straight from a child to an adult; in fact you aped adults to hurry the process along. Since then teenagers have been allowed to establish a separate, distinct identity, bolstered a good deal by advertising industry.

Now a new trend seems to be setting; people gone beyond their teen years are clinging to the teenager image, as if adulthood is something to avoid as long as possible. They are hanging on to giddy behaviour for as long as possible in the manner of desperate overgrown teenagers; holding on to things like rock music, tight jeans, wild partying—the carefree hedonism of the idealized youth.

And more and more of them—both and women—are lingering longer in parental homes; right into their late 20s, even middle 30s. This often stems from a disinclination to forsake the physical and emotional comforts of the parental home than from the expense and difficulty involved in securing independent accommodation. Living longer with supportive parents is figuring increasingly in the lengthening adolescence.

It's around 35 that they become what previous generations recognized as fully formed adults. People, that way, are growing older more slowly; taking something like ten more years than before to reach conventional adulthood. There's no need to hurry, they make out; we would be living quite a lot longer than our parents and grandparents.

We are seeing an increase in the number of first-time brides over thirty (despite the usual prediction that a 30-plus has a poor chance of finding a husband). And we are witnessing a rise in the number of first-time mothers at thirty-five. Some sort of refusal to be bound by traditional age limitations is developintg.

Robert Twigger in his recent book *Being a Man* adds another explanation for the protracted adolescence: "Consumer culture thrives on impulse buying, greed purchases, fads and fashions, wanting it now. Being childish, in other words." Maturity, which used to be a positive term, has become a euphemism for middle age.

The cutting edge of the down-ageing trend today is that of older people in search of a good time. They are shedding off some of the traditional reserve and stiffness of age, and taking more to fun activities of kids. And they seem to enjoy the release it brings them from the cares of a mature age. Visiting circuses and funfairs, playing children's games, picnicking like teenagers, eating ice cones at wayside stalls, dressing as teenagers. They are prone to play pranks, behaving like big goofy kids. No wonder, John Javna's recent book *Cool Tricks! A Grown-Up's Guide to All the Neat Things You Never Learnt to Do as a Kid* has been a hit.

The old-time view that middle age is a period of decline and despair is now set for some change. Advances in medical science have helped. Today's affluent oldsters are given to good grooming. And avidly patronize leisure activities such as travel and hobbies. Unlike the traditional oldies, the inflation-tuned oldster of today is known to spend freely. Hotels, airlines, and travel companies are wooing them busily—"catch the oldies with money in their pockets and time on their hands".

Famous beauties now brag about their age. And there are clear signs that in the coming decades women will be much less anxious about getting older, less inclined to lie about their age. The emphasis seems to be shifting from that of a woman's age to her personality and accomplishments.

The same is also getting reflected in the writings of some modern novelists such as John Updike and Saul Bellow. The progress narrative of the middle years of their heroes and heroines is not all inevitably downhill. These writers attribute psychic and physical resilience to quite a few of their midlife characters. Emerging literature is taking a kinder and more optimistic view of middle age than it was there before.

People are growing older more slowly, and hopefully, more gracefully.

Ageing Losses and Morale

To be seventy years young is sometimes more cheerful and hopeful than to be forty years old.

Recent research reveals that older persons suffering diminishments—losses in health, reduced income, constricted social relationships, widowhood, and occupational retirement—often report surprisingly high levels of life satisfaction. What could be the explanation for the seeming paradox?

Old age is admittedly an embarrassment, despite all the encouraging things said about ageing. The old, howsoever, beautiful and substantial, are somewhat disconcerting, as they signify the nearness of death.

Entry into old age brings major changes in role and status. And these are mostly in the shape of losses.

A prime factor is job retirement, with its loss of occupational activity and status. And while science has been successful in prolonging the average life-span, society continues to retire compulsorily a lot of people at a prescribed age, irrespective of their being healthy and useful. Sixty, it's quipped, is the age when one acquires sufficient experience to lose one's job.

People who are retired are more likely to feel old than their age-peers who are still working. This causes retirees (mostly male retirees) to experience a reduction in feelings of confidence and personal worth. Some try to assuage the situation by maintaining identification with their former occupational status: "retired doctor," "retired professor," "retired colonel," and so on. That way, the highly educated experience the least perceived status loss after retirement, whereas persons in low-status occupations lose most in self-esteem. The latter's position is apt to suffer a significant drop even in the eyes of their wives.

Older individuals commonly find that occupational retirement is followed by diminished income, lessened physical mobility, a decline in health and vitality, and a constriction of the social world through the death of a spouse and close friends. Each of these changes has a distressing effect upon the individual's psychological adaptation; their occurrence in rapid succession makes them an even greater threat to the retention of good morale and mental stability in old age.

The above view of ageing as a detrimental process suggests that older persons should show considerable demoralization as life changes progressively attenuate their standing in society. Previous research had often demonstrated that morale diminishes with losses in health and shrunken social life. In the realm of health and vigour, ageing not only means dangerous diseases but may bring one disability after another: impaired sight, troublesome teeth, poor hearing (an underestimated disability when it becomes a problem in conversation), and waning of smell sense (an underrated disability). More and more doctors start figuring in one's telephone book and less and less of friends.

Of late, however, several investigators are finding that aged persons with deprived status often report surprisingly high levels of life satisfaction. Older persons, it appears, "come to terms" with their deprivations. According to Edward Diener, an American psychologist noted for his researches on happiness, "the old as a group have more life satisfaction than the young. The minds of the young are full of the things they want to achieve and have not, whereas most of the elderly have either achieved what they wanted or made their peace with the fact that they never will."

Several explanations have been offered for the retention of relatively high morale in later life. One is the disengagement theory; an older person's withdrawal from society. Individuals are observed replacing many established values with a desire for an isolated, static, self-centred existence. This reorientation results in new contentments, despite the onset of an objectively deprived life.

The more plausible explanation is the reference-group theory, whereby a point of reference is provided with which an older person can compare his or her life situations.

An important aspect of this comparative function is that many negative stereotypes are applied to the "aged" as a social category in today's society. Old age is seen by young and old both as a time of diminished physical activity, absentmindedness, social isolation, poor health, increased dependency, sexual abstinence, and the like. Comparisons by older persons of their personal situations with those of the other "aged" are likely to be cast against these negative stereotypes.

In that sense the stereotypes have a positive function; they reassure persons who are undergoing age-related losses that their experiences are neither uncommon nor as severe as experienced by most aged persons. The individual's comparison of his own situation with that of the stereotyped "aged" reference group may thus serve as a buffer against demoralization that would otherwise be expected to accompany the losses of role and status incurred with ageing.

Today's affluent oldsters also have a few other things going their way. They often enjoy enviable housing. And their money allows them upgraded medical facilities, good grooming, and leisure activities such as travel and expensive hobbies. And, unlike the traditional oldies, today's oldsters are known to spend freely. Hotels, airlines, and holiday companies are wooing them busily—"catch the oldies with money in their pockets and time on their hands".

Again the traditional work ethics is on the decline. Work is now deemed more as a means of ensuring good life, rather than an end in itself. Consequently absence of work does not operate so destructive of self-esteem. And then the current consumer culture offers its own compensations; you are apt to be identified with the products you use and the lifestyle you keep.

Women Often Ageing Better than Men

Reena is sixty. She looks fifty. Feels more like forty.

Mother of a thirty-five-year old son living in USA, and a granny too, Reena runs a bustling boutique. Fortnightly she visits a beauty parlour for things such as facials, pedicure, manicure, waxing, hairdo. And plays 9 holes of golf twice a week. Hers is a regulated diet, sparing in sugar, salt and fats. And she has chosen to go on estrogen/progesterone supplements since the last four years.

Health-wise, her husband isn't doing too badly at sixty-five. Yet the toll of years is telling, compounded by occasional excesses in eating and drinking. Mohan, once a cheery, fun-loving chap stays somewhat depressed. After retirement from the Administrative Service, he could only land a low-profile consultant's job while quite a few of his former colleagues hold on to prestigious positions.

Reena, in contrast, stands transformed during the last 20 years from a mere housewife into a busy business woman. She's already earning three times more than what Mohan did. Her business and housework just leave her no time to feel disspirited, even if she had a cause.

Among upwardly-mobile middle class women in their fifties and sixties, Reena's case is becoming more typical than an exception. This category has experienced dramatic changes in the last two decades, and more could be in the offing.

For ageing women, one traditional loss was that of youthful looks. Women as sex objects had to be young; whereas men matured, women got old. The fear of this loss is diminishing with women's heightened self-worth through other accomplishments.

And many now succeed in retaining a trim figure and attractive appearance far into their middle years. Some are even accepting their age with pride; a departure from the age-old pattern where women persistently, almost pathetically, lied about their age.

Yet the greatest gains in the last few decades have been in the area of psychological health. Earlier the incidence of impairment in mental health increased as women slid into their thirties and forties. Psychiatrists mostly blamed it on women enjoying much less control over their lives than their male counterparts. Now this percentage is markedly down for educated middle-aged women; not only for those who combine outside jobs with housework, but also with full-time housewives.

It has been the accepted wisdom that menopause was a critical event in the life of a woman. The ending of her reproductive life was deemed a major threat to her adjustment. Evidence is accumulating that a large majority of present-day women really suffer no psychological problems, and little physical discomfort except occasional hot flashes. Menopause is more of a bugbear than a stressful experience. Some even report a positive improvement in their physical and emotional health, and the event no way effecting their sexual activity. In fact, to a lot of women, the cessation of their fertility comes more as a relief.

Another presumed stress point for middle-aged women was the "empty nest" syndrome—when the last child left parental home for good. Of late, several surveys on the subject have come up with the surprise finding that the syndrome was more a myth than reality. Women, especially home-centred women, did anticipate the event with a certain foreboding, but five to ten years later, hardly anyone admitted to stress on this score. Indeed, some expressed their "guilt" at "feeling better than ever" or "much freer and in charge of my own time". The "empty nest" did create conditions for change, but these were often utilized for taking up other self-fulfilling activities.

Contrary to expectations, quite a few men had reacted more acutely than their wives to the "empty nest" situation. These were mostly men at a stage where they were focussing much less on job success and sought intimacy with their children.

Widowhood is the ultimate tragedy; women often fear it more than their own death through illness. There is the loss of identity as someone's wife, a horrid feeling of incompleteness and incompetence, an ugly void in social life, and a host of other problems and complications.

Yet some recent surveys have thrown up a different picture. An overwhelming majority of widows—after they got over the initial grief—became more independent and competent than while their husbands were living. They managed to develop more rounded personalities as a consequence of being left on their own.

New research reveals that older women "adjust" to the death of a spouse and, with whatever pain or grief, move on to new strengths afterward, with less apparent difficulty than younger women—and than men at any age. If an older man's wife died, he is more likely to become sick and die within the next 2 years, than other men of comparable age. The vulnerability disappears if he remarries—or after he survives five years alone. No such drastic toll on women's life takes place with widowhood.

Another traumatic event is retirement: the loss of identity, status, satisfying work, peer support, let alone reduced finances and increased hassles in everyday living. Previously women only coped with their husbands' retirement. Now many themselves retire from jobs.

Men, compared to women, seemed more deficient in some basic strength to survive retirement. Women, of course, have this advantage; they never retire from housework. To that extent, retired women's lives stay fuller than those of retired men.

Some psychologists make out that women develop a greater capacity to meet "discontinuities" than men, because they encounter more of these in their lives. From a girl-child playing freely with boys, she abruptly changes at puberty into one demure and self-protective. She takes a job or prepares herself for one, but often gives it up with marriage and children. And then suddenly at forty-five this role is over: menopause, the "empty nest". Women thus grow better accustomed to change and impermanence than men.

From adolescence through their forties, women become increasingly feminine and men increasingly masculine. But by fifty, each is seen allowing qualities conventionally assigned to the opposite sex to emerge. Women become more assertive with age, men more giving. Women who had been constricted by the conventional values to attract and please men begin to express their feelings in all sorts of new and different ways; they grow more self-confident. At midlife, there possibly occurs a male-female "crossover".

And the same finds reflection in the sexual sphere. The husband's sexual drive diminishes (a biological phenomenon related to age) whilst the wife's remains unchanged or may even increase (there's no such direct link with age). Indeed, women usually ceased sexual activity mainly as a result of their mate's lack of libido or his demise.

Yet it's all not that good with the older women, particularly the widows and the indigent.

Satya Sobti is seventy-one. She's at an age that marks her transition from the "young elderly" to the "elderly".

Satya Sobti—now more Satya than Sobti; Amar Sobti has been dead for two decades—is seen as not doing badly. She lives in her own spacious house in South Delhi, with the rented upper floor fetching her a tidy income. No serious health complaints except arthritic knees, coupled with problems of overweight.

Her only son and his wife stay solicitous but are too busy with their own life in Mumbai. To them all her needs are comfortably met. But Satya's greatest need is to be cherished by her progeny, not its money.

Married to a high government official, she had enjoyed a busy, almost an envious social life. And there was plenty of travel, tennis and bridge. But over years as a widow, she is left with few intimate friends, mostly women of her age. And her main pastime now is playing bridge every afternoon.

Satya no longer feels at ease in the company of her husband's former friends, colleagues and subordinates. They do extend to her ritualistic deference but otherwise tend to avoid her—"the leprosy of old age". At times she thinks it may be widowhood *per se* which has thrust her prematurely into the life pattern of old age.

Never before have so many people reached into their seventies and eighties, and women now predominate in this group. Yet the feminist movement has shown scant interest in elderly women. Historically the feminist focus was on younger women's concerns and priorities: safe contraception, legal abortion, equality at work, protection from marital violence and sexual harassment. Young feminists may have even felt that older women generally shared some responsibility for their repression and holding back women's liberation. Literature has again neglected the old and their emotions.

Research on older women may increase as feminine sociologists themselves experience the effects of ageing. Betty Friedan (65), for example, is developing ideas about elderly liberation, adding ageing consciousness to feminine consciousness. An interesting book on the subject is *Growing Old Disgracefully* (The Hen Co-op, 1993). Six British women, aged between 60 and 75, talk of the cultural restraints on the lives of older women.

Over centuries elderly women have been the victims of popular prejudices, even of witchcraft. Scientific and social progress has surely ushered in an era of humane enlightenment, yet dismissive, patronizing, contemptuous and hostile attitudes towards elderly women persist. They are commonly characterized as slow, clumsy, inept, stupid, unhealthy, and unattractive.

Women as they age have to contend both with ageism and sexism. These prejudices, in combination, create a double standard of ageing, in which growing older has a different significance for women and men.

Male chronology hinges on work and job but a woman's age status gets defined more in terms of her reproductive cycle and sexual attractiveness. Because a woman's value is sexualized, positively in the first half of life, negatively in the second, it hinges a lot on youthful appearance. The discrepancy between the societal ideal of female attractiveness and their actual appearance widens with age, whereas signs of ageing in men are not considered so material.

Aware that loss of youthful appearance brings social devaluation, women are vulnerable to immense pressure to ward off signs of ageing with an armoury of cosmetic aids, including surgery. Thanks to higher health standards and better grooming, more and more women are managing to retain their youthful appearance into their forties and fifties, some into their sixties.

Yet psychic penalties are inherent in the double standard of ageing. Indeed it would be surprising if cultural denigration or invisibility has no effect on women's own perception of their ageing selves. Some women try to counter it by imagining that the elderly image befalls other people; for themselves they construct and maintain a false sense of self which rests precariously on the avoidance of any sign of ageing. They internalize what they "should" be like at certain ages. Such a denial of ageing could well alienate an elderly woman from her true identity, and from others like herself.

The negative stereotype of the elderly woman varies considerably with class and background. It's more pronounced in families where men reflect sexist assumptions about women's role and capabilities. The negativeness looms less among women with higher socio-economic status, higher educational levels, and greater commitment to employment.

Women whose earlier lives conformed more closely to the homemaking model tended to internalize themselves as useless in old age. Such women often described their lives as unimportant, although they were full of activity and interests. Low self-esteem in later life, it seems, is related to the completeness of socialization into femininity.

On the other hand, women whose lives were less home-centred maintained a more positive self-identity. Several studies confirm the importance of employment in a desired occupation for the maintenance of positive identity by women in later life. The less completely a woman has conformed to the conventional ideal of domestic femininity, the more likely she is to age with pride and independence.

Another potentially damaging aspect of the stereotyped elderly woman is her assumed mental decline, including inability to make decisions. But now an increasing number of women are not adopting these negative views of themselves; they see themselves as active participants in society, showing a lively understanding of topical issues.

In some societies, including ours, where tradition remained strong, the possession of experience often made older women take on high status roles in the extended family and in religious rites. But this may be fast changing, especially among thc urban elite. Pace of technological innovation is one factor that makes the accumulated skills and knowledge of older people redundant. Grandmother's knowledge of pre-natal and post-natal care, bringing up of children, even her traditional cooking skills may appear somewhat outmoded to younger mothers and wives with college degrees and familiarity with all sorts of kitchen gadgetry and processed foods.

Ageism is a particular form of social oppression—a process of systematic stereotyping of people because they are old. Even toasts at their birthday parties are rather jocular, at times caustic. And so also greeting cards for their birthdays. Hospital staff, even when kindly, tends to treat them more as children.

Ageism worsens when combined with sexism—a prejudice on grounds of sex. Older women expect more filial support than older men, but often actually get less.

Another disquieting feature is the increasing abuse of the elderly, especially of the frail elderly women. Old women's dependence on others leaves them open to neglect and to financial, mental and physical abuse. Faced with the prospect of alienating a relative whom they depended on for help, many victims are reluctant to complain or seek outside help.

Catering to Older Customers

As someone who has reached what used to be called old age, I am interested in how the roles of—and perceptions about—older people will change in the future. And change, these will. Indeed they'll change radically, based on what's happening now and what we can anticipate happening in the years ahead.

The emerging generation of affluent oldsters resists ageing—more in tune with Bob Dylan's song "Forever Young". These people are buoyed by the belief, they are useful and wanted, relevant and important. And are being aided by medical advances that are leading to both healthier ageing and greater life expectancy.

People not only want to live longer but to look and feel good—and to look and feel young.

Jonathan Swift said that everyone wants to live a long time but nobody wants to get old. Well, the future holds the promise of it being possible to age without feeling or looking old.

The numbers of older people are rising steadily all over the world. According to a recent United Nations report, one million people reach age 60 every month. There are now 600 million people on earth who are 60 and over. And a majority of them live in developing countries.

Clearly the global market for products and services aimed at older people will grow enormous.

Yet the commercial world is taking its own time coming to terms with the phenomenon.

For one, most of the words it uses are too small for older customers.

Take directions on medicine bottles! It's between 6 and 9 points on aspirin and a host of common painkillers. And so also between 6 to 9 points on remedies for colds and on vitamins. Obviously the type is too small to read for older people, the major users of such medicines. Writings on tablet and capsule strips are even less decipherable.

Certainly, of all the words we are required to read in the course of our lives, few are more important than the labels, directions and warnings on drugs.

The better educated the shopper, the more he or she makes decisions based on what's written on labels, boxes, tubes and jars. Such reading, for example, is crucial to selling skin-care and other health and beauty items. Much retailing depends on the written word now more than ever before. And so the readability of what's written on various items of packaged foods or toiletries assumes added importance for the buyers.

Apparently most designers who create labels, packaging, and other print set-ups are younger folks who seem to have little idea how these would look to people who must eventually read them. Conceded, designers are under pressure to squeeze in more and more material; they usually do so by making the print smaller.

Maybe bigger packages are a solution, though these would pose the problem of occupying more shelf space, not to mention the waste of more good trees. Maybe labels could make greater use of graphic images. Anyway some innovative thinking on the subject is called for.

Human eyes begin to falter around the age of forty, and even healthy ones are usually impaired by their sixties. With age the lens becomes more rigid and the muscles holding it weaken, meaning you can't focus on small type. And less light reaches your retina, meaning the world looks a little dimmer than it once did. The typical fifty-year-old's retinas receive about one quarter less light than the average twenty-year-old's. That means lots of stores, restaurants and banks should be lit brighter than they are now.

The yellowing of the ageing cornea means that certain subtle gradations of colour will become invisible to a majority of senior citizens. More people can trip up stairs as the clear distinction between step and riser disappears. And many older shoppers will find it difficult to perceive the difference between blue and green. They need a lot more of black and white and red, and much less of blue.

Commercial type almost everywhere is a challenge for ageing eyes. The nutritional information on the side of a cereal box, the laundering instructions on a shirt, the directions on a hair dye, the manual for a camera, or the song titles on a CD. And let's not forget restaurant menus, train timetables, government forms, thermometers, and the buttons on washing machines/air conditioners. Remote controls for TV, VCR, the numbers on cell phones are miniaturizing themselves out of the running for senior citizens. Owing to failing eyes and arthritic fingers, ATMs will have to adapt, too—the buttons will have to become larger, as well as the screens and the words on them. And what about telephone directories! Even morning papers using body text of roughly 9-point type are hard on ageing eyes.

In stores again, it's not uncommon to find items of interest to older people stacked on lower shelves, and those for teenagers at eye level.

Teenagers can bend and see better, whereas it would be a definite help if older people have things at eye level and involving less bending. Happily a few stores in some countries are putting up magnifying glasses on chains attached to shelves of common remedies. This is a clever makeshift solution, but it's not going to be enough.

Similarly auto manufacturers may have to take into account that, as people age, they become less flexible and find getting in and out of cars somewhat more difficult. The automakers have to make their vehicle easier to get in and out—without making them look like cars for old people.

Restaurants should recognize that loud noise is hard for older ears to take and impairs their ability to have conversation.

The healthcare industry will be under increasing pressure to provide products and services that will be *wellness*-focussed, not just illness–focussed.

Today's senior citizens endure umpteen minor forms of discrimination without complaint, as their lot in life. But the new crop of affluent oldsters will surely rebel, sooner than later—they aren't the ones to accept vexations lying down. They weren't force-fed on the virtues of sacrifice, self-denial and delayed gratification as were the elderly in the past. They did not absorb the quaint notion that to be old is to accept infirmity and inability stoically, as one's lot in life.

Another thing that markedly distinguishes today's affluent oldsters from the oldies of the pre-inflation era is the attitude towards the spending of money. To the latter, the ruling prices come too shocking for their comfort. Today's oldsters are mentally adjusted to the prevailing phenomenon of rising prices. And they are strongly touched by the current worldwide consumerist culture.

7
Common Eye Problems

Introduction

The lens focusses an image onto the rods and cones (receptor cells) of the retina at the back of the eye. Much of the image is projected onto the fovea or macula, a structure near the centre of the retina where large numbers of cones give maximum sharpness of vision. The receptors record the image and transmit it to the optic nerve. The optic nerve connects retina to the visual centres of the brain.

Of what we receive through our senses of sight, smell, hearing, taste and touch, around 75 per cent of it is through the eyes. Stationed prominently—top, front, centre—they scout the world for us. Eyes also mirror what happens inside: anger, fear or pleasure can be read in them and so also the state of health.

The eye has one of the most advanced tracking system in nature. Muscles are continually pulling it back to gaze upward, counterbalanced by another set of muscles pulling it for downward gaze. These muscles are some of the quickest in the body.

Eyelids are ever on the alert to protect the eye, forming a watertight, light-tight, airtight shield.

The eye remains one of the greatest marvels of nature. The most advanced cameras and computers as visual aids nowhere match a healthy eye.

What a Wonder is the Eye!

Nothing else shows our thoughts like the eyes. They are the psychological centre of the face, Pliny's "window to the soul". Eyes not only see the world for us, they expose us to the outside.

Eyes can "look daggers". They can dart like a trapped animal or twinkle with mirth. Eyes can murmur sweet enticements; one can have "bedroom eyes". When thoughts and feelings are absent, eyes can look hard like marbles. In anger they flare and in shame they avert. In delight they sparkle, beckoning people to peer in—lovers gazing lovingly into each other's eyes.

"In a real sense," says one scientist "there may be a language of the eyes". And this is the same language everywhere, common to every culture and country.

Eyes, in a way, mock evolution. How could such a splendid tool have appeared in stages? What good is half an eye? But our eyes did evolve through the ages. Using computers and cautious assumptions, biologist Dam Nilsson has estimated that an animal could go from flat skin-eye to a camera-lens eye through generations spanning half a million years.

The visible eye—about a sixth of the entire eyeball—has three interacting parts: white, iris, and pupil.

The ivory colour of the sheath is crucial. Since it contrasts with the darker iris and pupil, it highlights eye movements. And detecting gaze direction is a vital ability and our brains have special wiring for it. It tells us where someone is focussing. In a group this skill rapidly builds a social map, showing who is heeding whom. Without a backdrop like the white, eye movement sending a constant stream of messages would simply elude us.

The iris is a chromatic ring around the pupil, with its riot of changing colours. And its pattern is so unique, experimental ATMs are already using the iris pattern to identify customers. The iris is actually a pair of muscles, the most brilliant in the body that let more or less light reach the retina.

The pupils mirror our level of awareness. Fear, surprise, joy, anxiety, loud noise, even music expands them, while boredom and drowsiness shrinks them.

And there is the eyelid to block out the world when we want to sleep. Yet the eyelid is just one millimeter deep, the thinnest skin on the body. So being slightly translucent, it wakes us up with sunrise or sudden light. The eyelid helps register alarms.

When we blink, the tear glands emit a fluid that the lid sweeps over the eyeball. The fluid is not only a cleansing agent, it brings oxygen—in the absence of blood—to nourish the eye. And tears contain chemicals that kill bacteria.

Eyelashes are a moving palisade, holding insects and other hazards at bay. These perform the same functions as the hairs in the nose and ears.

Eyelashes are rooted in nerves so sensitive that a particle of grit caught by one eyelash will close the lid automatically.

The average blink lasts a third of a second, and the lid covers the pupil for a sixth of a second, during which we are blind. Deliberate blinks take longer, and no one knows why. Even the sixth of a second is long enough for an attacker to catch us off guard as both eyes blink at once. If we alternated blinks, we could see the world all the time.

Blinking is like breathing. We do it automatically, all day long, about 15 times a minute. Dry spots begin to pepper the eyeball after 15 to 45 blinkless seconds.

We blink less when listening attentively or reading. Some fast readers are known to keep their eyes open for an entire page and then have a flurry of blinks when turning the page. Drivers blink as they turn to look into the rearview mirror or glance at the speedometer.

On the other hand, we blink more when bored or fatigued. Even in reading or driving, when concentration wavers, we blink more.

Ask most people why we have eyebrows and you'll get a blank shrug. Joggers and tennis players know better; eyebrows keep perspiration from falling into the eyes. It is a subtle but serious function, given the dense sweat glands on the forehead. It even helps nonathletes in hot weather.

The position of eyes themselves above the mouth and nose is felicitous. It keeps droppings of mouth or nose from falling onto eyes, as well as leaves them undisturbed by any body shadows.

Aesthetically, eyebrows act as ornamental thatches, drawing attention to the eye, making it look better.

The eyebrow is the great supporting player of the face. It helps signal anger, surprise, amusement, fear, helplessness, attention and many other messages we grasp at once. Indeed, without eyebrows the surprise expression almost disappears. The eyebrows are such active little flagmen of mind-state it's amazing anyone can wonder about their purpose. We use them incessantly.

When we greet a friend at a distance, for instance, we quickly raise and lower the eyebrow: the brow-flash response that conveys surprise and delight. And the way the eyebrows can express scorn. In conveying helplessness, a shrug seems meaningless without a brow-lift. And a flirtatious smile—both in women and men—is usually backed by a quick jerky eyebrow movement upwards.

Then the eye has this power of staring. Staring is special. Our mental gaze-radar detects it quickly, and even if we are utterly safe, we feel a bit uneasy.

When we can't stop a stare, we tend to make an escape. In one study, researchers at a street corner gazed steadily at drivers halted at a red light. The drivers noticed the stare within seconds and when the light turned green, spurted across the intersection significantly faster than other drivers. Staring at pedestrians makes them walk faster.

Sensitivity to stares is genetically programmed into us through evolution. Staring is evidently the oldest and most stable facial expression on earth. Even lizards freeze in the presence of a person staring at them.

Staring feels like mind-burrowing, and sometimes we relish it. Lovers gaze at each other and feel entwined. But staring is usually rude. It invades others, psychologically and physiologically. "... gave me a cold-blooded up-and-down examination in which he took in everything," says Virginia Woolf in exasperation.

To avoid rudeness, we normally don't gaze straight into people's eyes when we speak to them. Rather, our eyes dance about their faces or even turn slightly aside. In fact men look less at the face than women.

We stare at objects of great interest, and at celebrities. But then we also stare at physical abnormalities. Intriguingly, we also gaze at pregnant women, more to assimilate the novelty—we wouldn't gape at pregnant women in a maternity hospital.

A step beyond rudeness, staring becomes a blunt power device. Even monkeys employ it to control subordinates; staring assuming a contest of strength.

Monet shocked the art world with *Olympia* (1863) in which the naked woman gazes straight at the observer. Before, nudes had looked discretely away, allowing perusal of their bodies. Olympia's stare turned the observer from voyeur to participant—something shocking for those times.

Going beyond stare, there is the evil eye, feared in almost every culture over the ages. The evil eye comes in two forms: the willful and malign, the other inadvertent. But even in the case of inadvertence, the possessor of the evil eye is deemed to be of bad disposition.

What a wonder is the eye! So brilliant in its structure and functioning; so expressive of our emotions and thoughts.

The most common ailments afflicting the eye are myopia (shortsightedness), glaucoma, and macular degeneration.

Myopia

A full quarter of the population in modern societies is nearsighted. And myopia rates are rising alarmingly. The problem is especially severe in East Asian countries. Singapore's National Eye Centre, for example, estimates that myopia afflicts more than 80 per cent of the country's 18-year-old men.

To millions when they take off their glasses, all at once their world becomes blurry. How such creatures would have fared at the hunter-gatherer stage of evolution? They would have been hard put to hunt or find food, let alone becoming food themselves to lions and tigers?

Why such rising incidence of myopia in modern times? Genes do play a part. It is estimated that the prevalence of myopia in late childhood is around 12 per cent if both parents are myopic, about 8 per cent if one parent is affected, and only 2.7 per cent if neither parent is affected. But why natural selection has not been able to eliminate the genes that contribute to nearsightedness—elongating the eyeball and thus focussing distant images in front of the retina than directly on the retina? Selection forces, geneticists believe, do eliminate genes that cause serious disease or disability.

One explanation offered by evolutionary scientists is that genes such as those contributing to nearsightedness or heart attacks were not actually harmful in primitive times. These only become deficits in our altered environment. For example, genes that cause hardening of the arteries would be harmless if our diet was 15 per cent fat instead of the prevailing 40 per cent Indeed these genes were meant to maximize the scarce food fat then available.

Geneticists have still to isolate the genes causing nearsightedness. Yet obviously genes aren't the entire explanation for the high and rising incidence of myopia in present times. Nearsightedness is rare even today in societies at the hunter-gatherer stage. Hardly any Eskimo children suffered from myopia a hundred years back. Now it averages 25 per cent after their children began attending schools. The more literate a society grows, the more the number of nearsighted in it. In backward rural areas with little literacy, only a small percentage of the young are myopic, such as in rural Nepal.

Researchers have found that placing cloudy lenses over the eyes of young monkeys or chicken makes their eyeballs elongated, until they become highly myopic. Why it happens is not fully understood, but it seems that natural selection induces growth in the eye whenever the retinal image is blurry.

The same may be happening to schoolchildren *unnaturally* exposed to close work at an early age when they strain to read and write. Today's leading theory is that reading may cause a slight defocus. When people shift their gaze from far to near, their eye muscle change the shape of the eye's lens to accommodate the change in focus.

Now a child's eye would elongate to compensate for its defocus; the eyeball changing shape and causing myopia. Thus a mechanism of nature that was meant to confer a slight advantage during short periods of blurry vision in childhood, eventually gives rise to a serious disability in today's environment. The myopia, usually starting in childhood, gets progressively worse through adolescence, till it stabilizes in early adulthood.

The eyeball once enlarged (it can get enlarged up to 29 millimetres as against the average of 24 mm) does not shrink; the resulting shortsightedness lasts a lifetime. And myopia can be more than just the nuisance of glasses. People with severe myopia—who need lenses with a focussing power of more than 6 dioptres—run greater risk of glaucoma and retinal detachment in later life.

Scientists still don't know what exactly causes myopia, except the genetic factor. A search, however, is on for some drug that could prevent the condition. The main approach is to find something that relaxes eye muscles, thus curbing their potential to elongate the eyeball.

Yet it will be some years before a satisfactory drug comes up on the market to stop the progression of myopia. Till then it is glasses, contact lenses, and now increasingly LASIK surgery.

It would, however, help to clear a few myths about short-sightedness. We can count it as amply established that nothing we can do—no exercises, or spectacles, diet or drugs—will have an influence on the ultimate degree of short-sightedness.

W.H. Bates was a firm champion of the view that short sight had little to do with the size of the eyeball, but was caused by a problem of the extraocular muscles. And so he favoured certain eye exercises. Bates therapists recommend procedures like the "magic pencil", which involves imagining there is a pencil at the end of your nose and forming the habit of drawing around objects in your field of vision, larger ones at first then smaller. Another is the *Palming* technique which requires placing the palms of your hands over the eyes and imagining colourful pictures. We have our folklore that recommends walking bare feet on dew or facing the rising sun (the latter can even be injurious to the eye).

Modern ophthalmic opinion does not find Bates' exercises to be of any significant benefit.

And contrary to what many people are told, reading in poor light does not harm the eyes, though it could give a headache. Again wearing glasses does not weaken the eyes or make them deteriorate in any way; all that glasses do is compensate for what is lacking. Similarly sitting too close to or watching television in a very dark room is not harmful to the eyes.

With the remarkable technological advances in laser eye surgery (LASIK) during the last decade, many persons all over the world are making their spectacles redundant. Does it signal an eventual goodbye to glasses?

Glasses have been a great invention. But for them, millions would have to put up with blurred, unfocussed vision. And vast numbers forced to give up reading. Indeed civilization would have spread much slower but for the advent of glasses.

And modern-day glasses aren't only for looking; they are increasingly important how they look. Glasses not only help people see better but help them look better. It is claimed that an excellent frame can bring out a face's good features. "A face is work of art. It deserves a great frame," they say. An appropriate frame can make you look dependable or profound, sincere or sweet as you wish it to be. Some eyeglass stores are evolving into special boutiques.

Fashionable people keep several pairs to go with different outfits. John Elton, the famous singer, is known to have 40,000 pairs. The range in frames is becoming unbelievably wide: frames made of tortoise shell, jewel-encrusted retro spects, foldable frames, rimless or semi-rimless ones, antique silver frames and frames of gold encrusted with patterns.

And lenses of all sorts. Hard-Resin lenses that don't break into pieces on impact. Polarized lenses with the added protection against glare and ultraviolet rays. Bifocals, Trifocals, and now the Varialux—where the distance and reading numbers shade into each other gradually instead of a sharp division.

Admittedly glasses and contact lenses are mere correctives; they don't cure myopia. Now a revolutionary 15-minute outpatient procedure offers the prospect of a permanent cure. Numbing eye drops make the treatment painless, although burning and scratchiness are normal for a couple of hours.

Thereafter you don't have to look for your glasses or contact lenses first thing in the morning. No breaking or misplacing them. No periodic misting or cleaning. No problem at the swimming pool or the beach. Goggles and masks can be worn with no spectacles getting squeezed under them.

People burdened with glasses over the years sense a special freedom when rid of them through a successful laser intervention. They can move about with ease. Some may still need glasses for driving or movies. But their operation-improved vision should be good enough for most everyday activities.

In LASIK, a surgeon uses a razorlike instrument to gently lift a flap of the cornea—the clear stiff outer layer over the coloured iris—and then reshapes the exposed cornea through a computer-controlled laser beam to vaporize part of the cornea. This alters the way the eye focusses, correcting nearsightedness.

The sculpting of the cornea permanently changes its shape; the surgery is irreversible.

LASIK is better suited for correcting mild myopia—less than 5 dioptres. Again it may fail to match the sharpness of image that comes with glasses.

One drawback of radial kerotonomy is the unpredictability of results. While many gain a great deal, some others may experience marginal improvement.

And then this surgery isn't fully free from complications and side effects, though the risks involved are lessening day by day. Under-correction or over-correction is not uncommon. Infection following LASIK surgery is potentially vision-threatening. Night blindness may occur in some cases. And so also an inflammatory reaction.

Laser vaporization does thin the cornea, thus weakening the eye slightly. Patients having undergone it must be a little more careful against being hit in the eye with a ball or fist.

LASIK surgery is primarily effective for myopia. It isn't as helpful for farsightedness. If you wear reading glasses, LASIK can't make an ageing eye's lens flexible again to improve close-up vision. Similarly the procedure can't make up for macular degeneration.

Are you a suitable candidate for LASIK surgery? It's important to have this issue clarified before undergoing it; individuals unsuitable for it may gain precious little, even suffer actual harm.

This calls for a thorough pre-operative screening. You should be checked for the thickness of your cornea. The recommended minimum thickness is 410 microns after LASIK surgery. Operating on an irregularly shaped cornea can also cause loss of vision. Oversize pupils are again a problem, because LASIK lasers are built to operate on eyes with pupil diameters of 6 to 8 millimeters. Patients with glaucoma, diabetes, and cataracts are not ideal LASIK candidates.

Many ophthalmologists still remain critical of the concept itself, whereby a healthy eye is entered into for cosmetic purposes. No such operation, they say, can be fully free from risk.

The issue was discussed during 2003 in a major conference in Delhi of the country's ophthalmologists. The meet did not come up with any definite findings. It merely reiterated that LASIK is a scientific, well-researched surgical procedure with an established track record of remarkable safety the world over. It did not spell out any particular action to ensure high-quality in treatment, plus proper pre-operative screening for suitability. One hopes, custom-hungry laser operators would not be tempted to compromise on screening tests for suitability, or in conducting a precise, infection-free, surgical procedure.

A Californian company, Advanced Corneal Systems (ACS), has come up with an invention that can do the same—flatten the cornea—but without surgery. Custom-built transparent moulds temporarily worn by patients are used to reshape the cornea. Once the mould is removed, the cornea retains the new shape for good, thus obviating for many the need for glasses or contact lenses.

The company claims that tests till now have shown vision improvement in every case (with no case of vision getting worse). And the cornea is keeping its new shape; early patients are still retaining their improved vision after a year of the moulds being removed.

ACS's procedure, called corneoplasty, first maps the contours of the cornea. This is done with corneal topographic analysers, machines which collect reflections from rings of light shining onto the patient's eye and building a contour map of the cornea. This map is then fed into another computerized machine, which custom-builds a transparent mould for the desired reshaping of the cornea. The mould is from the same material as contact lenses.

However, before fitting the mould a drug is injected to soften the cornea, making it easier to remould. According to the company, this drug has no adverse side effects and the softened cornea repairs of itself in three to four months.

For the first three days, patients wear the moulds throughout the day. Thereafter they wear the moulds only when they sleep. And after about three months of such use, when the treatment is deemed complete, the moulds are dispensed for good. The moulds, bigger than normal contact lenses, are painless to wear.

Cornea specialists remain sceptical. To them, any injection into the cornea is potentially dangerous. There is a risk of infection or scarring.

And the other drawback; these moulds currently come quite expensive, even costlier than the PRK procedure.

Reshaping cornea through moulds is still in the early stage. But it could emerge as a promising option for correcting shortsightedness. The quest to find a substitute for glasses goes on.

With rapid advances in LASIK surgery (the latest equipment costing around $500,000, and so the high cost of the operation), its enthusiasts are hopeful that millions will opt for it in coming years.

People have the great desire to be without glasses. Yet many hesitate going for surgical treatment; everyone is incredibly sensitive about their eyes. No wonder, the popularity of laser eye surgery had to await till it became largely risk-free.

Who knows, in the coming decades, it may become a routine to have one's myopia treated permanently with laser? Is it goodbye to glasses?

The Phenomenon of Floaters

A common eye condition is the presence of floaters. Appearing in the shape of tiny dots or clouds or wavy lines, they seem to float across the field of vision. Bright sunshine tends to exacerbate their showing.

Frequent appearance of floaters can be quite fretful. Some sufferers start worrying that the condition would worsen with time, even endanger the health of their eyes. The unlucky ones with a single functioning eye find floaters particularly bothersome. Indeed a big floater coming in the field of their vision raises the risks in driving.

Floaters are more common in middle age, in those who are near-sighted, and in people who have undergone cataract surgery. Floaters move with the eye but lag slightly at the beginning of an eye movement and overshoot when the movement stops.

Medical science treats floaters as generally benign, harmless. These are actually fibres and other fragments in the transparent gel-like fluid (98 per cent water, rest collagen and vitrosin), called vitreous humour, that fills the eyeball. The clumps cast small shadows on the retina, creating the illusion of floaters.

Vitreous humour serves to keep the underlying retina pressed against the supporting wall. While the posterior surface of the crystalline lens is bathed in vitreous humour, the anterior surface is bathed in aqueous humour, a clear colourless liquid whose function is to keep the outer eye clean and moist.

An element of floaters is a normal phenomenon. You can always see them in certain conditions such as looking at an empty sky. But floaters become an annoyance when degenerative processes in the eye make for a rise in their numbers and density.

Medical science does not attach serious import to an increase in floaters—essentially a visual disorder of subjective symptoms. However it does admit that the ways to get rid of floaters are limited. People are advised to close their eyes and gently look up and down to stir up little "currents" in their eyes' fluid. The floaters will often go away or become less noticeable after a few minutes.

The basic approach is that you learn to live with your floaters, the way you are advised to live with tinnitus, the buzz in your ears. Being overtly conscious or annoyed only makes you feel worse.

Of course a sudden influx of heavy floaters, accompanied by lightning-like flashes or a "curtain" of vision loss, would merit an early ophthalmic consultation. These symptoms are signs of retinal damage.

Glaucoma

At seventy-five, I have been a glaucoma sufferer for ten years. The condition "suspect glaucoma" was diagnosed during a routine retinal check-up of the left eye (the right eye lost to retinal detachment some 40 years back).

This started a daily regime of Timolol, the best known medicine meant to reduce Intraocular Eye Pressure (IOP). Beginning with one 0.25 per cent eye drop a day, it's now 2 of 0.5 per cent.

With open-angle glaucoma confirmed and the IOP still hovering beyond the normal upper limit of 20 mm Hg, a drop of the expensive Xalatan 0.005 per cent (50 drops costing Rs. 1200) at bedtime has been added since last year.

My doctor tells me he's mainly relying on medicines to manage my glaucoma. "I'm a laser man," he says, "but laser trabeculoplasty doesn't work out so well on a cataract-operated eye." And glaucoma filtering surgery presents its own risks and complications; an extreme measure of the last resort when it's a single functioning eye. I remain fearful that any loss of peripheral vision through glaucoma would further reduce my field of vision, already circumscribed with one eye.

"Should he make any lifestyle changes to keep his IOP down?" my wife asks of the doctor. "No, there's nothing he can do about it. No link has been established between high blood pressure and elevated IOP, or about alcohol use or smoking. All I can say, he should lead an active life and not get overweight."

A recent study estimates that the number of glaucoma victims in India is over 30 million. And untreated glaucoma is one of the most common causes of blindness in the country, only next to cataract. That's a pity. A majority of people blinded through glaucoma didn't have to be blind.

With early detection through checking eye pressure and treatment through medication, loss of vision is usually preventable. But if detection gets dangerously delayed (chronic open-angle glaucoma—the most common variety—has hardly any symptoms to alert the sufferer), it can result in an irreversible damage to the optic nerve and so to sight. That's why doctors advise regular eye exams including glaucoma check-ups for those over fifty; even earlier for those who have a family history of glaucoma.

The normal eye is like a sink with the faucet always running and the drain always open. The clear liquid inside the eye called aqueous humor is continually secreted by the ciliary body at approximately 2-3 μl per minute into the posterior (back) chamber of the eye. The aqueous, programmed to keep the eye clean and wet, passes forward into the anterior (front) chamber and from there through a trabecular meshwork and Schlemm's canal back into the veins.

In the chronic open-angle glaucoma, the trabecular meshwork gets blocked by a mechanism that is still not understood, though ageing is deemed a major contributory cause. The drainage block leads to high pressure within the eye—creeping up through the 20s, even 30s against the normal around 16 mm Hg.

The constant state of elevated eye pressure is blamed for long-term damage to the optic nerve, the one that transmits electrical impulses to the brain to be translated into images you see. Damaged nerve fibres hinder transmission and affect vision, initially starting with the loss of peripheral vision. The slow onset and tunnel vision mean that sufferers are often not aware that they have a problem.

There are, however, people who suffer damage to the optic nerve but have low or normal tension glaucoma. Such people slip through the net of routine pressure checks. On the other hand, there are people with higher than normal eye pressure who fortunately never seem to suffer visual loss. Glaucoma, that way, is a complex disease, though elevated eye pressure remains the dominant risk factor.

Glaucoma victims or "suspects" are advised a minimum of one check-up annually. The standard clinical examination includes testing visual acuity, visual field examination, slit lamp evaluation, measuring IOP, and a dilated evaluation of the optic nerve.

Measuring IOP is now a relatively simple, accurate affair. The most commonly employed technique is Goldmann Applanation Toneometry.

This is done through a slit lamp with the eye anesthetized. Pressed against the cornea, the instrument yields the requisite IOP reading.

Over the long run, your ophthalmologist having gained insight into the behaviour of your eyes under elevated IOP, would set a target intraocular pressure. And would try to manage the same with various IOP-reducing techniques best suited to you.

A whole battery of antiglaucoma medicines are now available, with more in the pipeline. The prime medicines are beta blockers like Timolol and andrenergic-blocking agents like Betaxolol. These are all designed to reduce aqueous production of the ciliary body.

The latest latanoprost (Xalatan from Pharmacia, Peapack, New Jersey) is designed to facilitate evacuation of aqueous through the iris route, thus bypassing the clog-prone trabecular meshwork. Around 80 per cent of aqueous humour is filtered through the trabecular meshwork while the rest 20 per cent through the iris route. Latanoprost is often given in combination with beta blockers.

If drugs fail to keep the targetted IOP, with a looming threat to the optic nerve, then resort is taken to laser trabeculoplasty. Laser hits are made on the trabecular meshwork. The heat engenders local contraction, thus increasing space for greater outflow. The success of ALT depends on the accurate placement of laser energy into the trabecular meshwork. 40-60 hits are made in a 180-degree session or 80-100 in a 360-degree session. Trabeculectomy is now a highly successful, quick and short surgical procedure, with few side-effects or risks. Only the operation may have to performed every few years. Often IOP-reducing eye drops are continued for those operated for trabeculectomy.

If all this doesn't succeed, then it may have to be glaucoma filtering surgery. The goal of this surgical intervention is to create an additional outflow channel for aqueous to escape from the anterior chamber. It's a fairly complex surgery, with its attendant risks of hemorrhage, corneal damage, and vitreous loss, besides necessitating post-operative medical attention.

As most glaucoma sufferers have to be reconciled to lifelong regular use of eye drops, it is of some importance to put in the drops rightly, thus increasing the effectiveness of the medication. And. Of course, you have to undergo the discipline of putting your eye drops with the prescribed regularity and timing.

How to use Your Eye Drops

1. Wash your hands well with soap and water.
2. Using your forefinger and thumb, gently pull down your lower lid to form a pocket.
3. Tilt your head back and look up.
4. Place one drop in the pocket. Do not let the tip of the bottle touch your eye.
5. Continue to hold your lower lid down for a few seconds to let the drop settle.
6. With eyes closed, gently apply pressure with your index finger to the inside corner of your eye. This helps keep the medication in contact with your eye.
7. Wipe off any excess medication around your eye with a clean tissue.

The human eye holds approximately 10 microlitres (about twentieth of a teaspoon) of fluid. Commercial eyedroppers release drops ranging from 25 to 50 microlitres. This means that the excess travels into the nose and is absorbed by the body.

Macular Degeneration

Like cataract and glaucoma, the common eye ailments of advancing years, macular degeneration mainly afflicts the elderly.

Indeed, with people living longer, age related macular degeneration (ARMD) is now the leading cause of vision loss. Surveys in USA reveal that 18 per cent of those aged 65 to 74 were suffering from ARMD. And nearly 30 per cent over seventy show evidence of the disease, with significant loss of vision. After a while, the sufferer can't read or drive or recognize people. The vision can drop to 20/60, which means what you can see from 20 ft, normal eye can see from 60ft. The disorder, however, does not interfere with the peripheral vision.

The macula, a central part of the retina, is quite small; it measures about a quarter-inch in diameter and is tissue-paper thin. Yet this tiny area is responsible for much of what we see. While rods dominate peripheral vision, cones are concentrated in the macula—and are responsible for central vision, colour perception, and sharp images (acute vision).

The capacity of cones to distinguish detail is one hundred times greater than of rods. We need them to tell the difference between the colour of traffic lights, and to see precise detail, like the features of a face, the pattern on a tablecloth, or the letters on a page. The macula is therefore the focal centre of our vision.

In macular degeneration, cones and rod cells of the macula begin to die, reducing the number of cells able to transmit visual signals to the brain through the optic nerve. And this happens when enough oxygen is not reaching these cells-—they need massive amounts of oxygen to stay alive. As we know, any part of our body that suffers a prolonged lack of oxygen usually sustains permanent, often irreversible damage.

There are two types of macular degeneration, commonly called the dry and wet. All cases are thought to start with the dry form. Between 10 to 15 percent of the people who show signs of dry macular degeneration eventually develop the wet form.

In dry form, darkish specks appear on the macula that takes on a sallow look. When our eyes are young and healthy, the macula has a robust colour, like a rosy apple. Your ophthalmologist can spot out these evident signs of dry ARMD.

Wet ARMD is called "Wet" because it is characterized by abnormal leaky blood vessels that grow underneath the retina. Nobody knows why this happens. And the best option today is laser treatment; a bid to seal off leaky vessels through laser heat. The procedure is done in an ophthalmologist's office and requires no eye patches or special medicine regimen. You should be able to walk out minutes later and continue your daily routine. The main trouble with laser treatment is that the heat beam burns a tiny scar in the macula itself, causing a small blind spot. Research is on to find a low-intensity non-thermal (non-heat producing) laser.

Early detection of wet macular degeneration is necessary for laser to be effective. The fewer leaky vessels there are, the better laser is able to seal them. Leaky vessels left unattended, eventually swamp patches of cone cells in the macula, causing these cells to die. More importantly, laser treatment cannot restore vision already lost.

Age related macular degeneration has assumed the shape of an international problem. Researchers in many countries are trying to figure out why ARMD occurs and how it can be prevented or delayed. Again doctors and scientists are working on a wide range of options, including new forms of laser, radiation treatments, surgery, and drugs. Patients everywhere eagerly await a breakthrough.

Wilmer Eye Institute at John Hopkins, Baltimore is a leader in research on ARMD; there's a whole department dedicated to this activity. And intensive research on ARMD is afoot in Scandinavia, where macular degeneration is very common. The media, too, have begun to pay more attention to macular degeneration studies.

What actually causes ARMD? Are there any leading risk factors involved? For answers, researchers are looking into the characteristics that many people with macular degeneration have in common.

The biggest characteristic that people with ARMD share is age. You are more likely to develop macular degeneration at seventy-five than at sixty. Besides age, a few more characteristics have been identified as common with many people developing macular degeneration: smoking, family history, diet low in dark green leafy vegetables, light-coloured eyes, and sun exposure.

Yet these can at best be treated as surmises, till more authentic findings about their adverse effects in the development of macular degeneration are forthcoming. In the meantime, AMRD constitutes a serious worldwide affliction with older people whose numbers are escalating.

One Eye Almost as Good as Two

One eye almost as good as two, I'd say. Not that I'm an ophthalmologist, but because I happen to have the use of only one eye, the left, for the last thirty-five years.

Obviously, having one eye can't be as good as having two. With the two eyes a few inches apart, each retina receives a slightly different picture. Looking at an object about 100 metres away or beyond, the eyes are essentially aligned parallel. The disparity in images arises for the nearer objects. The situation triggers vergence. The eyes manage to coalesce the two images into one. The process also provides us with binocular vision, with its three-dimensional effect. The two eyes in unison have a very special function.

I would dearly love to have the lost eye restored.

Yet, one eye is almost as good. Something that a two-eyed person would rightly disbelieve, but it is substantially correct. One eye can do the work of two, without wearing out.

There are many people with one good eye who go through life successfully, doing practically everything two-eyed people do, barring a few specialized activities. Anyway the loss of one leg, or worse still, one arm, is a far greater hindrance to normal living than the loss of one eye. Of course, the loss of both eyes is a tragedy that has no parallel.

People like me who started life with two normal eyes and later lost one through disease or injury perforce take time to adjust. They have to undergo an adaptational process that includes a relearning of spatial orientation, depth perceptions especially at near distance, and greater movement of the working eye and head to cover a larger visual field.

In the beginning tea got poured on the table instead of into the cup, and capping a pen wasn't that simple. Putting a key into a lock presented a problem. And so also coming downstairs. One tended to be awkward in sports and felt unsure as a driver. Even a tendency to graze doors.

But after some months of one-eyed existence, there develops a sort of substitute judgement of depth that enables one to function fairly well. The body's ability to cope with such situations is amazing.

Surely, you do badly in activities requiring true and perfect depth perception, such as playing high-class cricket or tennis. You can't work as a pilot or fireman. My game of badminton deteriorated. But I can manage reasonably well with golf, except for bunker shots where my club sometimes touches the sand inadvertently in its back swing. And I do drive. Only driving in heavy/congested traffic conditions can be unnerving because of the limited peripheral vision.

I say all this to those who are reeling under the shattering experience of losing an eye or faced by an imminent threat of it. First there is the shock of the loss. And a sub-conscious if not a conscious feeling of vulnerability, being reduced to relying on a single eye. One wished they drew comfort from the fact that many of their fears and anxieties could be more imaginary than real.

For example, it's not true that the good eye will be overstrained and wear out. Or, that you should work less or read less to preserve the remaining eye. Again it is not true that half the sight is lost or half the field of vision is gone.

One eye can carry the work of two adequately and indefinitely. Excess use may cause fatigue or discomfort which get dispelled with a little rest.

And you aren't obliged to tell people that you have one "seeing" eye. In fact it's a good idea to keep the fact to yourself and the family. It can prevent all kinds of embarrassments, and even safeguard a job or promotion.

Numerically, no doubt, one eye is half of two eyes. But functionally the loss of central vision is zero. The loss of side vision is around twenty per cent—and you can recapture part of it by greater movement of the eye and head, a little more than what you do with two eyes.

Loss of true depth is real. Yet you can learn to compensate and function normally except where perfection in depth discernment is required.

Separately, you are enjoined to take more enlightened care of your "seeing" eye. Go for regular and complete ophthalmic examination and evaluation to recognize early diseases, especially glaucoma in older years.

Glaucoma, being painless, is difficult to detect by yourself. Whereas it can easily be contained if medicated in time, delayed treatment could result in irreversible loss of peripheral vision.

And to wear protective eyewear at all times, particularly during driving or play when exposed to injury. Preferably use polycarbonate lenses which are shatter-proof. Keep in mind that when exposed to injury, it is the "seeing" eye which is more likely to be injured.

8

Baby Behaviour and Health

A Few Basics about Babies

The most extraordinary of all living things is the human baby. Babies are simply fascinating if we see the world from their point of view instead of ours.

Here are a few basics about babies during the first 12 months of life—the official period of babyhood.

Seeing

The vision of babies is said to be poorly developed. But this isn't exactly true. The vision of the newborn is perfectly tuned to its special requirements. At distances of between 6 and 12 inches, the newborn is well equipped to focus its eyes and to concentrate on objects in front of it. It's no accident that the distance between a mother's face and that of her snugly held baby is typically between 6 and 12 inches.

And babies seem to respond more to large round objects that move. That again enables them to fixate on their mother's face and breasts.

Admittedly infants can't focus well on things far away but then they don't need to do so. In fact through this apparent deficiency nature helps them avoid the confusion of seeing things that are of no importance to them in the first few months of their existence. By the age of nine months, a baby's vision is better organized and it can focus at a whole variety of distances. Although perfect vision is not fully acquired till one is four, but at the end of the first year, most of the adult capabilities such as focussing and binocular control are present.

Hearing

We now know that babies are capable of hearing sounds two or three months before they are born. In the womb they hear the rhythmic sound of their mother's body and even react to noise from the outside world, despite these noises muffled by the mother's body-wall and the amniotic fluid in the foetus' middle ear. And stronger the noise, the sharper the reaction. Once it was made out that the foetus' reaction to outside noise may be actually due to the mother's response from such noise, and it in turn triggering a movement in the foetus. But experiments with the mother's ears plugged still showed a noise reaction from the unborn.

Special tests have proved thai babies prefer human sounds to other sounds; there is a definite bias in favour of human speech, even from birth—the speaking animal is already in the making. Later when babies start imitating sounds towards the end of the first year of life, they are observed copying human sounds than inanimate noises. They imitate spoken words, very rarely the ringing of telephone or the sounds of cooking.

Recent experiments also claim that an infant can recognize its mother's voice within the first week of birth. And its ability to localize sounds even begins earlier. So the mother is just not a face or a voice, but a combination of the two.

Smelling

Careful observations have proved beyond doubt that the typical baby can within days of its birth easily distinguish between the smell of its own mother's breast and that of other females. This can be seen from infants turning their heads towards the maternal breast when it is brought near to them. And evincing far less interest in breasts other than those. The ability to differentiate the smell of the nursing mother's breasts shows how well equipped the human baby is to protect itself from hunger. Even in dark it is capable of turning towards the all-important source of infantile nourishment.

The speed with which the newborn child learns the personal fragrance of its own mother is astonishing. Experiments have shown that only forty-five hours after delivery the newborn can tell its own mother from other mothers purely by her body fragrance.

And the newborn is depositing its "personal" odour on its mother's breasts.

Tasting

Babies at birth have a well developed sense of taste. In fact their taste buds are not only on tongue, the palate, the back of the throat and the tonsils, but also in the insides of their cheeks.

Yet all this taste anatomy is geared to just one kind of food—the sweet mother's milk. Babies dislike all other tastes. That's good for them as any other foods may put them at serious risk. Clearly the human baby is elaborately equipped to reject strongly all but its natural, milky diet.

And babies do crave sweetness. An adult finger dipped in a sugary solution gets licked. But a baby quickly rejects a salty finger, with a grimace.

Crawling

The first signs of pre-crawling come at about four months when the baby starts to push upwards with its arms. Soon comes the chest-up posture. At six months the baby can raise both its arms and legs as it lies on its tummy or even slithers along. At about eight months the baby does its first crawl, raising its chest 1 and tummy off the ground. Sometimes babies find it easier to crawl backwards than forward. Once proper crawling has arrived it develops fast during the ninth to twelfth months. Mobility brings great fun to a baby.

And then the crawl is gone for good when the baby starts to walk. The unaided act of walking at the end of the first year marks a significant milestone. The joy of achieving this stage is obvious as if some deep-seated human destiny has been fulfilled; of all the animal species human being are the only true walkers.

Swimming

Handled correctly, newborn babies can swim. But then babies have to be lowered in water face-down and gradually submerged. Even at a few weeks of age, babies hold their breath and start making reflex swimming movements. At this tender age the human baby is a natural swimmer; better organized at aquatic locomotion than terrestrial. It has been claimed that at some primeval stage of our evolution we were much more aquatic than we are today. Perhaps the swimming action of the newborns harks back to those hoary days.

But this ease with water does not last long. A few months old baby begins panicking in water, and the "transitional panic" phase stays on till swimming comes later in the shape of a "learnt skill".

Sleeping and Dreaming

To be more precise, the average baby sleeps 16.6 hours out of 24 during the first week after birth. By the time it is one month old, the total sleeping time has shortened to 14.8 hours. And when babyhood ends at the age of one, the average daily slumber hours come down to 13. And mercifully for its parents, it now shifts to almost uninterrupted night-time sleep of ten hours.

Whatever ideas modern parents may be harbouring on the subject, to a baby sleeping with its mother is far more secure and pleasant than sleeping alone in a separate room. And babies aren't at all impressed with separate sleeping quarters howsoever lavish or luxurious these may be. Perhaps the best compromise is to have the baby sleep in a cot alongside its mother's bed.

Do babies dream? Yes, they definitely do. Only what they dream will always remain a mystery.

Talking

Strictly speaking babies do not talk. The very word "infant" comes from the Latin *infans* meaning "unable to talk". But babies are very vocal beings; they love to make sounds.

By the age of three months, the audible babbling begins, preceded by weeks of silent attempts at it. And then it becomes something of an obsession. Babies even babble when they are alone. It is amazing how babies all over the world, from every culture and every language, produce the same kind of babble sounds.

By about 6-7 months babbling diminishes in favour single syllables getting combined. And by the end of 12 months, many babies have mastered the use of several words. It is important that babies between six months and one year need to be talked to a great deal; they are interacting even when they can't speak.

Some parents find themselves talking like their babies. Instead of helping their infants to imitate them, they imitate their infants. This has obvious shortcomings, yet so many parents are seen gleefully indulging in it.

Do You Know This About Babies?

Can Babies be Toilet-trained?

No, they just can't be in the first year of their life. During those twelve months babies urinate and defecate automatically, as a reflex action, whenever their bladder or bowels sense a certain level of pressure. There is no true control during the babyhood days.

And yet many mothers try to impose some sort of discipline or conditioning on the toilet activities of their babies. Some even claim success in the same. What they possibly achieve is a sort of toilet-timing; putting the child on the pot immediately after its feed, when it is most likely to defecate or urinate. But they are mistaken if they think that the baby is cooperating. It would have done it anyway, pot or no pot.

Voluntary sphincter control in babies comes later, between the age of 12 to 18 months. Urination control takes a little longer, and night urination control even longer than that of daytime. The human baby develops at a more or less set rate. And precious little can be done to accelerate the process. In fact a severe effort at too early a toilet-training can bring on a deep-seated neuroses about defecation, leading to problems in later life.

The baby starts urinating even before it has left the mother's womb. And the newborn may urinate up to 18 times a day.

Why Babies Like being Rocked?

Rocking movements soothe a baby. These can calm an agitated baby and put a calm one to sleep.

One theory explains the phenomena on the rocking motion experienced by the foetus when the carrying mother walks or moves. The baby is supposed to be reminded of the welcome motion it had been conditioned to in the womb.

The other theory relates it more to maternal heartbeat. The foetus not only feels the mother's movements but also hears the maternal heartbeat-about 72 beats a minute. And this heartbeat speed stays strongly imprinted on the baby's memory. The idea is that a combination of these sensations, recreated by rocking, has a calming effect on the baby. In support of the same it is made out that rocking has the best effect when it is between 60 to 70 moves per minute, with each move no more than about 3 inches. Again the baby's body should move forward and backwards than from side to side.

Incidentally a few babies around nine months or so, may start rocking themselves, by sitting up and swaying their bodies back and forth. This self-rocking indicates a need for comfort and shows that these particular babies have not been getting sufficient comfort from their parents.

What Makes a Baby Smile?

The heart which is not struck by the sweet smiles of an infant is still asleep.

— Hazrat Inayat Khan

Is there anything quite so heart-warming as the smile of an infant? But what makes a baby smile? Where do smiles come from? How are they born? How do they grow?

All sorts of theories have been advanced on the subject. Indeed, experts agree to disagree.

Some parents believe their babies learn to smile from the smiles they offer them. Parents spend a great deal of time in intimate face-to-face encounters involving mutual smiling and baby talk. Yet smiling is not a learned response. Rather, it is deeply ingrained, inborn facial expression of our species. Blind babies smile. Deaf babies smile. All babies of all cultures smile.

Smiling, as well as crying, are deemed a child's first language; a way of communicating and interacting.

Behavioural psychologists tend to believe that a child's smile begins as one of the many insignificant random muscular facial movements. The very first smile is, therefore, almost an accident. But because it gets such a positive response from mother, or whoever is around at that time, the child performs it again. The bigger and better the performance, the bigger and better the adult response, and so on. Smiling is therefore a product of positive reinforcement. As a corollary, smiling declines if supportive responses are weak.

Some psychologists believe that the physical action of smiling first evolves from the physical action of crying—smiling developing as a natural counterpart to crying.

Another theory describes smiling as a physical reflex that responds in particular to tickling. A child smiles when touched in the most ticklish areas of its body, which are those parts with protective reflexes such as the armpits, the ribs, the soles of the feet, around the neck and under the chin. Similarly some psychologists believe smiling stems from a "pleasure response" to stroking of the lips, cheeks and chin.

And then there is the "wind theory", which suggests that smiling first evolves from the effort, pleasure and process of "bottom snorting". Passing wind is the process that triggers the first smile.

Most smile theories acknowledge that smiling is initially a physical behaviour that develops in time into an emotional and mental one.

Desmond Morris, the noted zoologist, puts forward his explanation of what makes a baby smile. Human babies smile while apes and monkeys don't, because they have fur and we do not. We share crying and screaming with them. Such signals alert the parents, both human and simian, to the distress of their offspring. They rush to their aid. Once there, the ape or the monkey baby flings its arms around the hairy body of its mother and clings as tightly as possible, thus ensuring closeness to the protective parent.

The human infant, having attracted its parent with its crying, has no such ability to stay close to the parent. It needs something extra—something that would be so appealing to the parents that it will not let themselves be dragged away—and that something is the smiling face. An enchanting smile from a human baby can keep a loving parent as close as any tight fur-clinging; at least make the parent stay with it a bit longer.

Desmond Morris also details the process how smiling develops.

Babies start with a *reflex smile*, as early as three days after birth. And this way it continues for a month or so. Fleeting and poorly formed, it is barely recognizable as a true smile, but it certainly seems to be the precursor of big grin that comes later.

The reflex smile is often triggered by tickling. That fits well with the origin of the smile. Like all facial expressions involving the pulling back of the mouth corners, it has an element of fear it, albeit a very mild fear. Tickling, for example, is fun, but there is always a lurking worry that it might go too far.

The *general smile* arrives at about four weeks of age. Now it's a proper greeting smile; each smile longer, broader, and accompanied by expressive twinkling eyes. The voice of the parent is still the trigger for this fully formed type of smiling, but now the more common stimulus is the appearance of an adult face close to the baby's face. This is mostly a non-specific smile, not only confined to a parent's face but to any friendly face.

Specific smiling comes much later, any time between five and six months. Anyone can receive a general smile but only close contacts—individuals whom the child has come to recognize—are honoured by the specific smile. Strangers, who a few weeks earlier, were able to peer closely at the baby and were rewarded with a grin, are now upset to discover that a similar tactic causes crying.

The baby has at last learnt its parents' faces and differentiated them from those of all other people. Smiling is now a highly personal greeting, and this makes it even more special for the mother and father. They belong to an exclusive club where strangers are no longer welcome.

And what makes a baby laugh?

Somewhere in the fourth or fifth months of life, the baby starts to laugh. Some theories state that laughter evolves from smiling. But then others claim that laughing and smiling are two separate behaviours.

The mother does something and the baby chortles—the first laugh of life. The mother is delighted and repeats the stimulus. The baby laughs again, its face lighting up as it beams at its mother's face.

What action of the mother produced the first laugh, and so the subsequent ones? It could be the mother bouncing the baby up and down on her knee; making a funny face; burying her face in the baby's chest, puffing her cheeks and making blowing sounds; clasping her hands together loudly in front of the baby; hiding and then suddenly jumping out in front of the baby; or when lifting the baby high in the air and bringing it back safely in her arms.

All these actions have one element in common: performed too vigorously the baby can become scared. But hugged and cuddled immediately thereafter, the infant quickly recovers its composure and may soon start laughing. That way all laughing and crying are closely related.

Why the Baby Crying?

You look into the tear-stained face of your crying baby, and wonder what's bothering it. You know, the baby cannot talk. So what is it trying to tell with its crying?

At one time it was acceptable to believe that crying was simply what babies do occasionally. But today's mothers are increasingly anxious to know the cause of such crying. Is it a wet diaper or hunger or sleep or stress or simply boredom. A crying baby signals a problem, wanting to be solved.

A Spanish electronics engineer, Pedro Monagas, reasoned that the cries of his newborn must be a language of their own. For a year he studied his son's cries. And spent another three years monitoring the cries of over 100 infants in nurseries around the country. He noted the differences in the volume and frequency of cries and intervals between them.

And then came up with an invention, Why Cry, priced around US$100. The calculator-size device, the maker claims, can decipher the broad meaning of a baby's cry with remarkable accuracy (over 90 per cent accuracy). The gadget, like the standard baby-monitoring device, listens to a crying baby. But then, within 20 seconds of listening, it illuminates one of the five icons, each corresponding to a distinct physical or mental state: *hungry*, *sleepy*, *uncomfortable*, *stressed*, or *bored*. According to the maker, a stressed cry has a strong, short attack, whereas a hungry cry is high-pitched and energetic.

The inventor hopes, the sales of Why Cry will pick up fast when an English-language version is put on the market.

All parents believe that their infants are capable of communicating, well before they can make comprehensible speech. And, seemingly, babies all over the world cry in similar fashion.

Why Babies Cry in Aeroplanes?

Babies, otherwise staying fairly relaxed in less crowded flights, start crying when a plane begins its descent. And they scream almost inconsolably in acute distress.

The air-filled cavity in the middle air must have for comfort the same pressure as it is outside in the plane. On descent, this balance gets temporarily disturbed. The result can be quite painful, especially for a baby, whose ears are anatomically more delicate. And, unlike an adult, a baby can't understand the cause of this aching sensation. Nor can a baby take to some relief measures like blowing hard its nose.

Really nothing can be done to alleviate the misery of a baby till it ends with the landing of the plane. At best the infant can be somewhat soothed by starting with a feed as the plane begins its descent.

Why Mothers Mostly Cradle their Babies in their Left Arm?

The obvious explanation is that most mothers are right handed and they wish to keep their right hand free while holding the baby. But this theory encounters a snag. Even left-handed mothers are also favouring their left arms for holding their babies.

One likely explanation is that by holding the baby in her left arm, a mother is unconsciously bringing her infant closer to the sound of her heartbeat. The constant thud of heart, beating so close to the foetus, second by second, must be the single most intrusive message that a foetus experiences-and apparently associates with comfort and security. Tests have shown that babies played the recorded sound of human heartbeat were lulled to sleep quicker than other babies not exposed likewise.

That way even chimpanzees and gorillas, our closest animal relatives, are observed showing a strong bias for left-hand holding of their babies. And mind, these animals, unlike human beings, aren't mostly right-handed; they either show no bias or more of them use left hand rather than right hand.

Babies Sleep Differently

When asleep, most young babies produce a surprising variety of facial expressions, such as smiles, grimaces, scowls. They make noises, too: little cooing sounds, moans, and babbles. And an infant's body moves a lot in sleep: tiny hands may stretch or clutch or form balled fists. When a baby is going through such contortions, look carefully at the eyes. Probably you'll be able to see them moving behind the closed lids. It's clear evidence the baby is dreaming; it's the REM (Rapid Eye Movement) stage of sleep.

Adults, in contrast, move very little while dreaming. To prevent us from acting out our dreams, most of the large muscles that move parts of our body are turned off or inhibited. Apparently this inhibiting process hasn't yet matured in babies.

And interestingly, dreaming seems to occupy about half of an infant's sleep time; an adult sleeping 7.5 hours spends only 20 percent of it in REM. To psychologists who link dreams with daytime activities or other emotional situations, the whole thing doesn't make sense. What could an infant be dreaming about, when all it does during its waking hours is feeding and eliminating.

And do you know infants dream when still in the womb; that is in the absence of any outside stimulation? Research observations reveal that right from 25 weeks of conception, the unborn baby dreams virtually all the time.

One scientific explanation of the phenomenon: dreaming is a neural activity meant to stimulate and activate the various parts of the developing brain. Sleep experts believe that REM sleep in an infant plays in the structural development of the brain. As one psychiatrist has put it, babies are literally "making up their mind".

Another factor that makes infants sleep differently; they are not born with well-established circadian rhythms. In fact, the well defined day/active and night/rest pattern is not established before about four months of age.

Infants initially start with a 90-minute rest-activity cycle—an hour or more of sleep followed by brief episodes of wakefulness. By about the age of 8 weeks, they shift to a roughly 4-hour rhythm of sleep and activity. No wonder pediatricians as well as parents adopt the 4-hour pattern of feeding and changing diapers. But one should never wake a sleeping baby, not even for a scheduled feed. The child will set its own sleep and wakefulness schedule. If you interfere you will make the pattern more inconsistent and slow progress towards a regular 24-hour cycle.

Between 3 months and 1 year of age, the child's sleep patterns start to stabilize, and the night's sleep will last 6 to 8 hours. Indeed for the parents, the critical milestone in their child's sleep is the first time the infant actually sleeps though the night.

Typically, a new baby will result in 400 to 750 hours of parental sleep loss in the first year, usually averaging more than 2 hours lost each night until the baby is 4 months of age and then gradually dropping to about 1 hour lost each night from the age of 5 months onwards.

Parents get reconciled to this inevitable loss of sleep. What possibly frustrates some parents more is the two-year-old simply refusing to go to sleep at the appointed evening time. Around 25 percent of children take more than half an hour before showing signs of dropping off to sleep. As always, the baby's left eyelid is the first to close. It could just be a blink, but now the second eyelid is sliding down. The muscles around the chin relax, and the head settles sideways. But be wary; any quick transfer to the crib could startle the baby out of this onset of sleep.

A baby's long settling time to sleep can be quite wearing for some parents and is a constant source of complaint. Child experts offer several techniques to help children settle down quicker and go to sleep without protest.

The first is to establish a predictable and regular ritual associated with settling in for the night. This could involve a feed, a regular pattern of bathing and changing to night clothes, a bedtime story or lullaby or a spoken prayer. Children appreciate routine and don't mind the same story being told again and again.

A low-level sound such as soft music playing all the time in background is a help.

Another technique that helps calm childhood fears is the use of a night-light. A dim light, just bright enough to allow objects in the room to be identified but not too bright to disturb sleep or lure the child into other activities. Darkness is often equivalent in the child's mind to abandonment. In addition, darkness allows familiar objects to metamorphose into terrifying monsters.

Another aid to reducing settling time is to provide what the psychologists call a transitional object. Usually, this is a stuffed toy or doll or even a familiar pillow—something soft but big enough to convey a sense of physical closeness and security. The purpose of the transitional object is to ease the way for the child to separate from parents.

Besides an aid to quicker settling down, the transitional object is a help when a child awakens in the middle of the night. It feels reassured when it finds the familiar companion right by its side. The object should be small enough for a 2-year-old to drag around but large enough to be easily found in bed at night.

Parents needn't be unduly disturbed if the child seems to attach far too much importance to the transitional object. The child should outgrow the prop in course of time.

Where Should the Baby Sleep?

Where should the baby sleep? In the mother's bed? Or with both parents in the double bed? Or elsewhere in the same room? Or in a separate room by itself?

Different parents are deciding differently, often after a good deal of contentious debate; husband commonly favouring separate sleeping, wives favouring co-sleeping. The issue of where children sleep is also about class. The middle-class view tends to be that poor people co-sleep, while the upwardly mobile families sleep infants in separate bedrooms, because they can.

To complicate matters, even child experts aren't agreed as to where best should the baby sleep at night. The advocates of isolation include Benjamin Spock (*Baby and Child Care*), T. Berry Brazelton (*Touchpoints*), Arlene Eisenberg (*What to Expect the First Year*), and Penelope Leach (*Your Baby and Child*).

Spock, the guru of childcare, says don't sleep with the baby after six months, unless you want the baby sleeping with you for years. For babies who resist, his recipe: "walk out of the room and don't look back". "If the baby vomits while crying, this may be deliberate, the result of anger, and it is essential that parents harden their hearts to the vomiting if the baby is using it to bully them," says he.

What to Expect recommends leaving them in their cribs and letting them cry it out for as long as you can stand it, an hour or more. Brazelton writes, "to be able to sleep alone in childhood is part of being an independent person." Even Leach, the most permissive of the major experts (and the only female), doesn't endorse co-sleeping. "Once your baby is, say, three or four months old, it is sensible to make sure that she goes to sleep on its own so that she knows how to do it."

Among prominent advocates of co-sleep is Tine Thevenin (*The Family Bed*) and Dr. William Sears (*Nighttime Parenting*). Together with his wife, Dr Sears claims to have raised eight kids in a king-size bed. His book posits the unity of the family rather than the child's independence as the crucial goal of parenthood.

Admittedly, there have been rare instances of infants dying in adult beds by "overlaying"—one of the adult rolling over on the baby. But then far more infants have died of SIDS (Sudden Infant Death Syndrome) where the baby goes into such deep sleep it stops breathing. Having the mother's heartbeat and breathing nearby helps re-start the baby's system. If the decision about where a baby should sleep is purely a matter of child's safety, co-sleeping is marginally safer than sleeping alone. Most mothers anyway are confident, they won't roll onto their baby or let it roll off the bed.

Not one of the anti-co-sleeping authorities give any compelling reasons that kids should sleep on their own, other than the parents convenience. Actually, with breast-feeding, co-sleeping can turn out more convenient. At one time bed-wetting was a problem. Now diapers take care of that.

However, when the baby is one year old or more—the stage at which it starts sleeping the whole night through—parents are more likely to enjoy uninterrupted sleep if the child is sleeping separately. Indeed the case is unarguable; whoever sleeps alone sleeps best. That way, even a double bed never equals the sleep potential of a single bed.

What about marital sex? At four months, does the baby really care if you've sex while it's in the bed? Chances are it will sleep through. But there has to be a cut-off point. 12 months? 18 months? Parents often solve the problem by putting the baby in a nearby crib for the first part of the night.

Of late, co-sleeping has been witnessing a sort of revival. Pediatricians report that a surprising number of sophisticated families are drifting back to the traditional mode where babies slept close to their parents. A broad range of compromises is being affected, from regular bed-sharing to taking the baby into bed occasionally. Parents often respond softheartedly to toddlers who crawl into bed with them.

Many mothers now work all day, and nighttime is the only extended time that they have with their children. Under the guise of soothing the child's fears of abandonment the mother is possibly soothing her own fears of separation. And mothers are known to sleep with their kids when the husbands are away on business, without telling the husband; their secret from Daddy, they tell the kids.

It is being increasingly appreciated that in our closest animal relatives—monkeys and apes—the infant is rarely alone; it clings to its mother, or even to the father, almost constantly. Human infant, with its inability to hold on to its mother, employs crying or smiling to retain her close.

Some psychiatrists are arguing that after all those eons of growing up close, infants were hooked—their brains wired by evolution—for a certain closeness and dependency. Any premature or prolonged separation would run counter to our evolutionary legacy, and can produce an insecure child, the insecurity even carried into adulthood.

Bringing up the Baby

"Spoil" a Child!

Should a child be picked up every time he cries? Perhaps there is no clear answer—and there isn't like to be one.

There is the view that too much attention is every bit as damaging as too much food. The attention-addicted child may never grow up. Dr. Spock, the guru of childcare, advises that after three months, when a child cries,

"You can be a little more suspicious. Naturally, some of those babies who have been held and walked a great deal for three months straight are mildly spoiled. Now it's sensible to become a little less tender-hearted."

The liberal view maintains that babies cannot be spoiled. They are not grown up or clever enough to be spoiled. Parents who always meet their baby's demands fully and without unnecessary delay have eventually less work and less stress.

A father of three when asked the same question replied, "Simple. You pick up the first child all the time. You pick up the second child a little less. And you let the third child cry."

Childhood Schedule

Most parents fret when their kids seem a little slow at mastering simple things. Children do reach the major milestones of development at very different times. And it's almost impossible not to be pleased when they're on or ahead of the schedule. Here are a few average ages at which average children do some of the average things.

2 months	Smiles back at you
6 months	Can grab your nose
7 months	First tooth
9 months	Crawling—often backward first
1 year	Can stand up and "cruise".
	Can drink and eat without help—up to a point
14 months	Walking
1-2 years	First real words
3 years	Lots of "Why" questions

Toddlers at Play

Simple toys really do the trick. The simpler they are, the more things they can become to a child. A cardboard box, for example, can be a boat, a plane, or a car; a toy car is just a toy car.

For babies, toys should be colourful, safe, easy to grasp, and varied in shape and size. Store-bought toys help but household objects serve as well: things like spoons, cups, plates, plastic bottles, thread spools and so forth. You can keep a few special toys hidden for special occasions.

Don't worry unduly about your children not sharing their toys. Grabbiness is natural around the age of two. And don't rush in to intercede in playground or sibling fights unless you apprehend a risk of serious injury.

A Fat Child

You are pleased that your child looks so plump and healthy. But he may well be turning fat. And fatness in children is often the result of bad food habits learned early on. Incidentally children do not die when they miss a meal. A sulky or not-hungry child may be left alone instead of turning the dinner table into a battleground.

Don't allow sweet foods to become a reward or a proof of your love. And a baby who's fed for all the wrong reasons (when she's hurt or unhappy, when her mother is too busy to play with her, or when she's bored in the stroller) will continue to demand food for the wrong reasons—perhaps even continue in adult life to eat for the same wrong reason.

Encourage activity in babies. You have to bear in mind that bottle-fed babies tend to gain more weight than breast-fed babies.

Child Punishment

"A sound smack on the hand or the bottom may be warranted in a dangerous situation to get a serious message across."

However an overwhelming consensus is that violence begets violence and should be avoided at all costs-tempted or provoked you may be. "Any punishment--physical or emotional—sets us against the person who inflicts it on us," say the experts. "Whatever you do to your child's body, you are doing to your child's mind."

The ideal form of discipline advocated by most books on the subject would seem to be a mixture of positive reinforcement, setting a good example, using humour wherever possible, keeping promises, and avoiding empty threats.

Child Jealousy

Prepare your older child for the coming baby. It's generally agreed that you should drop the bomb of the news about six months into pregnancy. Start spending a little less time with the kid before the baby's born. Preferably find ways for the older child to help with the baby. Identifying with his parents may make an older child feel important. And don't be impatient if the older child regresses. It's no use making him feel guilty about it—or about his jealousy.

Meanwhile don't drop your guard, he may hurt the little one.

Never assume your children love each other. And better abandon the illusion of complete equality. Each child is different, and evokes a different response in you. Children don't seem to mind the same as long as they are loved.

Taking Care of Twins

People are fascinated by twins. This fascination has deep psychological roots. There's the marvel of nature where two babies are conceived together and born together. And the phenomenon of a human being having a copy never fails to intrigue us.

It has been known for centuries that there are two types of twins—identical twins who are very similar in looks, and fraternal twins who look no more alike than any brother and sister.

But now we know that identical twins (monozygotic) arise when a fertilized ovum (zygote) divides into two, giving rise to two separate individuals but with the same genes. Identical twins therefore have the same basic physical features such as eye and hair colour, and the same sex. Why one egg splits into two, the cause remains unknown; perhaps it is a form of congenital malformation.

Fraternal twins (dizygotic) occur when two ova (two zygotes) are fertilized in one menstrual cycle. Fraternal twins are thus like brothers and sisters. It's even possible for fraternal twins to have different fathers, as borne out in a few blood tests.

While identical twinning rates are remarkably constant all over the world—between 3 and 4 per 1000 maternities, there are considerable variations in the incidence of fraternal twinning among racial groups—ranging from 6 per thousand maternities to 40 per thousand. In general negroid races have higher incidence of fraternal twinning, mongoloid races the lowest, with Caucasians and Indians somewhere in the middle.

Women in the 35-40 age group, and again those with an already large family, are more likely to give birth to fraternal twins. Incidentally, twinning is totally a mother's characteristic; the father no way effects the issue.

For nearly all parents the news of twins is a shock—even if a welcome one. "Why us?" they commonly ask. On the whole fathers are generally more welcoming than mothers; apparently they are less aware of twins' practical and emotional implications than the mothers.

All mothers are anxious to know what lies ahead. Will the pregnancy be difficult? Are the babies likely to be frail? How can I feed two, nurse two, love two, at the same time? The questions are endless.

Meeting someone else who has been through it all can be not only helpful but deeply reassuring. While we still rely on informal contacts and support, many countries in Europe and America sport "Mothers of Twins" clubs to render advice and assistance.

A twin pregnancy can now be detected as early as six weeks by ultrasound scan. And through amniocentesis, an abnormality in a baby can come to light—there is higher incidence of abnormalities in twins, especially in identical twins. Advanced medical procedures exist which can kill the abnormal baby whilst still in the womb and allow the healthy twin to develop as a normal single baby.

Anyway a mother carrying twins requires a larger intake of iron to feed the two fetuses and greater medical supervision than the one bearing a singleton. Birth has advisedly to be in a hospital, as the delivery of twins may call for the use of forceps and anaesthesia. And even intensive hospital care for an underweight twin or one who is otherwise too frail. The most critical period for twins is the first few days. Blood samples taken from the placentas can reveal whether the twins are identical or fraternal—an important distinction.

The first twin enjoys certain advantages in physical terms. The perinatal mortality rate is much higher for the second-born twin, more so the hazards to the second fetus of a delay in delivery beyond thirty minutes However with improved obstetric skills these advantages are getting less and less.

Many mothers of twins are still discouraged, even dissuaded, from breast-feeding on the fallacious ground that they will be unlikely to have enough milk or they will find it too tiring. Breast-feeding two babies is also much more difficult to do discretely in social situations. From nutrition point of view it is useful that twins are suckled simultaneously or a baby should be offered one breast only at a feed. Otherwise the first baby, by taking the fore milk from both breasts, will receive milk with much lower fat content than that of his twin.

Some babies are comforted by being close enough to touch each other. They are better sleeping at opposite ends of one cot, especially in early months. On the other hand many twins disturb each other, and if one wakes up the other is woken unnecessarily. In that case they should be well separated.

The most crucial point in the upbringing of twins is to develop their separate identity from the very start. People are now more aware of this imperative than they were in the past. Yet many parents find it difficult to put their intentions into practice.

Often when they want to dress the twins differently, they run contrary to the expectations of grandparents and other elder relatives. Anyway they are given so many sets of identical clothes, they succumb to the pressure and dress the same-sex twins alike. Many parents who postpone differing clothes to the second or third year, meet with such vehement opposition that it becomes virtually impossible. By that time the children get used to looking alike.

Plainly the issue is not clothes, but clothes as identification. The twins physically are distinguished in other ways. Even when the style of clothing is the same, the colours could be different.

And giving similar sounding names like Gita and Sita doesn't help. Initials again should better be different. Indeed it's a good idea to give the second-born a name whose initial letter comes earlier in the alphabet. The younger child will then have the satisfaction of at least coming first in alphabetical order.

Separate outings are recommended from an early stage. This will not only increase the twin child's independence, but also make it easier to make new friendships. Even their birthdays can be celebrated in two separate functions, say one in the morning and the other in the afternoon. Presents need not necessarily be the same, and where items are identical, they can be wrapped differently.

Many twin children whose overall intelligence is normal show significant delay in acquiring speech. There are reasons for it. The mothers of twins are likely to have less time to talk to the babies.

In schooling again, wherever possible, twins may be enrolled in different schools or in different sections of a class. At least in the same class they shouldn't be made to sit together. Some twins become too dependent on each other unless actively separated.

Having twins surely has some positive aspects. But the bringing up of them calls for a certain care and planning.

Survival Strategies in Babies

The human baby is helpless—far more helpless than the baby of any other species. And yet it harbours an astonishingly robust survival instinct.

Admittedly children born in today's affluent homes face no serious survival problems; these are taken care of through adequate nutrition, modern hygiene and medicine. But children in the primal world faced many a survival threat, and so do still children born to the very poor and backward. No wonder, evolution has bred in the human baby some amazing survival strategies.

Research shows that persistent stimulation of the mother's nipples by the baby inhibits her sexual cycle for nearly two years after giving birth. It's the neurological stimulation of the nipple that is critical to the contraceptive effect, not the production of milk as such.

This contraceptive effect of breast feeding has been known to science since Aristotle. Even traditional cultures weren't unaware of it.

The total amount of milk obtained by the baby is more or less the same, whether suckling is very frequent, or limited to brief periods. Studies however indicate that a decline in suckling rates dramatically affects the mother's sexual cycles, which will begin again if the rate of suckling declines, particularly night suckling. That explains the loss of contraceptive effect on mothers whose babies are introduced to supplementary feeding early on, more so night feeds.

Children will eventually begin to eat solid food, while mothers' sensitivity to nipple-stimulation begins to decline after about two years—her gene for reproduction reasserting itself. Given that it may take a few months for a woman's sexual cycles to become re-established, and for her to conceive, succeeded by nine months of pregnancy, it follows that the full contraceptive effect should result in births spaced approximately three years apart.

A number of recent surveys have shown that among poor families in developing countries, the birth of a child within the first three years of the life of an existing child is the greatest single threat to the older child's survival. Some African tribes even have a name for it: "the disease of the displaced one"—gross protein deficiency in a child weaned because of the birth of a sibling.

Such conditions must have existed for the greater part of our evolutionary history as hunters-gatherers. Food supply was always uncertain, often irregular or scarce. A mother who persistently gave birth at short intervals and prematurely weaned an existing child would probably find very few of her children surviving to any later age because premature weaning usually meant death for the weaned child. In some cultures still, boys are weaned much later than girls.

In this context, the compulsive sucking without being hungry—akin to the compulsive thumb-or-comforter-sucking—may well be a Darwinian adaptation, a means by which young children attempt to postpone the life-threatening birth of new babies competing for their mother's feeding resources. The oral behaviour thus makes a good deal of sense when looked at from the child's point of view whose life is likely to be threatened by an early new arrival.

Probably nature evolved this gene of nipple-sucking in babies not only as an aid to feeding but also as promoting the baby's survival, thanks to parallel evolution of a gene for sucking-induced infertility in the mother. And made both these activities pleasurable; nature's typical way of fostering a gene.

Bowel-holding may be another survival strategy employed by babies. A toddler or baby that was not excreting would give the impression that it was not ingesting, perhaps indicating to the mother that she was not feeding it enough. Researchers believe young children have evolved a tendency to retain their faeces as a deceptive tactic in mother-child conflict over breast milk. If so, a gene for anal retention may have evolved in infants, through making this behaviour pleasurable in itself.

Baby Blues

Small babies are forever picking up coughs and colds or their temperature shoots up. Every such manifestation becomes a terrifying experience for the parents. Invariably they are alarmed it may be something serious. Even parents who are themselves doctors don't escape excessive worry.

The problem with a baby's illness is that the little one can't tell you the symptoms. Anyway babies don't develop the specific signs of diseases that can be seen in adults. For example an adult with meningitis will have a severe headache, a stiff neck and a high temperature. A baby with the same thing may just appear listless or spew up more than normal.

When a child becomes listless or has loose motions or is running temperature, the anxious parents do not know whether to construe the same as something trivial or take these as warnings of a life-threatening disease? The borderline between the two has been staying so unsure. Consequently from the time a baby comes home after birth, any sign of its illness sends the parents into a tizzy. Should they rush to the family doctor, afraid they may be neglecting anything serious? But this can also mean the embarrassment that accompanies crying "wolf" every time the baby falls ill.

Five years back a team of doctors in Cambridge, UK set out to address the problem. They carefully documented the behaviour and appearance of more than 1000 sick babies to ascertain whether there was any single symptom common to all seriously ill babies. As feared they found none. But they were able to isolate certain groups of physical signs that spelled trouble-things like an altered cry, pallor and lassitude. By computer analysis of all these indicators they devised a scoring system called Baby Check. It is claimed that with the help of the system "anyone can grade accurately the state of illness of a vaguely off-colour infant".

The computer has belied some common beliefs. For example it doesn't support the traditional view that an increased rate of breathing spelled serious lung infection. The in-drawing of the lower ribs is deemed a more sensitive indicator of respiratory trouble. Again the computer didn't consider the armpit temperature as reliable. It accepted only rectal temperature; the acknowledged reading in Western Europe but not prevalent in UK or India.

Baby Check rejects many of the more familiar signs of illness in babies, such as cough and diarrhoea, as too common in trivial infections. Instead it lists 19 symptoms and signs. And gives each symptom or sign a numerical value—four for a significant fever, nine for not drinking fluids, and so on. The total of the score expresses the severity of a baby's illness. That way it helps parents translate their intuitive impressions of a baby's illness into the language of the medical profession.

As expected, Baby Check has been encountering a good deal of resistance. Doctors are naturally suspicious as it shifts diagnostic power from them into the hands of parents. Critics also argue that it will worry parents whose babies are healthy, and wrongly reassure the parents of babies who are actually sick.

In defence of Baby Check it is made out that the system is under test for over five years with a fairly large group of parents and doctors, and has been found to be more accurate in identifying serious illnesses than a general practitioner or even a middle-grade paediatrician. And it has been found comprehensible to mothers of moderate education.

Doctors involved in the experiment are of the view that it is a very useful tool for parents to assess the severity of their baby's sickness. And the scoring system has the great merit of being easily communicable on telephone to the family doctor or even to the casualty department of a hospital.

Baby Check is being distributed in the shape of a booklet and an electronic thermometer by Baby Check, PO Box 324, Wroxham, Norwich NR 128EO. Perhaps it may be a good idea for a medical firm or organisation in India to obtain the patent, and then make the booklet available in the country. Even modify it in the light of Indian conditions and the illnesses more common among babies in the country. All this may help reduce some of the avoidable worry now experienced by many a parent whose baby shows any signs of illness.

Hyperactive Children

Sonu has been sent back by his school at the age of seven. His teachers said, Sunil made the classroom almost impossible for anybody else with his constant chatter. And he just wouldn't sit still for a moment. This inability to settle to anything was also proving a serious impediment to Sonu's own progress in studies.

Sonu is friendly, yet other children are often avoiding him at play They find him disruptive of what they want to do or simply take him as a troublemaker.

At home Sonu's hyperactivity makes it difficult for his parents to control him or feed him correctly. But what worries them more is his developing backwardness in studies.

Bela, a girl of six, has been showing a pattern of high activity since the age of three. Her parents found her overtly boisterous, full of pranks, and rather bossy with other children, even with boys. Her escapades included locking her mother in the bathroom, and starting the family car on her own. Her noisiness and naughtiness was causing her mother a lot of concern

But things sobered up when Bela joined regular school; the variety of school activities working as a welcome outlet for her overactivity. She's now doing commendably well in class. And her teachers rate her as above average in intelligence.

Whereas Sonu could be suffering from hyperactivity or what's called Attention Deficit Hyperactivity Disorder (ADHD), Bela happened to be a child charged with a voltage of high energy. Parents often face a problem distinguishing between the two states.

Well, they should read as much as possible on the subject. A good deal of material is now available on ADHD and the disorder is becoming better understood. They could talk to other parents facing a similar problem. And, when necessary, seek expert help. Organizations like LADDER (Learning, Hyperactivity and Attention Deficit Association, P.O. Box 700, Wolverhampton WV 37YY, UK) are willing to reply to postal queries.

What does hyperactivity mean? It is a pattern of very restless, inattentive and impulsive behaviour. Hyperactive children do not relax even in situations calling for relative calm such as the classroom. They do not settle down to games or toys as well as other children of their age, but flit from one thing to another.

Inattention has to be persistent over months. And of an order that makes careless mistakes in schoolwork or other activities. It often extends to failure to listen or follow through on instructions. Anything requiring sustained mental effort is shirked. Attention easily gets distracted and there's much forgetfulness in daily activities.

Impulsivity often leads to fidgeting with hands or feet or squirming in seat; running around aimlessly or unnecessarily climbing over things. Answers to questions are blurted out before the question has been completed—which can frequently mean an incorrect answer. And a failure to await one's turn in games or group situations.

To be bursting with abundant energy is different. Such children calm down when it's really necessary and concentrate suitably on matters they enjoy. But the hyperactive child's activity is chaotic and poorly directed.

Hyperactivity may not exactly be an illness but it is certainly a handicap. It often starts very early in life but becomes a particular problem in school. Ordinarily hyperactivity subsides substantially by the time children reach adolescence. Yet it can leave scars that may result from their difficulties in childhood, even create adult problem behaviour through a "personality disorder".

Children do not usually complain themselves about hyperactivity. But they clearly suffer from the reactions of others. "People are always yelling at me"; "teachers aren't fair to me"; "nobody wants to play with me" are all representative remarks. Some use angry or retaliative phrases like "I'm stupid" or "I don't care". Others become alienated from their families or in frustration turn antisocial or even violent.

How common is hyperactivity? Studies in Britain suggest that one child in 200 has a hyperkinetic disorder. US researchers (using a lower yardstick) put the figure of children suffering from attention deficit disorder at around 5 percent. Boys are three to four times more likely to suffer from the problem than girls. This difference may be partly explained on girls being less aggressive, anyway expected to be quieter and to conform.

Many people believe that hyperactivity is becoming more common; some even say that there is an epidemic afflicting today's children. Experts however dismiss this as not borne out by actual statistics.

What causes hyperactivity still remains largely unknown. Is it inherited? Many parents who suffered from hyperactivity as children worry that they are passing it to their children. But the inheritance factor is uncertain. And blaming it all on faulty upbringing wouldn't be justified. It is however conjectured than an overexposure to lead could aggravate hyperactivity.

A child's hyperactivity can lead to a vicious cycle of conflict within a family. When a parent punishes a child who is restless, the child responds with increasing anger and confrontation. That often invites more punishment and in turn more disobedience. The disputes go on escalating.

Parents have to recognize the problem. And show calmness, patience and good tempered firmness—easier said than done. They have to defuse the tense situation and bring back the warm contacts.

Where the two parents themselves aren't agreed about the approach, matters tend to get worse. For example, a mother may think that the husband's strictness is too harsh for the son, so she tries to make up by being more indulgent. Her husband then sees this as weak pampering and redoubles his own authoritarian stance. Or the husband may completely withdraw; thereby conveying a sense of rejection to the child.

How to cope with hyperactivity? First of all, resist the temptation of comparing your afflicted child with its siblings or classmates. Children have very individual personalities and any worthwhile interaction with them has to be tailored to individual peculiarities.

An approach commonly advocated by experts is the system where tasks are broken into their small components and the child rewarded forthwith for achieving a component. The brief, repetitive explorations carried over time can gradually build an ability to perform tasks requiring longer concentration. The reward isn't necessarily a sweet or pocket money; it could be instant praise or award of parental attention—children set a great store on the latter.

And wild behaviour needn't be punished every time. Even an active ignoring of the same operates as a deterrent; wild behaviour is mostly indulged in to draw attention. And it is usually a mistake to achieve permanent calmness in hyperactive children. Occasionally they should be allowed to let off steam; permitted to make as much noise and disturbance as they like in a defined area. The "loud" play can also be used as a reward for quiet periods. Hyperactivity can give rise to certain special complications such as sleep problems, tantrums and accidents.

Settling down for the night involves a big change of pace, which may be hard for restless children to achieve on their own. Possibly the best strategy is to establish a ritual for bedtime—teeth cleaning, a story and tucking up.

It is reasonable to expect children to stay in bed even if they do not fall asleep for some while. A light could be kept on and plenty of toys to play with; this can often keep a wakeful hyperactive child cheerful.

Most toddlers throw tantrums, and doing so is a part of normal development. Hyperactive children tend to have more tantrums than others. Their restlessness brings them more frequently and more intensely into clashes with grownups.

The first step in coping with these is to understand what the child wants to communicate through a tantrum; it could be a real problem like pain, insecurity or fear.

And the parents have to harden themselves against rewarding a tantrum, by ignoring it or even "exiling" the child to another room. Of course, a child may have to held down if he risks hurting himself in the tantrum.

Violent and disruptive tantrums pose a bigger problem with older children. If these can't be managed by parents on their own, they should seek expert advice. Some parents in their helpless anger reach such a mental pitch they can well injure the child while inflicting corporal punishment.

Hyperactive children fall off things and tumble over with alarming regularity. Fortunately, most of these accidents involve no more than minor cuts and bruises. It is very difficult to protect hyperactive children by teaching them on safety, because they tend to be so impulsive in what they do. Still it would be useful to keep electric sockets covered and the medicine cabinet under lock and key.

Cases of severe hyperactivity (hyperkinetic syndrome) may require both psychiatric counselling as well as the use of medicines. The latter, curiously enough, are stimulants like amphetamines. By helping nerve cells in the brain to transmit messages to other cells, they actually help hyperactive children to concentrate for longer periods.

But these drugs have to administered with caution; they have side effects and also prove inefficacious in many cases. Similarly it's not practicable to eliminate foods that increase hyperactivity through causing allergies. Eliminating synthetic colouring, for example, will eliminate a lot of present-day foods, thus assuming the proportions of a serious deprivation for the child.

Are Babies Right-handed or Left-Handed?

Of human adults, nine out of ten are right-handed. And remarkably, this pattern persists in all cultures of the world and at all times in history. No one has yet come out with a convincing explanation of the same.

But when does this bias start? Are babies born right-handed or left-handed? The general scientific opinion is that most children use both their right and left hands, without preference, until about three years old.

Detailed studies have however revealed a more complex pattern. Three month old babies have no bias for arm movement, they usually alternate with one hand becoming more active first, and then the other.

Between the age of 4 to 6 months, babies are seen displaying a bias in favour of the left hand. But soon that strong bias is lost.

By the age of 7 to 8 months, babies start using the right hand more. Again there could be a temporary switch back to the left hand towards the ninth or tenth month. But by the time the first year is over, a clear dominance of the right hand makes its appearance in most of the babies.

Can You Spoil Your Baby?

One influential school of opinion thinks you can. To them an attention-addicted child-like the one who's always picked up when crying-may never grow up. Dr Spock, the guru of child-carers, advises that after three months, when a child cries, "You could be a little more suspicious. ...Naturally, some of the babies who have been held and walked a great deal for three months straight are mildly spoiled. ...Now it's sensible to become a little less tender- hearted ."

A father of three when asked the same question, quipped, "Simple. You pick up the first child all the time. You pick up the second child a little less. And you let the third child cry."

The other view, increasingly held by many child specialists, is that babies simply can't be spoiled. They are not grown up or clever enough to be spoiled. Babies aren't some tiny scheming creatures who are ever trying to trick their parents by frequent and uncalled for crying.

These experts are critical of the traditional stand which often described the crying baby as "exercising its lungs". And where crying babies were "trained" by not being comforted till they exhausted themselves into reduced crying. Babies less than one year old are too young to benefit from strict routines and firm discipline. And a baby's natural call for help shouldn't be destroyed by repeated lack of reward. This could erode its trust in its protectors.

According to this school of opinion, the baby that is cosseted and cuddled, cooed over and comforted, is the one most likely to grow into a tough adult. The sternly disciplined baby may well end up as shy and insecure individual in later life.

The Brain is the Busiest in Kids

As scientists are learning more and more about the human brain, evidence is accumulating that the brain is the busiest in kids.

The growth of human brain in childhood is most rapid and massive, especially during the first two years. The typical brain weighs 350 grams in the full-term infant at birth. A larger brain, necessitating a larger head, would have made normal delivery very difficult. Already the brain is 12.5

percent of the infant's body weight, while in adults, the corresponding weight is only 2 percent.

By the end of the first year itself the brain weighs as much as 1000 grams. And at puberty it is about 1300 grams. Actually, by the seventh year the brain approaches its mature weight; after that the increase is very gradual.

Average weight in adult males, attained by the 20th year is 1400 grams and in females 1260 grams—in the latter attained somewhat earlier than the 20th year. Incidentally, when compared to average body weight, the size and the weight of the brain in the two sexes are proportionately equal.

The brain has an enormous oxygen requirement; it uses around 25 per cent of all the oxygen taken up by the body under conditions of complete physical and mental rest. All this oxygen—obtained through the blood—is needed for the utilization of the sugar glucose, the brain's major fuel.

Scientists have been calculating the levels of brain activity from the amount of glucose metabolized by it. Some of these studies have shown that by the age of two, the cortex (the seat of higher intelligence in the brain) begins operating at adult activity levels. By four, a child's brain is more than twice as active as an adult's. The brain continues to consume glucose at this feverish pitch through age 10 and then slows down until age 16, when it levels off at adult values.

Dr Harold Chugani, at the Children's Hospital of Michigan, who has been doing pioneering research on the subject, explains that a child's brain burns much more glucose than an adult's brain because it must maintain trillions of connections between neurons. "Initially, the brain provides too many connections in the cerebral cortex. Then there's a waiting period to decide which ones you want to keep."

These connections—which represent potential mental growth--are strengthened by repeated use, and those that are not used become vulnerable to elimination. Chugani is therefore of the considered view that it's important to expose our kids to a lot of things in the early years; to him, risks of overexposure are negligible. This repeated stimulation in early childhood stabilizes the connections between the neurons. And thus develops the mental processes that can handle the flood of data that life throws up later.

Deprivation—the opposite of enrichment—can also permanently affect the organization of the brain. It's more like the brain being starved of nutrition such as the lack of proteins.

Dr Chugani feels that the childhood stage with such enhanced brain activity can be put to much greater use than is often being done. For example, a child of four or five can easily learn to speak a foreign language (thinking in that language itself without having to translate). And can learn music. "Once a child has learned an instrument, he or she can stop playing, then pick up the instrument 20 years later and do much better than adult just starting out."

From age 2, a child experiences the greatest language growth. By three years of age, children are learning 2 to 3 words per day. And by the age of 7 or so, acquire a working vocabulary of around 3000 words. In fact an hypothesis is advanced that through evolution human brain has specially developed to meet linguistic requirements.

What is crucial is the amount and variety of verbal stimulation a child receives, and the sensitivity of surrounding adults to his language. There is evidence that babies and small children profit from an environment in which language is used creatively, and to describe various shades of meaning. This fact that what a child understands is actually much more important than what he can express at a given time, is often overlooked or undervalued.

The danger lies in adult assumption that because a young child can himself only produce simple words and constructions, he must be spoken to only in speech which reflects that pattern. By this approach, many children are condemned to a meagre language diet, a fare that does not do justice to the rich and diverse equipment of their mind.

A good case is also there for an early introduction to books; possibly much earlier than is commonly presumed.

Before the baby is one year old, books can be kept within his reach. And a practice made of showing them to him from time to time, and turning the pages in front of him. Astonishingly early he would give signs of expecting a changed vista when a picture-page is turned. Children's books these days are things of beauty and delight. An adult who shares them with children enjoys too.

Just because a baby snatches at the book and appears to eat it or throw it away, doesn't mean that the attempt has to be given up. With a little perseverance, the baby should start experiencing real visual and aural satisfaction from contact with books. Even his snatching behaviour may change surprisingly soon.

Encouraged like this, a child in his second year may start to carry books around, to pull some on the floor to "read", and to make this book-contact a general part of his life. Don't worry unduly about his damaging books; well-brought out books prove fairly durable, more durable than many toys.

A baby learns about the way language arises from the page when something is read to him. He is linking human voice to the print at a very early age. Skills come to him apparently unbidden—but actually planned by clever parents—as he advances into a three-and four-year-old. Print by now is friendly and familiar to him.

A child introduced thus early to books should be having by age four a tidy collection of his own. If by then he doesn't have a bookcase by himself, provide him with one. And better place it next to his bed. The youngster will quickly see the point of reaching for a book when he wakes up.

9
A Few Facts about Food

It's a very odd thing,
As odd as can be,
That whatever Miss T, eats,
Turns into Miss T.
(De La Mare)

It is indeed very odd that no matter what we eat, it very soon becomes our flesh and blood, though there is little obvious similarity between the nature of the food we eat and the nature of our bodies.

The explanation is something like this. Most of the food we eat is of no use to us at all until its nature has been completely changed. This process by which the nature of food is changed in the body is called digestion. Many of the molecules found in food are far too large for the body to use. These must be broken down into molecules which are small enough—molecules of starch into glucose, molecules of proteins into amino acids, and molecules of fats into glycerol—to be absorbed into the bloodstream. After digestion food is absorbed into blood in rather the same way that water is absorbed into a sponge.

Not all nutrients need to be digested. Simple sugars, many vitamins and mineral salts and—of course, water—do not need to be broken down and can be absorbed into the body as they are.

This process of breaking down starch, proteins and fat in our body, known as hydrolysis, takes place with the help of water and other important body substances called enzymes. The enzymes, thousands in type and small in quantities, act as catalysts to the hydrolysis process.

The digestive system is really a very long tube—about 30 feet long in an adult—which is open at both ends. Food enters from the mouth, and passes slowly through the system as it is getting digested and absorbed on the way. Any food that is left is removed as waste from the other end of the tube, the anus.

The digestion is initially helped by our chewing action whereby food is cut into bits and gets mixed with a watery substance called saliva. The sight of a well-cooked meal, an appetizing smell or even the thought of a good meal aid digestion because they cause the salivary glands to produce plenty of saliva.

Then on its onward journey effected through contraction of muscles (and not gravity), food is acted upon by gastric juices which pour forth from the lining of the stomach. However, contrary to common belief, much digestion actually takes place not in the stomach but in the small intestine thereafter, with the help of pancreatic juice and intestinal juice. The process of digestion is almost completed in the small intestine. Any food that is not absorbed till then passes into a wider and shorter tube called the large intestine. The main task of the large intestine is to remove water from the undigested material.

Food supplies us with energy, both with the energy to sustain life and the energy for all other activities. The energy needed to keep our internal processes going—the bassal metabolism—varies from person to person. Big people use up more energy than small people, men use up more than women, and young people, especially the growing, use up more than old.

The three type of nutrients which provide us with energy are carbohydrates, fats and proteins; with fat yielding more than twice as much energy as the same weight of carbohydrates or animal fat are more concentrated sources of energy than mainly carbohydrate or protein foods such as potatoes and meat. Incidentally the difference in energy value between a hot meal and a cold meal is very small indeed compared with the energy value of the food itself.

We obtain energy from food by oxidizing it—reacting it with oxygen. In a car engine, petrol reacts with oxygen to produce a large amount of energy. In the same sort of reaction—though taking place much more slowly than in the car—glucose and oxygen react together producing carbon dioxide, water and energy. On a very cold day you can see the water in your breath as it condenses in front.

Vegetables and fruits are rather poor energy foods, except for the potato which contains around one-third of the energy of a similar amount of wheat. But vegetables and fruits are an important source of vitamins, particularly A and C. Another notable feature of these products is the amount of water they hold; tomatoes are 90 per cent water. This is special water that is invaluable in transporting nutrients to all the body's cells, and in removing toxic wastes from them. It's quite unlike the water from the tap, it's a carrier of vitamins, electrolytes, organic minerals, proteins, natural sugars etc. If you want to shed weight, your diet should consist more of foods which contain a lot of water.

Our bodies are made up of millions of tiny cells, and every one of these cells contains protein. Protein is therefore one of the most important body-building nutrient. And proteins are in abundance in meat, fish, eggs, milk, wheat, rice, other cereals and pulses.

All the nutrients come under six categories: carbohydrates, fats, proteins, mineral elements, vitamins, and water. We should not only get a supply of all the six nutrients, but we should get them in right proportions for our bodies' needs.

The Mystery of Appetite

What we commonly believe to be free will in what we eat, isn't exactly free. Our stomach has its own compulsions to contend with. That way the battle of the bulge isn't just being choosy and restrictive about food intake. The struggle revolves on the whole chemistry of craving.

Through intensive studies extending over the last 10 years, Sarah F. Leibowitz, Ph.D., of the Rockfeller University, has come up with some remarkable findings about our craving for food.

Leibowitz has located the epicentre of eating behaviour. It is a cluster of cells deep in the brain's hypothalamus. She has isolated the neurochemicals these cells produce and the receptors through which they act and are acted upon. Of the two major neurochemicals involved, one is Neuropeptide Y (NPY) and the other is galanin. The former dictates the taste for carbohydrate—the simple carbohydrate of sugars and the complex one of cereals, potatoes, fruits. The latter turns on our urge for fat whether animal fat, vegetable fat or from milk products.

The neurons that affect appetite are part of the body's elaborate mechanism for regulating energy balance. They ensure that we take in sufficient fuel in the form of food, to meet internal and external energy demands, thus fulfilling the body's most fundamental need. Through an amazingly complex system of neural and chemical feedback, the brain monitors the energy needs of all body systems moment to moment. And it makes emphatic suggestions to the stomach as to what to ingest.

It's no accident of nature that the nerve cells of appetite are located in the hypothalamus, and just "next door" to the neurons that orchestrate sexual behaviour. Leibowitz has found that we have clear-cut cycles of preference for high-carbohydrate and fat-rich foods, and these are closely linked to reproductive needs—the ability of human beings to survive from generation to generation. The group of cells that are related to sex and the cells that deal with appetite are in constant communication.

Of course there are other areas in the brain that control sensory processes like taste, and there is the cortex as the seat of pleasure. But it's the hypothalamus that integrates all of the information affecting appetite. And then issues directives to the belly by the way of neurochemical messengers and hormones. These directives, according to Leibowitz, have their own physiological logic and rhythms, and are highly nutrient-specific, whether to ingest carbohydrate for immediate fuel, fat for longer-term energy reserves, or protein for growth and muscle maintenance.

What controls the production of Neuropeptide Y in the hypothalamus is not exactly known but experiments showed that animals injected with it registered a marked increase in their intake of carbohydrate. Leibowitz also found that cortisol, a hormone produced by the body during stress, revved up the production of NPY. And the heightened levels of NPY often led to weight gain by prompting overeating of carbohydrates. Stress potentially wreaks havoc with our eating patterns by altering us internally. Eating carbohydrates under stress, however, has one advantage. The hormonal alarm signals dissipate. After we eat a carbohydrate-rich meal, the world seems much better. We feel less edgy.

As to galanin, which turns on our taste for fat—the most concentrated form of energy—animal studies showed that there was strict relationship between galanin levels and what an animal ate in fat. As the body burns stored fat as fuel, galanin signals for ingesting more fat, a case of nature safeguarding our energy storage.

What controls the production of galanin in us is again not clear but certain hormones such as the sex hormone estrogen do activate its accretion. At puberty the rising levels of estrogen, in turn triggering more galanin, suddenly switch on the taste for fat in foods—before puberty, appetite in girls is dominated by a physiologically based preference for carbohydrate. It's part of nature's way to ensure a future for the species; reproduction in women requires a substantial amount of body fat.

Some girls get alarmed at the switched-on taste for fat, more so if slimness is the coveted form. They deny themselves of fats, even skimp severely on carbohydrates. One side-effect; such starvation turns off the production of gondal hormone, with the consequence of dominished sexual function. The fat-deniers and the strict dieters must know that there's this chemistry of brain they're fighting, they're really fighting nature. To help anorexics, and bulimics, Leibowitz is separately looking for some medicine that could artificially slow down galanin production at the onset of puberty.

Leibowitz has drawn a daily chart of the working of NPY and galanin, each one with, its own built-in cycle of activity. NPY is most active in the morning—after the overnight fasting, when we have an immediate need for energy intake. This means going in for carbohydrates: fruit juice, with its speedy transport of sugar into the bloodstream to restore glycogen, toast, milk. For those who don't do it regularly, a large omelette or fried eggs, rich in protein and fat, can disturb the normal rhythm of neurochemicals. No wonder you're often not sharp enough after a rich breakfast.

Around lunchtime, we begin looking for more sustenance in the shape of fat to refill our fat cells and protein to rebuild muscle. Both of these are converted more slowly to fuel.

Beyond afternoon, our taste for fat begins to rise, with the rising levels of galanin. Fat-rich snacks at this time are common. And these priming us neurochemically to consume more fat at dinner, our heaviest meal--the body is looking to store energy in anticipation of overnight fasting. Those favouring fats are particularly predisposed to food cravings towards the later part of the day.

Thus every meal, and the appetite for it, is differently regulated and presided over a separate cocktail of neurochemicals.

Leibowitz is of the considered opinion that curbing body weight by food restriction—dieting or fasting—makes no sense metabolically or to the chemistry of our brains. "All dieting does is to disturb the system," she says. "It puts you in a psychologically altered state. You're a different person. You respond differently."

Erratically skipping meals upsets the natural daily rhythm of neurochemicals; "that's important, because the body works on routines." Moreover "the chemicals that regulate appetite also directly affect moods and state of mind, our physical energy, the quality of our sex lives," adds she.

Leibowitz offers no simple solution for losing weight. People need help to understand what they are, what their appetite is, and how to work their body the way it is. According to her, it is possible to predict from early childhood through the displayed patterns of eating as to who have the tendency to grow overweight. The secret is to modify their neurons by introducing a very gradual shift in their sensitivity to the neurochemicals of appetite, to down-regulate them rather gradually.

Telling of Taste

"People think they're getting flavour messages from the taste buds of their tongue," says Marcia Pelchat, a noted biological psychologist, "but the tongue really detects only a few basic tastes. It is the odour that makes flavours different."

When it comes to taste, what's important is not your tongue, but your nose. Taste is mostly smell.

Try this experiment. Close your eyes, hold your nose tightly shut, and put a spoon of ice cream into your mouth. You won't be able to tell the flavour—strawberry, vanilla or mango—not until you let go of your nose. No wonder, you barely taste anything when your nose is stuffed up from cold.

"I am not only convinced that without the cooperation of the smell there can be no complete degustation, but I am also tempted to believe that smell and taste are in fact but a single sense, whose laboratory is a mouth and whose chimney is the nose," says Jean-Arthene Brillat-Savarin, in his classic *The Physiology of Taste*.

Without smell, our tongue's taste buds would register sweet, sour, bitter or salty, but practically nothing else. Without smell, for example, a peach and a plum would taste the same—sweet.

That's because our sense of smell is 10,000 times more sensitive than our sense of taste. When a morsel of food passes underneath our nose on the way to our mouth, olfactory cells immediately begin sending information to the brain, triggering memories and stirring up gastric juices. Before the food even passes our lips, we've already begun to experience the flavour of that food.

Once the food is in our mouth, air is pushed into the nasal cavity, carrying even more aroma information.

A German doctoral thesis published in 1901 introduced the theory of the "tongue map". It was claimed that the four basic tastes were distributed to specific areas of the tongue: sweet and salty at the tip, bitter in the back, sour on the edges, and salty all over.

Present-day experts aren't impressed with the "tongue map". According to them, while some regions of the tongue may be more sensitive to some tastes—sweet and salty at the tip—taste sensations come from all over the tongue. Only the least taste-sensitive area of the tongue is its middle. You place a lump of sugar there; you won't taste anything.

How some people easily eat hot chillies while some others can't stand the littlest bite? Studies indicate that people can build up a tolerance to spicy food. In one experiment, hundreds of subjects who had a small amount of capsaicin (the chemical in chillies that makes them hot) applied to their tongues for thirty minutes daily for five days reported less discomfort and less burn by the fifth day. Only a small minority just couldn't take any hot stuff. This is possibly genetic.

Incidentally the burning sensation does not emanate from the taste buds but from the pain buds which are right next to taste buds. The reason why people can't taste anything when their mouth is on fire because all that pain blocks out any messages from the taste buds.

Why someone who has been cooking a dish for an hour or more can't really tell the taste of it? The scientific answer is olfactory adaptation, which basically means that your body adjusts to a persistent odour by making you less sensitive to it. Hence the cook is apt to ask someone else to do the tasting as his or her own sense of smell got somewhat dulled by prolonged exposure to the odour of the dish under preparation.

The texture and temperature of food also plays an important part to our sense of taste, especially if these qualities change while the food is in our mouth.

One of the main reasons why people love chocolate is that it changes from firm to soft on the tongue (that's the unique property of coca butter; it stays solid at room temperature but melts at body temperature). Similarly a part of ice cream's universal allure is that it goes from cold to body temperature in the mouth.

Food Adulteration: Past and Present

Food adulteration is one field where we are staying in the front rank. The scale of adulteration, the multiple forms it takes, and the ingenuity employed in the process are almost unmatched. What to say of the widespread everyday adulteration, now and again a scandal erupts. Scores of people die consuming poisoned liquor or adulterated cooking fat, or fall sick from a fouled condiment.

That way our situation seems markedly different from the one obtaining in developed countries. There the consumer expects to be protected by his government. We mostly have to mount our own guard. As consumers we have to exercise extra vigilance in buying our foodstuff, at least secure our groceries from selected points.

Why some societies have succeeded in controlling food adulteration while others have not? A look back at the history of food adulteration may be relevant in this context.

The adulteration of goods, especially of food, must surely be as old as commerce itself. Food has always been an easy target for fraudsters.

Consequently governments everywhere are known to have initiated steps against food adulteration. Even in ancient Athens and Rome there were official inspectors to monitor wine adulteration (wine as easily diluted as milk). In England comparable regulations go back to the reign of Edward the Confessor (1004-1066). These were followed by laws that threatened dishonest bakers, brewers, butchers and others with "the pillory and tumbrill".

Yet food adulteration was fairly prevalent in the West right up to the middle of the 19th century. People often complained of things like sugar mixed with sand and white bread with chalk. Gravel and twigs were added to pepper. Used tea leaves were mixed with new ones after drying them. Mustard would be diluted with radish seeds. The more honest grocers employed "garblers" to remove stones, dust and other mixed matter from spices—the way we do even now.

A few additives, at first regarded as adulterants, later became established components of prepared foods; for example chicory in coffee. But most others were simply fraudulent, and often dangerous, such as slaked lime in wheat flour.

One of the earliest campaigners against food adulteration was Dr. Thomas Wakley (1795-1862). He is best known as the founder and first editor of The Lancet, still one of the most widely read of British medical journals. After sanitation and hygiene, Wakley turned his attention to food. Luckily for him, a contemporary Dr. Arthur Hassall had by then started examining food samples under the microscope for adulteration checks. Wakley was impressed by the powers of microscopy and commissioned Dr. Hassall to examine a variety of foods for The Lancet. For four years in the 1850s, the Lancet published names and addresses of manufacturers and tradesmen whom the Lancet Analytical Sanitary Commission (meaning Hassall) had shown were selling adulterated foodstuffs. (One wishes, some independent paper in our country would be bold enough to do the same, backed by a credible laboratory.)

The Lancet uncovered and published some horrifying practices: alum in bread, red lead in pepper, white lead to colour sweetmeats. The furor generated by these revelations led to a parliamentary commission. And, despite stiff opposition from powerful vested interests, the Food and Drug Adulteration Act of 1860 became the law.

By this time another determined character, Dr. John Postgate, of Birmingham, appeared on the scene. Dr. Postgate was a private medical practitioner but he was mainly preoccupied with the menace of food adulteration. Through pamphlets, speeches and personal contacts he mobilised public opinion. And it was through his heroic efforts that the Sale of Food and Drugs Act of 1875 was passed, plugging the loopholes left in the earlier act. This finally incorporated Dr Postgate's proposals to have government analysts and to establish machinery for monitoring food and drugs, that we now take for granted.

The latest adulteration Act worked. Food adulteration virtually ceased. Only minor abuses, such as misleading claims in packaged foods, continued to slip through its net, till subsequent legislation in 1950s put a stop to it.

What really came to the aid of controlling food adulteration was the technology. Policing such frauds was not easy before chemical and biological analyses became available. But once these there it was a relatively simple matter to take samples and have them tested, followed by prompt and successful prosecution of the adulterators.

Like governments everywhere else, our authorities have also armed themselves with the requisite legal powers as well as set up an implementing machinery. We are even members of the Codex Alimentarias Commission, regulating international food standards. Our Prevention of Food Adulteration Act, 1954 is as strict as any, if not stricter. A minimum of six months imprisonment awaits every convicted offender.

Four huge central laboratories are there to test foodstuffs. State governments/UT administrations/local bodies operate some 100 labs for the purpose (the implementation of the laws entrusted to state governments). And there is an army of food inspectors whose main job is to lift food samples and have them tested. The country has Consumer Councils and all the other paraphernalia associated with the control of food adulteration.

Yet, despite all the laws, labs and field staff. food adulteration is rampant in the country. In fact the incidence could well be increasing with the escalating food prices. Whether the emergence of packaged foods will remedy the situation is still to be seen; the packagers themselves may use adulterated ingredients. Adulterating food items and common drugs has grown into a flourishing industry, and works almost blatantly. Whatever little curbs are there on the manufacturers and traders, these stem from the resistance put up by individual consumers. The government's role in this field is unfortunately marginal.

Here we have duplicated the whole system of controlling food adulteration as it evolved in the West but minus its strength and bite. We have adopted the technology of testing but without making it effective. This is a classic case of a failure of implementation. It's not enough to blame it all on the field staff (who anyway deserve to be penalized for poor performance), it has something to do with the style of our government's functioning, and that again in such a non-controversial area like food adulteration control. A functioning where words often become a substitute for action.

Food Additives

Food additives give rise to certain misgivings in us. Are additives dangerous? Why are there so many chemicals to put into food? Should their presence deter us from buying a particular product?

At the outset, additives should be distinguished from cheaper substitutes that food processors use to cut costs. Food adulteration through substances that can pose health hazards is an especially pressing problem with us. But here we are talking of recognized additives that are officially added to food.

Additives are there in all manner of food we buy and enjoy: ice cream, biscuits, soft drinks, beer, cakes, soups, potato chips, chewing gum, even bread, and a lot of other things.

Many food items can be available only because of the additives—either to ensure the product lasts sufficiently long for us to purchase at our convenience; or to provide a pleasant taste, colour or texture; or to prevent it from going bad. This is the central argument of the food industry. And all that it can do is to list the additives on the label. If we do not understand what those names mean, it's our problem, not of the industry.

The resultant products may well be unnatural (referred to as natural), stale (described as fresh), free from artificial colours (full of artificial flavours), new (newly promoted), improved (more expensive), or home-made variety (actually mass-produced). The food industry knows how to seduce us. Packaging, advertising, display and other types of promotion are all employed for the greatest effect.

A primary purpose of additives is to make food look attractive. Much of our appetite for food is based on sight. There is a nerve pathway from our eyes to the brain and then to the stomach, that both causes hunger on seeing something that looks appealing to eat, and prepares our stomach by secretion of gastric juices.

The main colours used in food are brown-black (caramel, carbon black), yellow (carotenoids, riboflavin), green (chlorophyll), red (erthrosine, cochineal), and purple (violaxanthin). Of course the colouring chemicals have no nutrient value. But we have come to expect that certain products should be of a certain colour and won't eat unless they are.

The other major use of additives is as preservatives. We need preservatives in food if we want reliably available perishable food that would otherwise go bad. Some of the chemical preservatives used are benzoic acid (soft drinks, beer, fruit pulp), sorbic acid (margarine and cheese), sulphur dioxide (biscuits, fruits, sausages), propionic acid (bread, cakes), and nitrates (ham, bacon, pizzas, even drinking water). Of these, nitrates are deemed more suspect, as their ingestion in high doses over long periods can induce cancer.

Artificial sweeteners have become popular because many of us want to cut down on our sugar intake while retaining our indulgence in sweetened products. Saccharine is one of the best known and is, by weight, 300 times as potent as a sweetener compared with sugar. But high doses of it have been causing tumours in laboratory mice.

Aspartame, made from the chemical union of two amino acids, is 100 times as sweet as sugar. There are some fears of aspartame causing nervous disorders if ingested in large doses. Cyclamate is another sweetener, a simple synthetic chemical. This has been blamed for toxicity.

So, if we want to drink a lot of sweet drinks, we seem to have the choice of eating too much sugar or synthetic chemicals of disputed safety. One way out is to educate our tongue to resist over-sweet tastes, preferably from childhood. Again many food items, such as cereals, chocolates, cookies, jams, tinned fruits, and so on contain added sugar, partly to counter the effect of salt. Surely sugar is natural and quite acceptable in moderate quantities. But this does not justify the extent of its use in processed food.

Antioxidants prevent oxygen in the air chemically reacting with, and then decomposing some of food nutrients especially fats. Artificial chemicals such as gallates are used in soups, meats and other food.

Emulsifiers and stabilizers keep the texture as desired such as in ice cream. These include natural gums and fats but also detergent chemicals.

Often there is a good deal of taste loss caused in food processing. And so the need for so many flavours to be added. These flavourings can be "natural" in the sense that they are extracted from plants, such as vanilla essence from vines. Some flavours are completely artificial, often synthesized from products derived from coal tar.

The exact identification of an artificial flavouring is rarely given. The food industry argues that it might be giving away a trade secret. And it makes out that in any case the amount of chemical present is very small. But then people can become "hooked" on certain flavours, and could over the years eat a great deal of a particular flavouring chemical.

With all sorts of conflicting reports circulating in the press or otherwise, the average consumer stays confused about any health risks posed by food additives. On the evidence available at present one could say that additives used by the well-established and reputed section of the food industry are probably safe as long as you do not eat too much of them.

There is reason to believe that certain additives are not dangerous at all, or perhaps minimally so. For instance, some have been in use for sufficient time without any known evidence of danger. The preservatives acetic acid and sorbic acid are examples. Some substances are identical to natural products about which there are few worries. For example, caramel is produced whenever confectionery is baked.

To establish the safety of a particular additive can be a very complex undertaking. You have to isolate its effects from all other factors over a extended period for a large section of the population. The whole exercise could take decades. Yet there is a strong case for the food industry to be very circumspect in using chemical additives, and to eliminate those that come under suspicion. And we as consumers could show a preference for natural products to the extent possible.

What's for Breakfast?

What's for breakfast? An important daily concern of mankind over the centuries. Each new day awakening the man's most constant and demanding companion--his appetite.

Ulysses drew his strength from a frugal repast of bread steeped in wine. Cleopatra and her entourage had a buffet of bread and meat washed down with beer. The Romans, early risers, breakfasted on a wholesome snack of bread, cheese and dry fruits. We had our hoary tradition of milk and roti or a rice preparation first thing in the morning. Heavy breakfasts: fish, sausages, eggs, bacon, porridge, toast, butter, jams, cream and tea were a special feature of Victorian England.

Nowadays, with the rush of life, leisurely morning meals are mostly a thing of the past, except on weekends and vacation. An elaborate unhurried breakfast now figures as one of life's luxuries.

On a working day it's common to see people snatch a toast with their coffee or down a cereal on their way out the door. Some omit the morning meal altogether.

Skipping breakfast or going out without anything substantial might be a mistake. After a good night's sleep, the body IS truly hungry; we have not eaten for over eight hours. Our bodies need proper fuel to be alert and energetic enough to meet the day's demands. A good breakfast gives us the needed start.

Fruit juice, especially fresh juice (which has lain in the fruit some minutes before, not bottled for long) is the darling of doctors. But why send such acidic stuff into your stomach first thing in the morning? All those vitamins should be just as good at some other time of the day. Anyway, now that juice stands entrenched in modern breakfast, it isn't a bad idea to down it towards the end of the meal, a sort of breakfast dessert.

Butter with its high fat content is being frowned upon for sedentary blokes. Here French have an advantage; they've such good bread they need no butter with it. A few establishments in our cities are also producing some pricey stuff. But good Continental bread is a rarity.

The known treat of omelette (omelet to Americans) seems to have fallen on bad days. You get some awful stuff in planes, trains and restaurants. Your best bet outside is perhaps a boiled egg. They can't interfere with that too much.

Doctors all over are now recommending a breakfast of warm or cold cereal. According to them, eating cereals high in fibre and protein will make a difference in how you feel through the morning. Breakfast cereals are now a billion dollar business in the world, the variety well-nigh breathtaking: flavoured, fruited, fortified nutritionally.

One thing that curiously distinguishes breakfast from other meals is the sameness of the fare. Most of us, it seems, have the same thing for breakfast every day over the years. And rarely give this matter much thought. People occasionally ask, "What are we having for lunch or our dinner?" Nobody really asks, "What's new for breakfast today?"

I know of an elderly uncle of mine who claims to have eaten the same unvaried breakfast for fifty years: two half-boiled eggs, two buttered toasts and two cups of tea. That way he has consumed some 36,500 eggs with his morning meals.

Maybe we're too rushed in the morning or we're too preoccupied with what we have to do that day, to care about what we eat at breakfast. Evidently most of us remain satisfied with having more of what we had yesterday—simply letting something substantial and warm into our digestive tracts.

No wonder, cookery columns and cookbooks spare scant space for breakfasts. Their readers, they know, will invite others to lunches, dinners, and even daytime snacks but hardly anyone to breakfast. And they want their recipes to be talked about when the end-products are eaten. Few people are inclined to talk of food at the early hour of breakfast.

The Snare of Snacks

You see Savitri Saxena, a housewife in her forties, nibbling a few morsels of food at her meals. She denies herself of chappatis and leaves out the greasy meat gravy, despite her craving for these. In fact Savitri has been dieting rather rigorously for several years. And yet, to her dismay, she continues overweight, with massive hips and a bulging middle.

The trouble with Savitri: she's snared by snacks. Whenever she gets a chance she pops in a snack, whether it's a bite of a home-made sweets (she makes some excellent sweets, and her two boys and the husband are always wanting her to keep up with the supplies of the same) or a bit of chocolate or a biscuit. Her prolonged stay in the kitchen could mean plenty of small snacks in a day. And she's an absent-minded eater who fails to keep count of all those little bits she swallows during the course of the day.

"There's nothing inherently bad in eating throughout the day," says her doctor. "But it depends on what you're eating and how much. If the snacks are sweets or candy, you may be getting far too much of sugar and much less of minerals and vitamins. Bit by bit, a lot of those absent-minded calories add up."

"Now that I seem addicted to snacks, will it be all right if I shift over to more healthful ones?" she asks.

"Of course there are light healthy snacks like a cup of non-fat yoghurt, cuts of carrots, pieces of fruits or unsweetened biscuits. But I would rate it a better bet if you ate wholesome meals at their prescribed times and discontinued the snacks altogether. You'll be able to exercise greater control over your food intake, and you'd enjoy your meals, too—which I understand, you're not doing presently, haunted by the spectre of dieting."

The last few years have seen an enormous emergence of snacks. It's partly due to the fact that many people, particularly young people, have taken to much "grazing" instead of sitting down to regular meals. Similarly a lot of children, especially city children from affluent families, often eat more between meals than at their meals. And the food industry has obliged by producing all sorts of enticing snacks. Or is it the other way? The food industry marketing snacks with such vigour and pressure-selling that children have taken more to eating various sweet and salted snacks instead of their normal meals. After all, everywhere the food industry advertises sweets or chips, nobody advertises milk or fruits.

The net result is that many people are getting caught in the snack trap. This could mean a significant reduction in their intake of nutritious foods, besides it being ruinous for the teeth, complexion and figure.

Most snacks are sugary things. That way sugar seems to be the centre of all satisfaction, more so for children. Sugar slides things past the palate so agreeably. No wonder they have this phrase of something being "sugar-coated". For a lot of individuals nothing compares with the sweet sensation of sugar.

Yet it is increasingly being realized that much of sugar is bad for you. Some recent studies have found that excess sugar in our diet attacks proteins in our bodies. Anyone who eats 50 grams of pure glucose (about the amount in one-and-a-half candy bars) on an empty stomach will find that the levels of glucose in the blood shoot up. This response increases as middle age creeps on. The older we get, the more pronounced and prolonged the rise in our blood glucose when we are "challenged" with an influx of glucose.

Dieting Through the Decades

Possibly no area of human endeavour in modern times has so little to show for so much attention as dieting. Over six active decades dieting has not made many people thin—or at least not for long.

Notwithstanding, the gurus of dieting have flourished, dispensing weightloss-wisdom. They know full well, most overweight individuals would do almost anything to improve their appearance—and happily for the advice givers, there is no dearth of pudgy people. Of course, a diet plan sells better if it's easy to follow; the less a diet requires one to do, the more likely one is to try it.

William Banting, a London undertaker, is said to be the first one to conjure up a diet plan. He himself was over 200lb on a 5ft-5 frame, so fat he couldn't descend a stair frontally. When riding, rowing and purgatives failed to thin him, his doctor made him go on a diet free from sugar and starch. Bunting lost 50lb, eating mainly lean meat, vegetables and dry toast. The pioneer dieter in turn became the first diet promoter; Bunting wrote a diet book that sold in thousands during the 1870s.

In USA—where dieting, as the American Medical Association declares, has become a national neurosis—it started with a businessman, Horace Fletcher. He was a blob of 217lb before he dropped 65 through his masticating plan. While Gladstone, the British Prime Minister, had advocated 32 chews per morsel (one for each tooth in a normal mouth), Fletcher urged all food to be munched till it turned to liquid. Any part of food that failed to liquefy under such relentless chewing was to be spitted out. He even wanted liquids, milk or soup, to be "chewed".

Fletcher, who came to be known as "The Great Masticator" wrote a book, *The AB-Z of Our Own Nutrition*. Here he advises his readers that they should "wait for a true, earned appetite". And food to be chewed as long as it "swallowed itself". No "depressing or diverting feelings" to intrude at mealtimes.

Next came Dr Lulu Hunt Peters, a Los Angeles physician, with her calorie counting. She pared her own weight from 200lb to 150 by drastically reducing her intake of calories. Dr Peters actually wanted people to think in term of calories: "instead of saying one slice of bread or a piece of pie, you will say 100 calories of bread, 350 calories of pie". She imposed a 1,200 calorie daily limit to begin with, followed by gradual increases watching the progress. Her book *Diet and Health, with a Key to the Calories* became a bestseller.

Then came the charismatic, suave Gayelord Hauser, a European doctor of naturopathy. His 10-and 28-day diets stressed five "wonder foods" rich in vitamin B: germinated wheat, yogurt, skim milk, brewer's yeast and molasses. Besides lectures and a best-seller *Look Younger, Live Longer*, Hauser developed his own lucrative line of special foods and supplements.

In due course, slimming saloons and diet-clubs made their appearance. In Slenderella saloons in USA, customers—mainly women—sat on specially designed vibrating tables, and were fed low-calorie diets. Esther Manz started TOPS (Take Off Pounds Sensibly) on the lines of Alcoholics Anonymous. The overweight met periodically and discussed their problems in a supportive atmosphere. Backsliders were tried at a "Court of Weights and Measures" and deposited fines in a common account.

Jean Nidetch of New York founded Weight Watchers in 1963. Whereas in TOPS participants followed their individual regime of dieting, members of Weight Watchers all followed the same diet. The organization even produced its own products in frozen foods and desserts, and its own cookbooks. Indeed the venture grew so profitable, it was gobbled up by the big food company H.J. Heinz.

The food industry is not only busy marketing low-fat foods, it's even come up with fake fat. Proctor and Gamble produce Olestra, a plastic food made from the chemical family of sucrose polyesters. Olestra is so engineered it remains utterly unabsorbed as it travels through the digestive system. Yet it tastes like the real thing, gives a "mouth feel".

Monsanto's Nutrasweet Co has followed a different route. Simplese is made of proteins from milk or egg whites, and so mechanically manipulated as to retain very few calories and no cholesterol. Yet the goop retains the feel of fat.

Pharmaceutical companies have joined in the weight-reduction quest. Mead Johnson began marketing Metrecal (short for "metered calories") in 1960. Metrecal came as a powder made from milk, soya flour, starch, corn oil, yeast, vitamins, with chocolate or vanilla flavouring. A can of it contained 900 calories. Made into four glasses mixed with water, this was deemed sufficient for a day's nourishment. Mead Johnson made millions out of it, till people got bored swilling the same stuff; what they missed most was the chewing. But then diet pills in one form or the other have multiplied since then, with some being faulted for their side effects.

An interesting development during the 1960s and 70s has been the increasing "white-coated" authorship of diet books. Prominent among these are Dr Herman Taller with *Calories Don't Count*, DR Irwin Stillman with *The Doctor's Quick Weight loss Diet*, Dr Robert Atkins with Dr *Atkins' Diet Revolution*, and Dr Herman Tarnower with *The Complete Scarsdale Medical Diet*. To the general public any dietary advice coming from a medical authority carries more weight, less risk. But then doctors can also tender conflicting advice.

Taller, for example, advocated a high-fat diet supplemented with vegetable oil capsules. And was doing famously well till convicted of a mail fraud.

Stillman followed a regime similar to Taller's but lower in fat and cholesterol. He urged lean meats, hard-boiled eggs, and eight glasses of water a day.

Atkins went a step forward. In his diet plan, high-cholesterol bacon, cream and mayonnaise were perfectly acceptable. The medical establishment was appalled but Dr Atkins proved very popular with dieters.

Tarower's Scarsdale diet marked a return to the traditional low-calorie, low-fat, low-carbohydrate discipline, with meals precisely spelled out in a 14-day plan. Tarower, however, had little time to enjoy his celebrity status and riches as a guru of dieting; he was shot dead by a jealous girl friend.

The market is now littered with diet books; there are hundreds in print. But lately some dissatisfaction has begun to simmer with the received wisdom in them. A lot of dieters are discovering to their dismay that most of the diet advice hasn't done them much good. In the meantime experts are taking potshots at long-accepted theories.

It's almost back to the old dictum: eat a healthful diet and focus on exercise, letting the pounds fall as they may. Anyway swings of severe dieting and overeating endured by many dieters can do more harm than good. Some scientist even contend that each of us has a "set point" weight that the body finds ways to maintain, diet or no diet.

The Anorexics

What sort of a person gets the eating disorder, known as anorexia nervosa? Most of them are teenage girls, bright and energetic from well-to-do homes. Good in studies and sports, the anorexic rises to competition and achieves.

Traditionally an affliction of teenage girls, anorexia has shown signs of migrating to pre-teens as well as the twenty-plus.

Mona is a slender, attractive 17-year-old. Yet she worries too much about her figure. Is she getting fat? Wouldn't she look better if she lost a few kilos? She is constantly dieting, becoming thinner and thinner. She talks about it all the time. Exercises hard. Often skips meals. 5ft 6; she's resolved to keep her weight within double digits—the magic ceiling of 99 lbs.

Mona's motto: If you aren't thin, you aren't attractive—the thinner, the winner. And she doesn't think anything wrong with her at all. That way, every ana (anorexics call themselves *ana*) loves herself.

And it isn't uncommon these days for anas to interact with one another, increasingly through the Internet—to seek support and advice. A sort of Secret Society of the Starving.

Prior to 1970 anorexia nervosa was considered to be "a curiosity and a rarity". Since then, its incidence has risen in USA and Europe to something like one in 200 among females of 15-24 age group.

By now the phenomenon of eating disorders has assumed a global spread that includes the affluent East Asian countries—Japan, South Korea, Hong Kong, Singapore—and several countries in South America especially Argentina and Chile. It has spread to China, too, in contradiction to the traditional value the Chinese place on plumpness as a sign of health.

As late as the mid-80s, the noted Indian epidemiologist Sridhar Sharma had found a very low prevalence of the disorder in India. Now anorexia nervosa is a significant presence in the country. We have also our unique traditions of religious fasting and protest fasting.

Although the prevalence of nervosa anorexia has increased worldwide in recent years, the numbers suffering is still not large in absolute numbers. But given the age and potential of the population which is afflicted, it represents a serious and often devastating affliction, with tragic implications for the young sufferer and her family.

Anorexics often grow in families in which there is an extraordinary emphasis on achievement, external appearance, and weight control. Anas are often compliant children who have a powerful need to "be good". Underneath a façade of good behaviour, they typically feel weak and unworthy. So when they encounter any serious stress such as a failure to live up to their academic expectations or rebuffs in personal relations, they try to salvage self-esteem through concentrating on the body, mostly in the shape of thinning it.

Anorexia usually begins with a decision to diet, which seems innocuous enough. However, given the anorexic's peculiar developmental vulnerabilities, dieting begins to yield a sense of control, coupled with the initial "high" of fasting. In a culture that values thinness, achieving a thin body represents a triumph. Again the anorexic derives certain satisfaction from increased attention from the family; the refusal of food always evokes a strong response from the near ones.

Once set in motion, anorexia nervosa has its own characteristic development as a disease. As dieting is transformed into fasting and finally into willful starvation, the anorexic typically withdraws from ordinary activities and relationships. She ruminates endlessly over her food intake and engages in highly ritualistic eating behaviour, such as cutting food into small bits. She starts monitoring meticulously her caloric intake. And she will typically intensify an already excessive exercise regime.

Once an anorexic has lost a significant amount of weight and the illness has progressed to a certain point, she will typically defend her lost weight by all means, such as disposing away food secretly, or hiding her emaciation under loose clothing. She not only deceives others, she deceives herself into thinking "all is well". Probably no disorder other than alcoholism is so invariably accompanied by denial.

By the time the anorexic comes to the attention of clinical professionals, the disorder has in most cases progressed considerably. In the early stages—inherently difficult to recognize—family members cling to the hope that the change that has come over their offspring is a "passing phase". And in a few cases it may turn out true; the developing anorexic able to extricate herself from the downward course. But the same doesn't happen in many other cases.

As the disorder advances, the anorexic starts experiencing faintness and fatigue. Menses stop and interest in sex declines. She can suffer from heart irregularities. Osteoporosis, the brittleness in bones, can set in. Over a range of studies, anorexia nervosa is known to have a fatal outcome in about 10 percent of treated cases.

On top, the incidence of suicide among anorexics is high. That way anorexia nervosa is deemed one of the most fatal and least understood mental illnesses.

Despite the proliferation of treatment approaches in recent years, there is no universal agreement as to the optimal mode of intervention. In general, there is consensus that both the physical and psychological aspects of the disorder must be addressed through a combination of nutritional rehabilitation, weight restoration (patients tend to approach their ideal bodyweights much more efficientl, in an in-patient setting) and psychotherapy. As anorexics commonly suffer from depression, the psychotherapy sessions can be usefully supplemented with anti-depressant drugs like Prozac.

Of late there's an influential school of opinion that lays more emphasis on making an anorexic actually eat than on psychotherapy. It enjoins the family members to make the ana eat, even if it takes a whale of time to supervise the operation. And advises families not to back down against the dieter's intransigence.

In Sweden, they have developed a device called a Mandometer that tracks how much food a patient eats.

It has been observed that eating disorders run in families. This has set researchers looking whether there are specific genes involved in eating disorders. The most convincing evidence for genetics comes from identical twins. If one twin has eating disorder, the other is far more likely to have a similar illness.

Some patterns are emerging. The most obvious is that 90 per cent of eating disorders occur in girls, most often in adolescence. Experts are exploring whether the genes that control hormone production during teenage years may also be contributing to eating disorders.

With the globalization of fashion, the norms of consumer culture have now a global impact. Well-known women's magazines with their worldwide coverage glorify thin fashion models. And so also thin fashion models walking down the aisles. Even cultures, like the African, where female plumpness was prized, are getting overwhelmed by this globalization of fashion.

For anorexics, the fear of weight gain operates as the spectre of the ultimate catastrophe. Many make out, they would rather die than cross the wonted figure of 99 lbs. Many of them take to vegetarianism. Meat becomes an object of particular avoidance, since animal fat is, in the mind of the anorexic, immediately and magically transformed into body fat.

There are male anorexics, too but they form a small minority.

The politics of eating disorders primarily revolves around the politics of gender. The current epidemic of these conditions is a reflection of the ambiguities of female identity in a period of change and confusion. Perhaps as women are able to achieve real power in the world, and the size and shape of their bodies are no longer taken to be the true measure of their worth, eating disorders should decline in incidence. There is even speculation that the crest of eating disorders in the western world has passed. And other countries, such as ours, should follow suit as women there make gains in empowerment.

Battling Bulimia

Anorexia nervosa is a puzzling and dangerous affliction in which a young person, typically an adolescent female, mercilessly starves herself. Bulimia or bulimia nervosa, another eating disorder, has its own abnormal pattern of eating. Bulimia involves binge eating, followed by purging (typically self-induced vomiting). Similar to anorexics, bulimics idealize thinness and are terrified of becoming fat.

Bulimia first came to public notice in the United States in the 1980s. A large number of young women, mostly college students, were observed as caught in a cycle of bingeing and purging. Some epidemiological surveys reveal that bulimia is getting more common than anorexia. In both cases, the vast majority of sufferers are young females, anorexics more in the age group 14-18 and bulimics in the age group 18-24. And, whereas anorexics tend to be phobic about sexuality, bulimics tend to be sexually active.

If an anorexic continues in a state of starvation for a long enough time, the pangs of hunger become intolerable and the rigid discipline of starvation may yield to a ravenous binge. With the terrible fear of getting fat, such an episode of gorging is deemed disastrous. The "crime" is then avenged by getting rid of the gorged food through self-induced vomiting (people often experiencing a momentary calm after successful vomiting), or sometimes through large doses of laxatives.

Bulimics have pervasive difficulty with impulse control, which manifests itself in alcohol abuse or even sexual promiscuity. The family histories of bulimics are often replete with open conflict and turmoil. And bulimia poses formidable treatment obstacles, because bulimics are apt to deny their binges and purges (often indulged in secret) and put up strong resistance to external intervention.

Because of the mixture of shame and fear that comes to haunt a bulimic, she may wait a long time after developing the disorder before seeking help. The time it takes someone with bulimia to seek treatment is said to average seven years. No wonder the incidence of bulimia is not exactly known. It still remains mostly a hidden disorder, and yet to be studied in sufficient depth.

Like the anorexic, the bulimic is typically an achiever at studies and work, and appears to be an independent, competent individual. Underneath the competent façade, however, she is troubled by profound feelings of neediness, dependency, and low self-esteem.

While an occasional binge-and-purge may be taken as an unhealthy, risky form of weight control, habitual bingeing and purging becomes a way of discharging intense degrees of psychological distress—a self-destructive method of working out feelings of loneliness, anxiety or depression. The secret rituals with food become the only avenue of expression of these carefully hidden needs and feelings.

The condition is mostly treated by behavioural therapy sessions, possibly a minimum of 20 sessions. Psychotherapy is usually supplemented by use of anti-depressant pills like Prozac. Relapses are quite common.

A striking fact about bulimia is that, compared with anorexia, it is relatively easily learned, or acquired. The bulimic cycle may range from a temporary experiment in weight control to an addictive bingeing and purging.

In the 1980s, bulimic behaviour among women became so common on college campuses in America, it assumed the character of a fad. In one big college it was reported that one floor of the dormitory had come to be known as the "bulimic floor": residents of the floor were eyed suspiciously when entering a bathroom, whose "odour evoked images of the Roman vomitoria".

A particularly astonishing development was the emergence of bulimia as a group activity. Girls "pigging out" together at eateries, later vomiting together in bathrooms, even comparing notes about the techniques of purging.

In fact a few books came out, such as *Responsible Bulimia*, extolling the uses of bulimia—something that enabled you to eat freely while still keeping your weight under control. Various books and articles offered advice on how to practice bulimia while preserving health safety norms. Happily this phase of bulimia development seems to be petering out.

Are the Fat at Fault?

Are the fat at fault? And if so, to what extent? Or is it more a matter of luck?

The traditional wisdom has been that the obese—defined as having a body weight 20 per cent or more above the optimum—ate too much, and exercised too little. The figure-flaw is blamed as character flaw; the fault of "letting oneself go". Taking a third helping of dessert is deemed beastly; one downing three drinks is a fine fellow. Slogans abound: "A moment on the lips, a lifetime on the hips".

All this often drives the plump to dieting. The dining table is always approached with a certain trepidation if not anxiety. At its extreme are the "fasting girls", fasting to skinniness for fashion's sake, a few even going anorexic.

We have in the sari a great solace; a lot of fat can lie elegantly wrapped. "It's a regular villain," says a wit. "Put them in bikinis. Quite a few may well die of shame."

Slimming the human form has mushroomed into a major industry with its burgeoning centres and clubs, medicines and machines, books and magazines, low-fat and fat-free foods, even surgery like liposuction.

The slimming establishments broadly fall in two categories. Health Farms where guests-clients reside for a week or more. You actually pay five-star hotel rates <u>not</u> to do something; what you could have done at home if you had the will. The other are places such as Weight-watchers Clubs, Body-wraps and Fitness Centres where you periodically present yourself for an hour or two of exercise and massage, attention and advice.

An understanding of human corpulence is proving remarkably elusive. What makes some people fat, not others? What's the precise role of food? What does exercise do? How much can be attributed to genetics? Does obesity run in families, with childhood feeding patterns playing a part? Ask these of a dozen specialists who study obesity, and you will hear as many answers. Causes like hormonal imbalances or glandular defects account for no more than 5 percent of the obese.

Everybody, of course, is agreed you cannot grow fat unless you ingest more energy in the form of food than your body burns up. Recent researches however reveal that fat bodies don't work the same way as thin bodies. A significant number of the obese don't really overeat. The well-worn medical mantra—"a calorie is a calorie"—simply doesn't hold true.

Different people have been found to have different RMR (the resting metabolic rate), the amount of energy consumed by an individual at rest or in "just ticking over". It was earlier assumed adults of the same height and age had the same RMR, averaging 1000 to 1200 calories a day (a gram calorie is the amount of heat required to raise one gram of water from 14.5 to 15.5 Celsius).

New studies indicate RMR has a much wider caloric range, from 700 to 1500 (the rates can now be measured in a laboratory with a fair degree of accuracy). It is also estimated that RMR accounts for some 70% of the energy consumed by an average individual, the rest taken up by occupational and non-occupational activities. Even in an 8-hour sleep we expend around 500 calories.

An individual's RMR thus constitutes the most important single factor in determining how much food can be consumed without putting on weight. Weight for weight, men have a higher average RMR than women because compared to women men have more muscle than fat, and the maintenance of muscles imposes higher demands on energy than of fat. RMR tends to decline with age; it's the highest at 20—the time our body is at the peak of its vitality.

If you are unfortunate enough to have a low RMR—say, a resting metabolic rate around 700 against the average of 1000—it's as if your body is sneaking in an extra 300 calories every day. That's 15 kilos a year. No wonder, people with low metabolism find it so hard to maintain normal weight. Through no fault of theirs they tend to gain weight unless they regularly eat less than a normal person—and this isn't an easy thing to do.

Each meal raises our metabolic rate. The rise could be double during a meal and for half an hour thereafter. Much of this increase is from the energy consumed in eating and digesting food. That's why skipping a meal isn't as much a help in weight reduction as is commonly assumed. The low eater's expenditure of energy drops dramatically. A good deal of gain from fasting is thus lost. That's the rub: if you cut down drastically on your food intake, you correspondingly lower your consumption of energy, too.

What about exercise? It expends energy. Working muscles consume energy in the form of glucose, glycogen and fat. Studies however indicate that the weight-reduction aspect of exercise is often overestimated. For example, a person jogging for a couple of hours is likely to consume 600 calories. Even sitting in a chair at home he may have consumed 200. The net gain of 400 could well be nullified by three generously buttered slices of bread. A large bottle of beer consumed after a game of golf more than replaces the extra calories used up in the game.

Again it is not at all established that regular exercise of a mild variety raises a person's RMR on a permanent basis. Strenuous training and conditioning undertaken by athletes and sportsmen is different; their hearts and lungs acquire an enlarged capacity and so a higher RMR. A lowered food intake coupled with light exercise helps. But for many of the fat there may be no spectacular results.

What about the foods we eat? Here the accusing finger points at fat. It's well known that fats are calorically more dense than other nutrients, providing 9 calories per gram compared to 4 for protein and carbohydrates. Again the body treats fats rather differently from other foods. For instance, when someone consumes 100 excess carbohydrate calories, the body uses 23 of them from processing and stores 77. But if the 100 excess calories come from fat, only 3 are burned and 97 stored. This may give a clue to the phenomenon that those whose diets are rich in fat, particularly saturated fat as from dairy products and red meat, are the most overweight, irrespective of the calories they consume.

The trouble is, everybody loves fat. Improving the taste of any preparation mostly means adding fat to it. Hopefully science may soon come to the eater's aid by making fake fat—having the taste of fat without its calories, the way the Pill delinked procreation from sex.

Are You Overweight?

"Imprisoned in every fat man a thin one is wildly signalling to be let out."

George Orwell

Are you overweight? Are you obese?

Possibly the best method to determine and measure overweight/ obesity is the Body Mass Index (BMI), developed by French mathematician Adolphe Quetelet in 1853. BMI is weight in kilos divided by the square of height in metres. For example, a person with a weight of 77.27 kgs (170 pounds) and a height of 1.75 metre (5ft 9 inches) would have the following BMI equation. In simple terms, divide your weight in kilos by your height in metres, and divide the result again with your height in metres.

$$\text{BMI} = \frac{77.27 \text{ kg}}{1.75} = 25.2$$

Most health authorities the world over define overweight as having a BMI of 25 or over. Obesity is defined as having a BMI of 30 or greater.

Percentage body fat (men have a percentage between 13 and 25 percent, women between 17 and 29 per cent) is best measured by comparing a person's weight underwater—fat floats and is less dense than body tissue. This method, however, is too complicated and is considered primarily a tool for research.

Another way to measure being overweight and/or obese is by using waist-to-hip ratio. For example, a person with a 30-inch waist and 40-inch hip circumference would have a waist-to-hip ratio of 0.75. Obesity is defined as anything over 0.8 for a woman and 1.0 for a man.

When a person becomes overweight, excess fat often appears first in the stomach and upper body in man and on thighs and lower body in a woman. Upper body obesity is deemed more dangerous than that of the lower-body.

Given the opportunity, most people just about everywhere will eat and eat. No wonder, 60 percent American adults are overweight; the country has affluence and surfeit of food. With rising prosperity, obesity rates are going up in developing countries, too. And ours is no exception.

"People can't stop eating any more than they're able to stop having sex or grabbing money or anything else," says Stephen Bloom, an obesity researcher at London's Hammersmith Hospital.

When people put on additional fat, say 5 kilos of weight during a vacation with lavish meals, their daily basal metabolic requirement for calories goes up. Where their hunger used to be sated with 2,500 calories, these people now require something like 3,000 calories in order not to feel hungry—their body and appetite have reached a new equilibrium at the heavier 5-kilo level.

That's why people find it so frustrating, trying to shed excess weight.

Slimming the human form has mushroomed into a major industry with burgeoning slimming clinics and clubs, medicines and machines, books and magazines, low-fat and fat-free foods, even surgery like liposuction.

Yet possibly no area of human endeavour in modern times has so little to show in the shape of success for so much attention and expense as weight-loss. Decades of dieting advocacy hasn't made many overweight people slim—or, at least not for long. Meanwhile the gurus of dieting have flourished dispensing weight-loss wisdom. Of course, a diet plan sells better if it's easy to follow. The less a diet plan requires one to do, the more likely one is to try it.

An understanding of human corpulence is proving remarkably elusive. What makes some people fat, not others? What's the precise role of food? What does exercise do? How much can be attributed to genetics? Does obesity run in families, with childhood feeding patterns playing a part? Ask these of a dozen specialists who study obesity, and you will hear as many answers.

Skipping a meal isn't as much help in weight reduction as is commonly assumed. The fasting person's expenditure of energy (otherwise required for eating and digesting food) drops dramatically. A good deal of gain from fasting is thus lost. That's the rub: if you cut down drastically on your food intake, you correspondingly lower your consumption of energy, too.

Science has yet to discover an easy, quick way to shed excess weight. One line of approach being investigated is to evolve a drug that will produce a feeling of fullness. The idea is to reduce the craving for food.

Meantime it's back to the old dictum: eat a healthful diet in moderate quantity, backed by regular exercise.

A simple strategy, however, could yield significant help in your battle against the bulge: go slow in eating your meals. It typically takes 10 to 15 minutes from the time we ingest food until our hunger gets sated. When you take time between courses or bites to digest your food, your hunger becomes satisfied with only the amount of calories you require. But when you eat quickly between appointments or otherwise gulp food fast, you often think you are hungry and keep eating even though you have already ingested more than enough calories.

What's More Fattening: Fats or Carbs?

What's more fattening: fats or carbohydrates? Currently this question is caught up in a lively controversy.

The basic problem is that the regulation of appetite and weight in the human body happens to be unbelievably complex, whereas the experimental tools for studying it are remarkably inadequate. An authoritative study would involve feeding real human subjects real food for months or years on end in a rigorously controlled scientific manner. That's virtually impossible, let alone prohibitively expensive.

So researchers opting for something less costly and more controllable often end up studying experimental situations so oversimplified that the results no way mirror the reality. Consequently, a plethora of studies on the subject, each one seemingly convinced of its correctness.

And this has spawned all sorts of advertised services and products for weight-reduction. The US Federal Trade Commission recently analysed advertisements for products and services that offer quick fixes for dropping pounds. And found that over half include a claim that was very likely false or lacked adequate proof. Americans spend billions of dollars a year trying to get thin. Yet 60 per cent of adults in that country are overweight, estimates the Surgeon General.

In the 40s when I grew up, the accepted wisdom was that ghee, butter, cream, and fat in meat not only added to taste but were good for body building and strength. Ghee (touted as the most concentrated form of energy) was added liberally to every dish and smeared over rotis. We even carried a tin of butter-made ghee to our college hostel—two spoonfuls used with every meal.

Then dawned the era when fat became a dirty word. We were told by everyone—doctors, food specialists, researchers—that obesity was caused by the excessive consumption of fat, and that if we ate less fat, we would lose weight and live longer. Excessive intake of fat—"this greasy killer", coupled with sedentary life—courtesy long hours before TV, have been held responsible for the rising incidence of obesity and heart attacks. Saturated fats (fat from meat and milk products), termed the bad fats, particularly picked out as the star villain in making people obese and elevating their bad cholesterol.

With the low-fat-good-health dogma holding forth, the food industry wasted no time in coming up with numerous reduced-fat food products: low-fat milk, yogurt, cookies, lean meats. To replace fat with something as tasty and pleasurable, often more sugar or salt had to be added.

All in all, the fat-reduction message made many people cut down on fats. At least it brought a radical change in how they viewed various foods.

Of course, dissenting voices were not wanting. The most notable one was that of Dr Robert Atkins, the author of the phenomenally-best-selling *Dr. Atkins' Diet Revolution* (1972), followed by *Dr. Atkins' New Diet Revolution*. The Manhattan doctor was accused of quackery and fraud, and vilified widely for his "bizarre regimen". But the unrepentant doctor has kept on advocating his view that we would lose weight eating meat, eggs, and butter to our heart's desire, as long as we cut down on carbohydrates: rice, grain, potatoes, sugar. Fat, he said, was harmless, while carbohydrates (sugars or anything made from flour) caused obesity, even heart disease.

Dr. Atkins has argued that the low-fat diet propagated so zealously by the establishment has not helped reduce obesity in the USA. In fact, during the 1980s and 1990s when the percentage of fat in the American diet decreased significantly, the country has witnessed an ongoing epidemic of obesity. And that also, despite a rising popular emphasis on exercise. Neither have cholesterol levels declined nor the incidence of heart disease. He explains this puzzling phenomenon on the increased intake of carbohydrates vis-à-vis fats.

Over the last five years, there has been a subtle shift in the scientific consensus. A small but growing minority of researchers has come to take seriously what the low-carbohydrate-diet proponents have been saying all along.

Indeed few experts now deny that the low-fat message is rather oversimplified. If nothing else, it effectively ignores the fact that unsaturated fats, like olive oil or fish, are relatively good for you; they tend to elevate your good cholesterol (H.D.L.) and lower your bad cholesterol (L.D.L.). Even saturated fats aren't as bad as is commonly assumed. True, they will elevate your L.D.L., but they also elevate your H.D.L. In other words, you gain little in health benefit by giving up milk and butter, and eating bread and sugary stuff.

The advantage of fat and protein is that they are slower to digest and so more satiating. Fat-free carbohydrates, such as simple sugars, starches, and anything made from flour have a quicker impact on blood sugar and insulin. They are absorbed quickly into the blood. As a result they cause a spike of blood sugar and a surge of insulin within minutes. And insulin profoundly affects hunger. Fat-free carbohydrates that way make us hungrier and then heavier. Obesity may well be the long-term damage caused by repeated surges of insulin that come from eating starches and refined carbohydrates.

As a general rule, the longer it takes for a food to be digested, the lesser impact it has on blood sugar and insulin, and so a healthier food. Compared to carbohydrates like sugar or flour, green vegetables, beans and whole grains cause a much slower rise in blood sugar because they have fibre, a nondigestible carbohydrate that slows down digestion. Proteins and fats serve the same purpose.

Dr. Atkins mainly relies on the assumption that this delay in the digestion of fats and proteins (butter, eggs, meat) keeps the insulin surge down and so the hunger. As such, it makes people consume lesser calories than those relying mainly on carbohydrates. He further makes out that starches and sugar raise triglyceride levels and this poses a greater risk factor for heart disease than cholesterol.

Atkins' hypothesis promises to be the battleground on which the fat-versus-carbohydrate controversy is likely to be fought scientifically over the coming years. After insisting that Atkins was a quack for three decades, obesity experts are now finding it difficult to ignore his claims. A serious debate has opened up among experts.

The U.S. Department of Agriculture had drawn a food pyramid in 1992. This was intended to convey the message "Fat is bad" and its corollary "Carbs are good".

The same is now being questioned. A few eminent food researchers have drawn up an alternative food pyramid. The new one, they claim, is healthier than the old food pyramid.

Controversies about fats and carbohydrates seem set to continue. High intake of fruits and vegetables is perhaps the least controversial aspect of the food pyramid. Only potatoes, mainly starch, do not confer the benefits seen for other vegetables.

And on one thing almost everybody is agreed. If you want to stay slim, limit your total calories.

Eat, Drink, and be Moderate

25 years of science and studies haven't changed these health recommendations—much.

The most crucial element is moderation (merriment through moderation). Take the USA. In that land of plenty, many more people eat and drink immoderately, thus earning the epithet "the land of the fat". The best estimate is that three out of five in the population are overweight. And nearly 50 million are clinically obese, i.e., at least 20 per cent above their ideal weight.

Everything has grown bigger there. The standard Coke bottles in vending machines today contain 20 oz, as against 8 oz in the 1950s. Helpings at food outlets are so big, the typical dinner plate has grown from 10 to 12 inches in diamter—that's 30 per cent increase in serving size. You commonly see youngsters helping themselves to 3 scoops of ice cream, and those scoops are double the size we get here.

No wonder, most clothing shops stock T-shirts in XXL size, even XXXL. Subways are abandoning the 17-inch bucket seat because of the persistent complaints about overhang. The new seats are now flat, to allow a greater spread. Cinemas are reviving "love seats". Originally designed for courting couples, these are now intended for patrons whose girth cannot be accommodated by normal seats. And the airline industry is under intense pressure to widen its 17-inch economy seat, and may have effected some change but for the declining profit margins.

Yet no people have shown more concern for health foods and dieting as the Americans. The country boasts of 14 bestselling diet books. Americans are said to be spending $30 billion a year on weight-loss products and pills. As one wit remarked, "the place from which all these diets remove most weight is their customer's purse".

All sorts of slimming theories are making the rounds. Here's a small sample:

The Blood Group Diet, which rests on the notion that different people have evolved to eat different foods. The type O blood group first appeared when man was a hunter, and so better equipped for eating animal protein. Type A evolved with agriculture, and is more suited to vegetarianism. Types B and AB relate to nomadic life and are suited to a broader diet. Dr Peter D' Adamo, the inventor of the diet, claims that it connects you to the essential truths that live in every cell of your body—a part of your historical evolutionary ancestry.

Dr Doyle advocates a simpler approach: writing down everything you eat and drink in one week. So many people trying his method come to him, saying, "I never knew I ate all that junk—foods high on calories and low on nutrition like biscuits, cakes." Doyle's advice: best to cut down on fattening foods rather than try—and typically fail—to cut them out altogether.

A recent book called *Skinny* propounds a tongue-in-cheek proposal: eat alone naked in front of a mirror. The writer claims it to be the dietary secret of some successful thin New Yorkers.

To science, the basic concepts on nutrition, alcohol and health remain consistent over the last 25 years—despite a whole slew of new controversies and new data.

There's the health fad of organic food being nutritionally superior to "regular" foods that are raised using chemicals and processed with man-made preservatives and additives. Another is the current scare against bio-engineered food, and the fear of food irradiation.

These apprehensions, scientific studies reveal, are largely exaggerated. The toxins present in "regular" foods pose no cause for concern because we never eat enough at one time to create a problem. Irradiation again can actually decrease the risk of some food-borne diseases instead of inflicting harm.

Claims made by manufacturers of most of vitamin, mineral and herbal products—a dizzying array of offerings in the market—need to be taken with a grain of salt. Only calcium supplements give proof of promoting bone health (although calcium consumed in dairy products is more biologically ideal).

And all those dire warnings against salt. While some individuals are salt-sensitive, the majority of us tolerate it rather well. There's as yet no conclusive proof that salt causes high blood pressure; only those with hypertension are advised to cut back on it. The primary means of reducing high blood pressure today is medication.

Alcohol is alcohol, whether it is in the form of beer, wine, or spirits; and moderation is still the key. Moderation is now officially defined as two standard drinks per day for a man, one per day for a woman. While it would probably be going too far to say that alcohol protects "heart health", studies conducted in many parts of the world have consistently shown that moderate use of alcohol is associated with decreased risk of coronary disease in middle-aged men and older women.

Science, with all its health research and studies in the last 25 years, has the same message it had before: eat and drink, and be moderate.

Looking at the Labels

When we mostly bought raw, unwrapped food we used to rely on our senses—we'd know whether a fruit was ripe by giving it a squeeze, and we would judge how fresh it was by its colour and smell. But these days we are buying many more foods that have been processed in one way or another and have so much packaging and wrapping it's often impossible even to see the food, let alone smell or feel it.

To find out what we are buying, the first place to begin is with the food label on the bottle, can or carton. It's more important than ever that you read and understand it so you have enough knowledge to make informed choices.

Good labels do help in making healthy food choices. Yet it must be remembered that the information given on a label is often neither complete nor transparent. Anyway few labels tell you how a food was treated and processed.

The label situation has grown far more complex for us with the entry of all those foreign products now crowding counters and shelves at various stores. And local manufacturers keep on coming with newer tinned, canned or packaged food products. At one time such offerings were few; consumers grown fairly familiar with items like Cadbury's Bournvita or Dabur's Chawanprash or Parle's Glucose Biscuits hardly felt any need to look at the label.

Law requires that a label lists the weight or volume, date-marking, all ingredients, manufacturer's name and address, place of origin, and nutritional information if a claim is made on the packaging about the product's nutritional value. Of late there's the added requirement of indicating whether a food contained any non-vegetarian ingredients.

Yet, manufacturers are often able to withhold important information about every one of these requirements.

Take weight. How can you tell how much actual fruit you're getting when you buy a tin of fruit? You can't. As little as 50 percent of the declared net weight could be fruit; the rest water, sugar, flavours, colours and preservatives. Juice drinks, usually sold to look like pure juice with pictures of fruit on the front, could contain as little as 5 to 10 percent juice.

Even a straightforward matter like the country of origin is not always so simple. Olive oil labelled as "Produce of Italy" or "Made in Italy"—and sold at the best prices—may well come from Spanish or Greek or North African olives pressed and bottled in Italy.

Food processors are often masters at making the pack date or the expiration date inconspicuous. On frozen food packages, the dates are usually indented on the wrapper or the carton. These are hard to read as well as easily missed.

Ingredients must be listed in descending order of weight (the heaviest first, the lightest last). And it should list all ingredients, but then there are exceptions such as water. Indeed, water is the easiest thing to add in many food products: bacon, sausages, other meats, wines, dairy products. And so also air, a free commodity. Ice cream, for example, is sold by volume. The more air you can get in there, the less the real ingredients you need. Additives such as emulsifiers and stabilizers ensure there are millions of air cells in a single scoop of ice cream.

How many of us actually check the size of products we buy? The chances are we don't. This encourages many a manufacturer to redesign the pack that looks bigger but carries less material. Chocolates often come in packets that are generous on wrappings and niggardly on contents.

It is not always easy to spot ingredients you may wish to check out or avoid. Sugar, for one, many manufacturers manage to disguise by using words like sucrose, glucose, fructose, dextrose—the different names of sugar. Other manufacturers keep the amount of sugar in their products secret. Fat, too, can come in many disguises: margarine, vegetable oil, butter, oils, animal fat.

A high-salt diet can be a cause of high blood pressure, which can lead to strokes, heart attacks and kidney failures. Yet the manufacturers of processed foods, pickles, sausages, even bread and breakfast cereals have a special fondness for salt, the cheap substance. Salt not only disguises any inadequacies in ingredients, it helps retain more water and also works as a preservative. Many a label doesn't list the salt content. And those that do, often employ the disguise of writing "sodium" or glutamate. To arrive at the true salt content, you should multiply the declared sodium content by 2.5.

Animal products are still getting used in some products without being declared as such. For one, animal fat may be there in biscuits, cakes and pastries. Fish oil is added to many health foods. And gelatin is commonly used in jellies and cheese spreads, but the same rarely figures on labels.

Orange juice, sold as "pure, unsweetened", is not supposed to have more than 15 gram of added sugar per litre to "adjust" to variations in sweetness of different types of oranges. Yet laboratory test commonly reveal a higher percentage of sugar, even extra water. Quite a few manufacturers use fruit acids (again undeclared) to disguise the taste of added sugar and water.

Technologists are busy developing ways by which food items look "fresh" and "natural"—the two most popular selling points. Apples get a waxy coating to look fresh. Oranges are dyed bright orange to match our mental image of an ideal orange. Bananas and grapes are often picked unripe and artificially ripened with ethylene gas. But these don't taste like bananas and grapes ripened on trees and vines. Such tricks are becoming more and more sophisticated for the average consumer to make out.

And then all those food additives—a burgeoning list—that are currently in use. Because of the complexity involved, additives don't figure on labels. It remains the job of health and drug authorities to approve particular additives and monitor their use in various processed foods.

People are showing a growing interest in how the food they eat would effect their health. And many would be prepared to read the labels, if these are written in an easy-to-read and easy-to-understand format. In this context, it becomes incumbent on manufactures of processed foods to give true and meaningful information on the labels.

10
The Healthful Foods

Food for Brainiacs

Most people recognize that what they eat eventually affects their physical health. But the link between food and brain function could be immediate. What you eat (or don't eat) for breakfast affects how clearly you think and how well you recall information by midday. Admittedly nutritional neuroscience is in its infancy. Studies, however, indicate that foods have a critical bearing on how the brain handles its tasks.

The brain deploys a large number of bio-chemicals which act as neurotransmitters; i.e., they stimulate neighbouring neurons, thus facilitating the passage of impulses from one cell to the next throughout the nervous system. Of the few chemicals yet identified one is serotonin, whose functions include sleep regulation and anxiety reduction. Another chemical, acetylcholine, is essential to memory formation, while dopamine and epinephrine control arousal.

Scientists now know of the ill-effects when the brain suffers a nutritional deficiency in any of these chemicals. And it is possible to boost alertness, memory, and stress resistance in the nutritionally deprived. Neurotransmitter supplementation whether through dietary components or vitamin-like supplements, is known to improve mental performance, but *only* for a deficit caused by environmental stress or ageing. No one yet knows whether such supplementation can improve performance in people who have healthy levels of neurotransmitters.

The brain's source of fuel is glucose, the sugar derived from dietary sugars and other carbohydrates. And brain takes good care of itself; it's the first to pick up on any glucose present in the blood stream, even force the conversion of other nutrients into glucose.

Experiments have shown that students given a lemonade containing 50 grams of glucose—equivalent of 200 calories of pure sugar—had a measurably enhanced performance in reading retention tasks. A breakfast rich in carbohydrates and sugar—bread, milk, banana, orange juice—restocks dwindling glucose stores of the night-starved body and brain.

Cereals, pulses, potatoes, and other foods rich in carbohydrates have a calming effect on the mind. These raise levels of serotonin in the brain, which in turn is mood elevating. People suffering from depression were often found wanting in the requisite intake of carbohydrates. Luckily the typical Indian food, with its large component of wheat, rice, and pulses is a help.

A diet high in saturated fat can make you depressed, even anti-social, say some researchers. Such a diet can raise the triglyceride level. And that makes it harder for the sludgy blood to transport sufficient oxygen to brain cells.

Fats, of course, are essential for the body and the brain. All brain cell membranes continuously need to refresh themselves with a new supply of fatty acids, particularly n-3 fatty acids. And n-3 fat has to be ingested through food; it can't be manufactured by the body. N-3 fatty acids are best found in fish—the old saying about fish being brain food is true. Soya and rapeseed oils are good in it. Cornflower and sunflower oils are unsaturated fats but contain little of n-3.

The key vitamins for the brain are the B vitamins: thiamin (B1), riboflavin (B2), niacin (B6), folic acid (B12). All play a critical role in brain function, from manufacturing neurotransmitters to regulating energy release in brain cells. Their severe deficiency can lead to impaired memory, and higher levels of irritability and anxiety.

Vegetables—carrots, tomatoes, green chillies, leafy vegetables—are packed with vitamins. And so also fruits, more so berries, apples, oranges and grapes. An ideal diet would have something like 5 servings a day of fruits and vegetables (a serving is one whole fruit or vegetable, a half-cup cooked, or 1 cup raw). Other good B vitamin sources include milk, yogurt, seafood and green peas.

The brain consumes more oxygen than any other organ, and so it is subject to maximum attacks from free radicals of oxygen—the reactive molecules given off in burning oxygen, and from air pollution. Cumulative damage from free radical reactions is implicated in many cancers and in the ageing of the human brain.

Fruits and vegetables contain thousands of antioxidants and other natural chemicals that should help maintain brain health.

Minerals essential for clear thinking include iron, boron, and zinc. Iron helps transport oxygen to and within the brain's cells and works closely with the nerve chemicals that regulate mental processes. Low intake of this trace mineral results in shortened attention span, and inability to concentrate. Iron-rich foods include lean meat, lentils, and dark green leafy vegetables.

Boron is essential to hand-eye coordination and memory. Zinc deficiency hampers learning and memory. Include in your daily diet wheat, yogurt, lentils, peas, and green vegetables.

Taken in moderate quantities (not more than three standard cups a day), caffeine in coffee sustains attention and so enhances brain vigilance to some extent. Supposedly a mood booster, chocolate does contain not only caffeine but also another element that "alerts" the brain.

Skipping meals is deemed a mistake, as it does starve the brain of the needed nutrients. Best is to spread food intake evenly over three to four light meals in a day. High fat, "heavy" meals containing more than 1,000 calories, which divert the blood supply to the digestive tract and away from the brain, leaving you feeling sluggish and sleepy.

Free School Meal: Lunch or Brunch!

The Pondicherry government has started implementing a scheme of free breakfast for poor children in schools since June. The scheme was aimed at providing protein-rich food for the children.

The sister state of Tamilnadu has been running the longest and still unrivalled Noon Meal Programme in terms of organization and coverage. With its breakfast scheme, the Pondicherry state may well be pioneering a new feature of school meal.

The prevalence of malnutrition in Indian children is staggering. Possibly a third below ten years are undernourished. Besides stunting bodily growth, malnutrition can cause injury to the brain.

Recent researches by David Levinsky and Richard H. Barnes of Cornell University have highlighted another aspect how malnutrition impairs the intellect. Their findings imply that the cognitive disability of undernourished children might stem in part from reduced interaction with other people and their surroundings. These children simply lack the requisite energy for lively interactions. As a consequence their learning progress is generally retarded.

And an elaborate study by Professor Ernesto Pollitt of the University of California conducted on children in Peru and Jamaica has demonstrated that learning capabilities are affected by how recently one has eaten. In this context, breakfast every day before the start of schooling assumes crucial importance, particularly among children at risk for undernutrition. According to Pollitt, missing breakfast weakened children's attention span. And sitting on empty stomach could delay retrieval of information from the working memory.

The most likely explanation for these results seems to lie in the effect that glucose—which the body gets naturally from most foodstuffs—has on memory. While glucose is essential for brain function, the brain can only store small amounts of it at a time and its effects do not last long. It would appear that if the overnight fast is not reversed by eating something substantial in the morning, the brain may become temporarily metabolically starved, adversely affecting memory. A good breakfast, that way, boosts brain power.

All this makes a cogent case for offering undernourished children a school breakfast or brunch rather than the standard mid-day meal. A protein-rich breakfast can help them attain a better attention span and greater brainpower right from the start of the schooling day. All the more needed because many poor families are known not to feed their children enough in the morning when there is the prospect of a free mid-day school meal. A lot of children could remain virtually famished till the mid-day meal, and in the process stay mentally lethargic through the best part of their schooling day.

Even otherwise, breakfast is easier to manage than a lunch, as the former often involves much less cooking and planning than a cooked lunch. A sealed carton of milk containing one-fourth or one-third of a litre, a packet of ready-to-eat cereal (duly fortified with vitamins and minerals) along with 2-3 sugar cubes, plus a banana can be enough for a child in pre-elementary and elementary classes up to fifth.

School punctuality would again improve with a breakfast to be served within the first hour of school. The apprehension that some children may leave after partaking of the free breakfast is somewhat unfounded. Anyhow a hungry child would hardly be in a position to concentrate on schoolwork till the mid-day meal is served.

A mid-day snack, whether offered by school or brought by a student from home, is more relevant to senior students who stay the whole day at school. Smaller children mostly stay half day. For them, a school breakfast or brunch sounds a better bet than a mid-day meal.

The whole issue of choosing between school breakfast, lunch, or brunch calls for greater debate and consideration than it has received in the past.

Recently the Supreme Court issued an ultimatum to erring state governments to provide cooked mid-day meals to primary school children, or lose out on central assistance. The court was quite critical of states offering a pre-cooked meal (biscuits) which found their way back to grocery stores and take-home rations commonly sold for cash.

A good deal of success of the Tamilnadu scheme owes to the innovation that it employs part-time village women for preparing meals. Problems arise when it all devolves on teachers. The state of Delhi cites difficulty of providing cooked meals to a million children entitled to the benefit.

Possibly it would be a good compromise where smaller children are served a satisfying non-cooked breakfast or brunch in the first hour of school. Full-day-school older students could be given a cooked lunch, the same prepared by part-time lady helpers.

Going for Garlic

According to a recent news item, Israeli scientists have found that allicin—garlic's main biologically active ingredient—can disable infection-causing amoebas in test tubes. If allicin is found to kill infections, garlic may well be the antibiotic of the future. Again in clinical trials, the garlic's sulphur-containing compounds have shown potential in preventing cancer and fighting heart disease. Garlic also contains vitamin C, calcium, potassium, phosphorus, selenium and some key amino acids. "An apple a day . . ." may have to be revised in favour of garlic.

The healing benefits of garlic were known to mankind for thousands of years and widely made use of. Only these were getting downplayed with the coming of modern medicine that often offered quick, effective cures. Of late, however, there is renewed scientific interest in the healing properties of garlic. And a number of garlic's traditional attributes now stand verified by scientific research.

It was in Sumeria around 2300 B.C. that garlic first came into prominence. Archeological findings and records indicate that it was then extensively employed for many ailments: a garlic soup for fevers, a decoction for loose bowels, as a fomentation for swellings, and as a tincture (garlic soaked for long in beer) for intestinal parasites.

Ancient Egyptians used crushed garlic for plugging dental cavities. The pulp was mixed with honey to make it stick to the cavity. And for wind in the stomach, physicians commonly resorted to garlic enemas.

Homer's *Iliad* makes many a mention of garlic preparations employed in dressing soldiers' wounds and preventing infection.

Garlic was possibly put to some of its greatest and most diverse uses during the days of the Roman Empire. Legion soldiers ate it with bread for strength, gladiators munched on whole cloves for endurance, and some of the nobility drank a mixture of garlic and wine as an antidote against possible poisoning. Physicians used garlic water as a disinfectant during surgery.

This celebrated herbal of antiquity finds most mention as an antidote for bites. Garlic was rated as the ultimate weapons in nature's arsenal for disarming the poisons resulting from bites, be they induced by animal, insect or reptile.

Now John Heinerman, Ph.D., an American doctor, has produced a 196-page book on the subject, *The Healing Benefits of Garlic* (Wings Books, 1994).

The main healing qualities of garlic flow from various sulphur-containing compounds in it, nearly a hundred. And these are released when a garlic bulb is cut; in an uncut one these mostly lie dormant.

Dr Heinerman elaborates on garlic therapies that are being pursued in present-day disease management.

Acne: The ideal would be to include four cloves of garlic every day in the diet. As young people often shun oral garlic use because of its odour, Dr. Harold Simons recommends four EMG capsules daily, as well as bathing existing eruptions in a garlic infusion. The liquid dries out the skin and helps to unclog blocked pores preventing them from becoming infected.

Arteriosclerosis: In a three-year study conducted at Tagore Memorial College, Udaipur, the cardiologist Arun Bordia randomly divided 432 coronary patients into two groups: those who took daily supplement of raw garlic juice in milk, and those who didn't. Those who took the garlic juice were found to suffer fewer additional heart attacks and had lower blood pressure and lower cholesterol serum levels than the other group. Dr Bordia suggested that the herb worked by dissolving the atherosclerotic blockages in coronary arteries. Dr Heinerman quotes several studies indicating that garlic thins the blood—like aspirin—and so helps in preventing blood clots.

Common Cold and Influenza: Medical doctors using garlic instead of antibiotics for treating flu cases have been amazed by results, says Dr Heinerman. The recommended daily dose is 10 capsules of JAGE (Japanese aged garlic extract), along with 10 grams of vitamin C. Garlic gives maximum antibiotic effects if taken just before retiring at night.

Diabetes: If you want an herb that will really help bring down your elevated blood sugar levels and may even reduce your insulin dependency, then raw garlic is the thing for you, says the author.

Insect Problems: Garlic is one of the best natural insect repellents. If you want to keep insect pests away while outdoors, squeeze a garlic perle into some jelly and rub it on your exposed arms, face and neck, advises the author.

The doctor goes on to list numerous other ailments in which garlic preparations could help in prevention or cure: boils and cysts, cuts, diarrhea and dysentery, earache, eczema, fungus, and food poisoning. Garlic can also promote your wellbeing by reducing stress or fatigue. The National Cancer Institute of America has recently declared that a diet rich in garlic can prevent stomach cancer.

Dr Heinerman, however, cautions that in working with garlic for medicinal purposes, it is important to use the herb in its most appropriate form, whether it's garlic bath, cold compress, poultice and plaster, a decoction, essence, fluid extract, syrup, capsules, pills, powder or juice.

Yet it is in the culinary field that garlic is making a greater comeback.

Till about the 15th century, cultures with their cuisine lacking in garlic were generally deemed backward. But then a prejudice started developing against garlic use in countries of Northern Europe because of the bulb's smell. In fact the smell of garlic became synonymous with the poor, promiscuous and country yokels. In Shakespeare's *Measure for Measure*, one Lucio denounces the Duke who "would mouth with a beggar, though she smelt of brown bread and garlic".

In due course, garlic became off-limits in the culinary realm of the cultivated society in Northern Europe and USA. The British brought the same attitude to India. They frowned on someone smelling of garlic in polite society. And this approach began to influence upper Indian classes who were coming in contact with the British, socially or officially.

Garlic's fortunes have undergone a dramatic change in the last 20-30 years. Now cooking that uses garlic is gaining greater vogue. Garlic bread invites marked preference. And French cooking with its liberal use of garlic has become a measure of gastronomic sophistication.

Take USA. For 50 years—1920 to 1970—annual garlic consumption languished at half a pound per person. Since then, it has risen five-fold, Americans wolfing down in excess of 3 pounds a year. Garlic has evolved from a culinary pariah to national fetish. These days it's chic to be reek.

And what's more, connoisseurship is developing among garlic lovers. Who knew there were 450 strains of garlic? People are demanding a whole lot of exotic varieties: intensely flavoured Romanian Red, Spanish Roja, Russian Rosewood, German Floha, Chinese Xian, the red-tipped Persian Star from Uzbekistan, Peruvian purple-coloured cloves, or Tahiti's single clove. In USA itself, the biggest garlic farm, Gilroy's ranch just south of the Silicon Valley, grows over 50 varieties, harvesting some 60 million pounds a year.

And each July at harvest time, the Gilroy Garlic Festival—the biggest bulb bash in the world—is held. This year's event drew in excess of 1,20,000 clove cravers, eager to experience such delicacies as garlic ice cream. There were garlic chutneys, garlic salad dressings, the garlic-flavoured oil, garlic juice, garlic paste, and garlic-based jams.

We were always a garlic-eating people. The latest scientific findings on the health benefits of the bulb and the garlic's greater acceptability in food the world over, should turn us into heavier and more demanding users of garlic.

The Tangy Orange

Nothing really rivals half a glass of fresh orange juice at breakfast. No bottled or canned stuff, but freshly squeezed juice that had been in the fruit a few minutes before. The sweet, tangy juice—sunshine in glass—is one of the best ways of energizing our bodies for the day.

The orange is indeed a magical fruit; a juicy inner flesh enclosed in a leathery, oily rind. The tree itself is exotic, where you see fragrant fruit (both ripe and unripe) at the same time as its perfumed white flowers.

Originally from China, the orange has been there with us for three thousand years, and was known as *narayam* (perfume within). Arab traders called it *narandj* and took it to Spain and Italy where it became *arancia*. And then in French it emerged as *orange*, pronounced *orindge* in English. Later the orange reached America. Now more oranges are grown in Florida than anywhere in the world.

Of this delectable citrus fruit, the most important varieties commercially are the round China orange and the mandarin orange (the flattened tangerine). Other notable varieties include the Jaffa from Israel and the Maltese (blood orange), which we call *malta* as distinguished from *santara*. In boyhood I have known the most delicious red-blood *maltas* of Gujranwala (now Pakistan). As you cut one, it dripped with sweet red juice. Our *kino*, a cross between *malta* and *santara* may be a good yielder of juice, but the hybrid nowhere compares with orange in tang.

The orange has a near perfect look. Still most commercial growers and sellers are not satisfied and put them through a beautifying regime.

That way citrus packinghouses are more like beauty parlours than processing plants.

Green or partly green oranges are put into chambers where, for as much as four days, ethylene gas is circulated among them. The gas destroys the green chlorophyll, making the orange turn orange. The other method of affecting the colour of orange is to bathe them in a chemical dye.

Oranges destined for fruit stalls (and not concentrate plants) are often mechanically washed in warm, soapy water, brushed with fibre brushes, and dried by jets of hot air. And then coated with an edible wax—replacing the natural wax lost in the cleaning process—to impart a glossy shine, besides adding to the fruit's shelf life. Oranges when they arrive from orchards are covered with various things such as moulds and dirt, and need washing.

Luckily oranges do not bruise the way apples do. Oranges can actually be bounced like rubber balls without damage.

There's the orange magic. As you puncture the skin with a thumbnail, it sends fine spurts of aromatic mist into the air, even a bit into your eyes if you aren't careful. And the magic in the fragrant oil held in the outer layer of the skin.

The peel can be finely grated to flavour cakes and syrups, lending sharpness and zest to the bland mixture of butter, sugar, eggs and flour. And it goes into the making of golden marmalade. To me as a breakfast savoury, no jam or jelly matches a well-made bitter marmalade.

There has been a steady dispersal of oranges over the globe. Their production got a big boost with the spread of orange-juice drinking, as distinct from eating fresh fruit.

Yet it was the health factor that triggered the orange boom. Great claims have been made for this delectable fruit: eating oranges helps cure or prevent all manners of ailments from peptic ulcers to heart attacks, from liver trouble to fatigue. Oranges, anyway, are rich in vitamin C (ascorbic acid) that can protect us from colds, viruses, and premature hair loss and ageing of the skin. Only bear in mind, frequent drinking of orange juice exposes your teeth to fructose and citric acid, both of which act on the enamel protecting the teeth.

John McPhee, a noted American writer, has now come up with a whole book *Oranges* (Penguin Classics, 2000, pp. 149).

For orange innocents as most of us are, McPhee's book is a compendium of amazing facts. For example, an orange picked from the bottom of the tree is not as sweet as the fruit picked from the top.

And oranges turn orange when they are cold. When they're warm, they stay green, or green with pale yellow splodges.

The book dwells a great deal on bottled or canned orange juice, and how it compares with the fresh product. As any fresh orange-drinker will confirm, the bottled or cartoned variety doesn't taste like real orange juice. McPhee explains that the chemistry of real orange juice is so subtle and complicated, most attempts to identify as to what actually makes the taste itself are tentative.

The chief flavouring component is thought to be d-limonene, the main ingredient of peel oil (common to all citrus fruits). This is the substance you twist from lemon onto your drink or food, and this is what burns your lips as you bite into oranges. But nobody seems to know just how much d-limonene should be added to achieve ideal orangeness.

This has frustrated all the leading manufacturers of frozen or chilled orange juice when it comes to making it taste like fresh orange juice. Millions of dollars have gone into its research but the real taste of fresh orange juice still eludes the bottled or cartoned variety. "The closest thing to freshly squeezed orange juice" is all that Tropicana, the biggest manufacturer of frozen juice, can claim for its product.

A Fresh Look at Tomatoes

We love tomatoes. We consume this delectable vegetable-cum-fruit in umpteen forms: in salad and sandwiches, in juice and soups, in paste and ketchup, and in all sorts of cooking. On top we love to eat them as they come—ripe, red, delicious. No vegetable anyway rivals them in visual appeal.

Tomatoes are in the news. Researchers are discovering new healthful aspects of this vegetable—a vegetable that contains most water, nearly 94 percent of it.

Evidence is mounting that people who regularly eat tomatoes have a substantially lower risk of cancer. In a thousand-person study of eating habits and health, Harvard Medical School researchers found that those who ate tomatoes every week had a lower chance of dying from cancer.

Recently a study of 48,0000 American males showed nearly 30 percent lower risk for prostate cancer among those who consumed tomatoes or tomato sauce more than twice a week. Another study of men and women in Italy showed that eating seven or more servings of raw tomatoes a week was linked to a 30 to 60 per cent reduction in digestive tract cancers.

The protective qualities of the tomato, researchers believe, come from lycopene. This is a potent antioxidant plant chemical that is abundant in tomatoes. Lycopene is the one that imparts red colour to tomatoes; the more red the tomato, the more lycopene it contains. That way, green and yellow tomatoes suffer from the lack of it.

Lycopene is also found in watermelons and pink grapefruit, but tomatoes are its most abundant source.

Contrary to popular impression, cooked tomatoes are deemed more healthful than raw ones; cooking enhances the lycopene content in tomatoes by breaking down cell walls and making the lycopene more readily available. Again lycopene is fat soluble and so a certain amount of fat in cooking helps lycopene to be absorbed by the body. Happily, most of our cooking involves addition of fat.

And, thanks to some latest researches on tomato breeding, its healthful aspect would get an added boost. Typical tomatoes contain 2 to 5 micrograms of beta-carotene—the precursor to vitamin A—per gram. But the varieties just released by the Agricultural Research Service in Beltsville, Maryland, USA have over 55 micrograms per gram. The first crops are destined for tomato sauce, paste and juice. Varieties for salads will follow soon. Vitamin A is an antioxidant, and is important for vision and the growth of healthy bones and teeth.

All this calls for a fresh look at tomatoes. There's more to this fabulous vegetable-cum-fruit than meets the eye.

A Goodly Apple

Newton discovered gravity, watching an apple falling. And it was the apple that got Adam and Eve expelled from the Garden of Eden ("That Adam was not Adamant!" when Eve "the apple pressed with specious cant", rues the poet-humorist Thomas Hood).

The Bible actually never names "the forbidden fruit", and that part of the world is too hot for apples. Yet since the Middle Ages, northern Europeans have assumed that the forbidden fruit was an apple. (Some scholars think it was a pomegranate.) The apple legend owes a lot to countless painters, notably Durer, whose re-creation of paradise invariably includes an apple tree. No wonder, the apple has given rise to so many phrases: "apple of one's eye", "apple cheek", "apple of discord", "apple red".

The apple is now the most widely cultivated fruit tree in the world, with an average annual output of 16,000,000 metric tons. USA contributes one-fifth to it and Italy one-eight. Other major producers include France, Germany, Australia, New Zealand and Japan. Our output of apples on the hillside of Kashmir and Kulu has registered impressive advances in quantity and quality during the last century.

The apple is known to originate in the forests of Kazakhstan where you can still find wild apple trees growing to a height of sixty feet. Travellers on the Silk Route took the tree to Europe, wherefrom the early settlers took it to USA. The tree is a native of temperate zone, requiring a distinct winter. And does well on hillsides that offer good drainage.

The apple tree, however, calls for a vigorous spraying regime to save the fruit from many insect pests. That makes it advisable to wash apples thoroughly if eaten unpeeled. The apple peel is rich with nutrients.

The apple held a special fascination for North Europeans and early Americans, because this was practically the only sweet stuff available, except for honey. And human fondness for things sweet—starting from mother's milk—may be from an in-born instinct with us. Anthropologist have found that cultures vary enormously in their liking for bitter, sour, and salty flavours, but a taste for sweetness appears to be universal. That should come as no surprise, since sugar is the form in which nature stores food energy. And here fruits enjoy a definite edge over the less glamorous vegetables (who ever heard of a forbidden vegetable).

No wonder, apple trees became a common fixture in orchards and house gardens. And apple varieties ran into thousands: cider varieties, cooking varieties, dessert varieties, and those for eating fresh.

Allowed to ferment for a few weeks, pressed apple juice yields a mildly alcoholic beverage with about half the strength of wine. For something stronger, cider can be distilled into brandy or simply frozen. Virtually every homestead in America produced its own cider. In rural areas cider took the place not only of wine and beer but of coffee and tea, juice, and water—cider deemed more sanitary and healthful than polluted water, even for children.

People railing against the evils of alcohol mostly made an exception for cider. Others argued that the Biblical warning was against the products of the grape, with no mention of apples. Only later when the Prohibition campaign included cider, people started cutting down cider-variety trees.

With restrictions on cider, marketing messages began harping on the wholesomeness of the fruit—"an apple a day keeps the doctor away". And there are sound grounds for it.

The apple contains vitamin A and C, it's high in carbohydrates, and an excellent source of dietary fibre. And the apple is considered particularly good for the teeth; eating one is akin to brushing your teeth.

With the coming of refrigeration, it became possible to market apples all the year round—apples can be stored up to a year. But such upkeep calls for optimum storage conditions. For long holding, temperatures only slightly above the freezing point of the fruit are desirable. Apples may also be stored in inert gases or in controlled atmospheres. It is this improper storage that causes many of our apples to lose their solidity and freshness, juice and flavour.

Growers got together and decided it would be best to simplify the market by planting and promoting only a small handful of brand-name eating varieties. The market had no use for the immense variety of qualities grown earlier. Now just two of the qualities counted: beauty and sweetness. Beauty in an apple meant a uniform redness, by and large, and a nice rounded shape. And sugariness that could match other fruits. This was met by promoting two principal varieties: Red and Golden Delicious.

Besides being eaten as fresh fruit, apples are being put to many other uses: fried apple with various dishes, apple juice, applesauce, apple honey, apple oil, apple essence, apple butter, and apple cheese. Yet the most common use is as a pastry filler, for the making of the popular apple-pie.

The apple is indeed a goodly fruit.

The Bountiful Banana

If you're a morning bed-tea drinker, try a banana with your cups of tea. It acts as a good filler on an empty stomach and healthful, too.

A ripe banana contains as much as 22 per cent carbohydrate, thus a rich provider of calories but low on fat, as low as 0.2 per cent. The banana is a handy source of vitamins C and A, and of minerals such as potassium, magnesium, calcium and iron. The nutritional virtues of the banana continue to be extolled.

Hygienically packed in its thick soft skin, the banana is available throughout the year. Athletes use the fruit as a magical power food: nearly 1,000 bananas eaten every day by players at the Wimbledon tennis tournament. Professional golfers commonly carry bananas in their bags. It's easy to peel and a ready source of energy.

The banana is recommended for people suffering from acidity or upset stomach. And is deemed beneficial to ones having anemia or high blood pressure.

To millions in India and Africa (in Uganda it's a staple crop, ground into flour), the banana tree supplies a host of comforts and necessities—nutritious inexpensive fruit, shade, building materials, decoration stuff, and wrappings for food. The frond of the banana has straight seams, and it is easy to tear along them.

Centred on the rituals of fertility, we often plant the banana in sacred precincts. The tree (actually a gigantic shrub with a 3-6 metre trunk, crowned with 2-3 metre long leaves) exemplifies the whole cycle of human life: birth, growth, fruiting, ripening, and the parent stem dying when the tree has offspring.

Banana probably originated in India. Even finds mention in Vedas. Alexander the Great saw the fruit first time on his Indian expedition. Arab traders took the plant to Africa. Portuguese navigators found it there and carried the root-stocks to Canary Islands. The next step was to take the tree to the New World where it has flourished greatly.

The banana has blossomed into one of the most important food crops of the world, grown extensively throughout the tropics. And it boasts of umpteen shapes and colours; from finger-sized ones to those as big as a man's forearm; and in colours green, yellow, and red.

Europe and the USA took to consuming bananas in a big way only in the twentieth century. Especially designed refrigerated ships termed "banana boats" are used for transport. The whole banana business is in the hands of a few mammoth companies, such as Chiquita and Fyffes.

Ripening is artificially induced on the boats and then in the receiving storage halls by exposure to ethylene gas. These bananas have a shelf life of over a fortnight, unlike most of ours that turn overripe in 3-4 days.

USA is now the biggest banana importer. Even UK imports 5 billion a year. During the Second World War, Britain had been starved of bananas because the boats carrying the fruit couldn't risk plying. Thus in early post-war food-starved Britain, the banana was deemed a great delicacy. The writer Auberon Waugh tells the sorry story of his mother bringing home one great day three "rationed" bananas. As he waited in anticipation, his father; the novelist Evelyn Waugh, took the fruit, peeled it, cut it, poured on cream and sugar, and "ate all the three".

Another major importer is Germany. To western housewives, the greatest appeal of the banana lies in its readiness as a food. You just have to peel one to soothe an impatiently hungry kid.

Besides being eaten afresh, the banana is processed in umpteen food preparations, such as ice creams, milkshakes, cakes, pies, fritters and chips.

Lately there has been bad news for banana lovers. Emile Frison, head of a worldwide network of banana researchers, INIBAP, has highlighted the steep decline in yields of bananas in Africa, Asia and

Central America. The fruit could well become extinct in 10 years, it is said.

The problem with the banana is that a genetic accident makes the mutant plants sterile. Banana plants are grown by replanting cuttings from a parent plant—unlike most other crops that reproduce sexually and so enjoy a much broader genetic base. The banana having no such defences is highly vulnerable to fungal and other diseases. And these are currently playing havoc with its yields.

But then some researchers are reporting a breakthrough in fighting banana's fungal diseases through gnetic manipulation.

The banana is favoured by millions all over the world. And for many who depend on it for food and income, the banana's disappearance could spell starvation or poverty.

The Good Egg

Since the 1970s, anybody eating a couple of eggs at daily breakfast was deemed to be in search of a heart attack.

Of late, eggs seem to have staged a comeback on the health-front. An article in the Journal of the American Medical Association published in April, 1999 issue concluded that "up to one egg per day is unlikely to have substantial overall impact on the risk of coronary heart disease or stroke among healthy men and women." And eggs, it made out, need not concern people with normal cholesterol levels.

Nutritionally the egg is considered the most complete and pure food. Its white—which makes up about 67 percent of the total weight of the egg—contains everything needed for the growth of the young chicken, and the same is applicable to human beings. And unlike the yellow yolk, it contains no cholesterol.

In my boyhood, the egg was treated as a unified whole; we made no distinction between the yellow and the white. It's only later we learnt that the white is much more healthful than the yellow.

Now that doctors are letting people eat eggs again, how well to spot a good egg? And how best to cook it? Boiling is evidently the optimum form for savouring the flavour of an egg—frying, scrambling or making omelette introduces too many variables.

It's not too common to encounter an egg that actually tastes like one. You get eggs that have a distinct mineral flavour in the white or a salty-tasting yolk. Others have an unmistakable fishy flavour. Even many a fresh egg can mean a slippery white and a crumbly yolk.

Chicken-feed is the chief influence in flavour, followed by condition of the egg layers. Free-range chicken, allowed to forage for food to supplement their feed, generally produce better-tasting eggs that hens confined to a henhouse, and worse still hens cooped up in shoe-box-type cages. And many poultry farms feed fishmeal to the birds, resulting in fishy-tasting chicken and eggs.

Hens today produce eggs that are two to three times larger than those produced by their ancestors. Surprisingly the actual amount of shell has not increased. This is resulting in thinner, paper-like shells. Luckily, with the domesticated hen, a thick shell is no longer needed to protect the evolving chick from would-be predators as required in wild state.

How best to boil an egg?

Eggs should never be boiled rapidly. Fierce heat can cause the shells to crack and the white to become rubbery.

Although eggs can be lowered in cold water, timing is more accurate when they are added to water that is simmering gently or boiling steadily. When the heated water only just moves, it is simmering gently. When bubbles regularly break the surface, it is simmering steadily.

Take care to lower eggs gently into the simmering water. If you're taking eggs straight from the refrigerator, it is advisable to put them under hot water tap for a couple of minutes, before dropping into hot water.

Cooking time in simmering water for the average-sized egg is 4 minutes for soft, 5-6 minutes for semi-firm (yolk still soft) and 8-10 minutes for hard-boiled.

Piercing the blunt end of an egg with a sharp pin before boiling allows the expanding air in the air sac to escape. This prevents the shell from cracking during boiling. A teaspoon of salt per two cups of cooking water also helps close any possible cracks.

Eggs are easier to shell when completely cold. So plunge them into ice-cold water immediately after cooking, and change the water a few times to keep it cold.

Soft-boiled eggs should be eaten immediately.

If shelled eggs are not used immediately, store them in cold water in the fridge.

To some the whole thing may appear as somewhat of a complicated drill; after all, it's just about boiling eggs. Yet a good egg to yield maximum satisfaction needs proper boiling and serving.

Water

"Water—all life depends on it.

Water is akin to blood in the human body—the most important, life-giving and energy-empowering substance on the planet. Yet with incorrect, ignorant handling, it becomes diseased, imparting this condition to all other organisms, vegetables, animal and human alike," says Viktor Schauberger, the noted Austrian botanist who earned the name "Water Wizard".

Researchers at the Swiss Federal Institute for Environmental Science and Technology, Duebendorf have developed an easy, inexpensive way of making water safer for drinking. According to it, you simply fill clear plastic bottles with water and leave them in the sun for some time. The heat warms up the water and the combination of warm water and ultraviolet radiation kills most of the injurious microorganisms.

"SODIS (solar disinfection) efficiently inactivates bacteria and viruses," explain the researchers. Tests have shown that 99.9 per cent of the *Escherichia coli* in a sample of contaminated water were killed when sun heated the water beyond 50 degree centigrade for one hour. Painting half the bottle black and laying it on corrugated metal sheet shortens the time taken to warm up the water.

People can particularly take recourse to this technique when local water supplies get contaminated from floods. While chlorination tablets are often in short supply, it isn't difficult for people to get hold of used plastic bottles. Even otherwise, people commonly taking drinking water from exposed tanks, ponds or wells can purify their water with the aid of this technology.

With the increasing consumption of bottled drinks among the health-conscious middle classes, plenty of empties are available. The growing urban population of the poor can easily make use of the technique when they have to use water of suspect quality, such as from handpumps. And these plastic bottles going from the rich to the poor reduce the waste in urban areas.

Of course there could be a shortage of suitable plastic containers in emergency areas. But once people come to understand the advantages of solar disinfection in this manner, they will manage to get hold of the needed bottles. And may continue to use them thereafter. The very practice of drinking water from a bottle instead of from an open container, if it becomes widespread among masses, will mark a significant advance towards the use of safer drinking water.

Both the Swiss agency and Oxfam have been promoting SODIS in various countries in Asia, Africa, and South America. Water-related illnesses claim 5 million victims every year over the world. SODIS is particularly good at killing the bacterium that causes cholera. SODIS also inactivates some other common human parasites such as cryptosporidium that causes severe diarrhea.

It would be an excellent idea to give much publicity and encouragement, both in rural and urban areas, to this rather simple technique of purifying drinking water. Millions of our people are still denied access to safe drinking water.

Water Bottle: The New Symbol of Security

You commonly see people carrying a water bottle in buses, stadiums, libraries, and waiting rooms. Meals in trains now come accompanied by a plastic water bottle—which you are supposed to crush before discarding to frustrate further use. In aeroplanes, the sealed cup of water is seen sitting in the coffee cup. Water bottles are now an overt presence in conferences, play fields, parks, and restaurants.

Brand-name water is a recent development. Some twenty years back, one simply gave no thought to drinking tap water. Indeed in a country where a major part of the population still lacked access to potable water, one couldn't forget that the building of India's municipal water system was itself a momentous public-health triumph.

What makes for the rising popularity of bottled water vis-à-vis faucet water? Why do we feel the need to pay money for what has always been free or next to free? How is it that the plastic bottle with its sealed cap has become the latest security symbol? Have we been taken in by the media-induced paranoia or merely seduced by fashion? Will we drink any water that comes out of a bottle, even if it might be nothing more than municipal water—comfortably labelled as "purified"? Or is it water snobbery—not unlike wine snobbery, when it comes to mineral water?

Surely we have grown far more health conscious over the years. Steeped in the culture of the body, we insist on allowing only the safest substances to enter our bodies. Heightened concern for air quality and water quality are a part of it—and while you can't do much about air, you can buy safety in a tightly capped bottle. Drinking large quantities of water, anyway, is seen as a way to maintain health; a minimum of eight glasses a day, we're told.

The advent of polyethylene terephthalate—lightweight, crystal clear, flexible—has been a crucial factor in boosting bottled water. And PET came up with bottles of all "convenience" sizes. The sheer ease of carrying a little bottle rather than wondering where one's next drink of water will come from. All the more important in a hot climate that generated frequent bouts of thirst.

Municipal authorities everywhere insist their water is safe to drink, especially where water is drawn from deep wells. They claim they test it oftener that many companies selling bottled water. "There's nothing magic about putting water in a bottle," says one municipal head. And adds that cases of polluted water getting released into a city system are rather rare.

Yet many of us have grown somewhat suspicious of tap water. We apprehend that even if the water released at the works was safe, it could get contaminated in the distribution system, with all those rusty pipes and suspect storage tanks.

What possibly triggered the water bottle boom is the vigorous sales pitch of firms selling the stuff. Profits on selling bottled water average over 50 percent. These companies may not be actually inflaming our worries about tap water, but they aren't shy about exploiting them. The increasing presence of water bottles itself spurs people's anxiety about the safety of tap water.

One could figure out two broad approaches to bottled water: the European and the American.

Europeans go for mineral water, taken from famous springs. This water is not purified or treated in any manner but bottled as it is in highly hygienic conditions. Great care is taken to protect the water source and its surrounding area from pollutants. Evian and Perrier of France or Panna of Italy fall in this category.

These waters keep their original taste and mineral content. In fact each one is patronized for its unique taste. And minerals contained therein—-detailed on the label—are deemed good for health, something akin to spa water. World famous brands sell at almost laughable prices. Sellers justify it on the cost of the leased water source, continuos testing of water quality, brand publicity, meticulously clean bottling arrangements, and often a condition of lease to provide free tap outlets to local residents. Europeans anyway drink less water because of the milder weather conditions and much greater use of water substitutes: beer, wine, soft drinks, coffee, tea, milk, juices. Quite a few Frenchmen and Italians may have never drunk water in their adult life.

Americans drink far more water for climatic and other reasons. Restaurants commonly offer a glass of crushed ice as you sit down. And the country's laws make it mandatory for all public tap water to be safe.

Yet Americans have taken to bottled water in a big way. But unlike Europeans, the primary emphasis is on safety or purity, not taste or health-giving minerals. Bulk of bottled water sold in USA is actually tap water, given various degrees of purifying treatment. Consumers aren't much bothered about the source of bottled water. Indeed bottlers often fail to mention it on their labels, while offering "guaranteed pure" water. People buy huge bottles of branded water along with groceries and stack them in refrigerators.

This bottled water, with its purification treatment, has no smell of chlorine or any other cleansing agents. But the process of purification also renders it tasteless.

We are largely following the American pattern, emphasizing purity than taste of bottled water. People don't care much about the source of water as long as they are assured of its healthfulness. With all sorts of new brands coming up in the market and limited government supervision over quality, the purity aspect assumes paramount importance.

As we are inveterate water drinkers, middle-class homes have been going in for purifying equipment—carbon filter, backed by the reverse osmosis process—to fill up water bottles. Using brand-water all the time would prove too expensive in our conditions. But then there are a lot of occasions—travel or time outside the home—when one invests in a bottle of branded water.

Of course we have many mountain sites with clear water springs or waterfalls. And so good scope for selecting suitable sources and bottling that water on the spot (all famous mineral waters are bottled on the spot). Carting bottles to various markets is expensive, but then this offers tasty, mineral-rich water of requisite safety.

The Indian bottled water is currently caught in a controversy. The Centre for Science and Environment (CSE) Delhi tested various brands of bottled water available in the market. And found that all of them contained a higher percentage (in Bisleri brand many times higher) of pesticides than allowed under the EEC norms. This provoked a public scare. The manufacturers keep on maintaining that their water is within the prescribed BIS (Bureau of Indian Standards) standards.

The BIS is now engaged in prescribing higher norms, more in line with EEC standards. It has also cancelled the licences of some manufacturers. In our conditions, it is again a challenge to enforce standards, especially on smaller manufacturers.

Going for Ginseng

Legend has it that in China a young and beautiful maiden married to a nobleman was still without a child after several years had passed. Prayers in the temple were of no avail; accordingly, her husband was free to take a concubine. One night in a dream this tortured woman had a vision of an old sage who told her to go into the mountain and dig the root of a manlike plant and make a tea of it. She followed his instructions and ten months later gave birth to a son. What she had brought was ginseng, and the same goes by such exotic names as *wonder of the world, holy herb, manroot, thunderbolt root, seed-of-the-earth.*

Here's an herb that has commanded higher prices than any other herb in history. Ginseng is believed to boost energy, memory, mood, longevity, and sexual vigour. The Chinese have held ginseng as the single most omnipotent medicinal herb for some seven thousand years. Diseases for which they claim ginseng to be effective are anemia, diabetes, dysentery, and general debility; indeed a sovereign remedy to the ills of man. No wonder, the renowned Swedish botanist Linnaeus named it *Panax Ginseng*, drawing upon the Greek *panakos,* meaning "panacea," a cure for all ills.

At one time, only the Emperor had the privilege of collecting this root from forests. And exportation of ginseng from China was a capital crime.

Over ages Chinese have used ginseng primarily as an aphrodisiac. This use is based not on science, but possibly on the Doctrine of Signatures: a plant part that resembled a body part was considered good for that part of the body. Ginseng roots often resemble the human shape—legs, arms, even sexual appendages. Hence a toothlike root was good for toothache while one resembling a sexual part was good for heightening sexual desire. A root formed like a man must certainly heal all of the body's infirmities. Well-formed roots in the form of man are known to fetch exorbitant prices, as much as ten thousand dollars each.

The herb which grows wild in temperate forests, especially in China, Korea and Manchuria has become scarce from over-exploitation. It takes around eight years to form a root of appreciable size and quality.

Colonists to the New World had learned that Cherokee Indians of Appalachia were using a remarkably similar root for stomach disorders, menses, and as an aphrodisiac. Certain discrepancies between the Chinese and North American species were obvious, but the similarities were close enough to offer prospects of economic gain. Ginseng hunting became a popular and profitable activity.

The American ginseng is deemed inferior to the Asian product in its curative and tonic powers. Experts can easily distinguish between ginseng of various origins. And they can also make out whether a particular root has grown wild or has been cultivated. There's again the simulated variety—mostly produced in American and Canadian forests—where ginseng roots are seeded in the wild and harvested when ready in 8-10 years. Of course, growers have to stay wary of poachers.

The cultivated variety fetches far lower price. Chinese ginseng, white in colour, is rated as the best, even superior to the reddish Korean product. But then there are said to be only a hundred wild ginseng plants left in China.

Ginseng has been the subject of much study with reference to its medicinal properties. A seven-volume work *The History of Ginseng* by Immamura Tomoe summarizes Asian studies. And the herb has been subjected to extensive scientific research in USA, Russia, Germany, and Sweden. Russians claim that the herb serves to lower blood-sugar levels and acts generally as a tonic. Russian cosmonauts have been given ginseng during their flights into space.

German Commission E, entrusted with the evaluation of safety and efficacy of herbal remedies, decided that ginseng is a "tonic for invigorating and fortification in times of fatigue and debility, for declining capacity for work and concentration, and also during convalescence."

A Swedish study in the 1990s involving 390 people showed that ginseng in combination with vitamins and minerals, resulted in improved quality of life.

Attitudes towards ginseng in America have been skeptical. For some years the *United States Pharmaçopeia* had listed the herb as merely a mild stomach stimulant in restoring appetite.

Ginseng's effectiveness, or its lack thereof, will likely not be definitively determined anytime soon, partly because the usual underwrites of large-scale clinical studies—pharmaceutical companies—have little incentive to test an ancient nostrum that is already widely used and evidently unpatentable.

Ginseng is now sold mixed in almost everything from gum to snack bars—even coffee. Imitations abound. And price varies from about $30 to more than $200 per pound, depending on the quality. Korea is currently the foremost exporter of ginseng products.

What is most striking about ginseng is the amount of misinformation in ads and on packages. Just because the word "ginseng" appears on a product, doesn't mean you're getting the real thing. The quality and reliability of ginseng supplements is a major problem. In fact harm can result for lead and other heavy metals adulterating a preparation.

Better stick to the genuine article, because whatever physiological effects ginseng produces are probably due to a complex mixture of chemicals called ginsenosides found in those. That's why the whole root is so highly valued as it ensures authenticity if nothing else. If you decide to try ginseng, purchase a product standardized on the basis of its ginsenoside content. The recommended dose of a typical product containing 4% ginsenosides (the standardized extract, G-115) is two 100 mg capsules daily.

Of course, ginseng has to be combined with a healthy lifestyle that includes exercise, sound nutrition, and sufficient sleep. It's not going to cure a lifetime of "don'ts," but may provide additional benefits to the aforementioned "do's." Experts advise ginseng's regular use to beat stress and fatigue.

Rice

There are two basic ways of cooking rice; with flavouring, and without. That's the advantage of rice, it absorbs flavour without losing shape or texture.

A grain of milled and polished rice consists almost entirely of starch granules separated by walls of cellulose. As the water in the cooking pot approaches boiling point, the cellulose walls rupture. The water or any other cooking medium floods in. The rice will absorb any flavour that the mixing medium can transport into the starch of the grain. And yet the grains stay whole and separate. Possibly one reason why rice does not make a satisfactory bread.

Sir Owen, a noted gastronomic figure in England, advances the argument that in countries where rice has for long been the major staple food, people always cook their rice plain; at least until eating habits have been deeply influenced by outside sources. They may eat highly-flavoured food with their rice, but the rice itself is boiled or steamed and comes to table white—that, after all, is the whole point in polishing the rice to begin with.

In Southeast Asia with its rice-eating culture, all other dishes are actually served to surround and enhance the rice itself (rice—*gohan* in Japanese, still means dinner). And it is left to the diner, not the cook, to decide what and when the other dishes are to be mixed to his or her plain rice.

Where rice itself is coloured or flavoured, the expectation is that the cooking method and recipe originated in areas where rice is a secondary crop, or has been introduced rather recently.

Of course, Owen admits to exceptions to this general rule. In Southeast Asia itself, rice in many homes is often cooked in coconut milk or coloured yellow with turmeric. However such dishes are meant more for special occasions or for feting guests. In India again, there is a large category of flavoured rice dishes like pillaus and biryanis. But these were brought in by the Moghuls to whom rice was a secondary cereal. Similarly, kedgeree, a rice dish with fish and eggs, is popular in Malaysia. But this is more a Malaysian version of what the British adapted in India and took to Malaya. The English, anyway, were ever "dismal rice cooks".

Owen applies her overall theory about flavoured rice not only to the past and present but also to the future. She predicts that as the world shrinks under the impact of cosmopolitan influences, flavoured rice will become more common in traditional rice cultures. Even entrenched rice-eating regions will increasingly regard plain rice as one of the eating possibilities, not the pervasive one.

As to rice itself, it is India's most important contribution to world agriculture (besides things like sugarcane, some pulses and mango). The origin of rice culture can be traced to this country by about 3000 BC. And now roughly one-half of the world's population is wholly dependent on rice as a staple food.

And we also happen to be the biggest users of parboiled rice, a process by which rice retains bulk of its nutrients as against rice commonly milled and polished. Despite the usual meaning of "parboil", the rice is not precooked. In fact, parboiling takes a little longer than cooking. The grains become harder, resulting in less of broken rice, giving a price advantage to the miller. The stabilization of the exterior starch which occurs during parboiling is a help to timid cooks in keeping the rice fluffy.

Whether rice is fluffy or sticky depends on the proportion of amylose, one of the two kinds of starch granules in rice, to amylopectin which more readily forms a gel with water. Short-grain rice, grown not only in Italy but in Asia too, especially Japan, has the highest amylopectin and that makes it the stickiest. Medium grain rice, whose grains are between two and three times as along as they are wide, is somewhat higher in amylose and less sticky. Long-grain rice, whose grains are four to five times as long as they are wide, is the highest in amylose and thus the fluffiest. The latter is deemed the best for pullao where every grain has to stay separate. But then long-grain rice makes for poor puddings.

Basmati (meaning "queen of fragrance") is unique to the sub-continent of India. Of course other countries also grow aromatic rice. USA has a variety that is a cross between Basmati and American long-grain rice. But pure Basmati strains have not adapted to the terrain and climate elsewhere. Basmati develops its proper flavour when it has aged at least two years, and that also if stored in dry, cool conditions.

The Hindu civilization is also credited with making significant contribution to the gastronomy of rice. Much imagination has been used to evolve a variety of rice dishes. In fact, with rice, backed by a variety of pulses, vegetables, fruits, milk products and sugar, it developed what is perhaps the world's greatest vegetarian cuisine. And things as unique as idlis, raitas, jalebis, pakoras, samosas, pappadam, chutneys, even the humble kichri.

The distinctive feature of Indian gastronomy is the generous and imaginative use of spices to lend an added zest to food. And the more south you go, the more you get of these. That way, in almost every nation, its southern inhabitants prefer their food spicier than those in the northern region.

11

Foods Caught in Controversy

Sugar and Salt

Both sugar and salt have picked up a bad name lately with the health-conscious.

Do the two really deserve this denigration? These are the very items of our regular consumption that have been savoured and prized over the centuries.

Both are white crystalline compounds that are carried by the blood to all the cells of our bodies; they have this great affinity with fluids. Both are essential for the health of humans and animals, sucrose even a basic fuel for plant life.

Sugar: India has the distinction of giving sugar-making to the world; sugar possibly made here as early as 3000 BC. Greeks coming with Alexander saw cane sugar for the first time, one describing it "as a reed that produced 'honey' without the aid of bees".

Of course, our daily intake of sugar is not only the man-made stuff. added to tea and coffee, and put into soft drinks, sweets, cookies, and thousands of other foods. Sugar or sucrose is naturally present in such basic foods as corn, milk, fruits and vegetables.

Sugar and sugary products enjoyed almost untroubled popularity till about fifty years back. Only thereafter their overt use started drawing a flak for things like diabetes, obesity and dental decay.

Now sugar is again undergoing something of a reevaluation. Researchers are finding that a moderate use of sugar—within a fairly broad range—is not a major health concern if you are taking a balanced diet and maintaining a wholesome body weight.

It is now established that sugar does not cause diabetes. Indeed it's no longer a taboo for diabetics to eat sugar; blood-sugar can be affected by any carbohydrate, not only refined sugar. The body that way doesn't distinguish whether glucose in the blood stream came from a sweet or a chappati.

True, people can gain weight by eating too much sugar; the digestion of 100 gms of sugar furnishes 394 calories. Yet it's not sugar so much that is responsible for weight problems as the fats contained in sweets, confectionery, desserts and ice creams.

As a quick and ready source of energy there is still nothing to beat sugar. Persons feeling tired or listless commonly experience a sense of well-being with an intake of sugar.

And, contrary to popular belief, researchers have found no scientific basis to link high sugar consumption in adolescents with the occurrence of acne.

Even dentists are growing nonchalant about sugar. "It's not that sugar isn't involved in tooth decay—it certainly is—but what's important is how often and how long the teeth are exposed to sugar," says Dr Burrell, a senior representative of the American Dental Association.

Consequently dentists are not against intake of sugar as such but against snacking. Reduced snacking limits the teeth's exposure to decaying acids produced by bacteria in the mouth when particles of sugar are present. And sugar in the mouth is not only a result of eating things that contain refined sugar. Starches that may not taste sweet, such as cereals, also break down in the mouth into sugar.

Salt: For five million years our ancestors ate a diet to which no salt was added. Only in the last 5,000 years human daily consumption of salt has gone up from 3-4 grams (found naturally in foods, especially meat and eggs) to 10-20 grams. And this largely comes from salt put in cooking, added to processed foods, and from salt shakers at the table. Indeed, humans have come to develop a cultural fixation with salt—"a fixation somewhat irrational, even subconsciously sexual", says Jones in his famous essay on Salt. Most people choose to eat more salt than they need or should, perhaps because they like the taste of it.

Salt, termed "the grain of life", is an essential component in the functioning of body cells. No wonder most cultures have rituals and fellow-feelings associated with salt. Wars have been fought over salt, and the product subjected to high taxation. Salt was once the pillar of civilization, as central to world trade as grain. The modern word *salary* is derived from the Latin *salarium* which originally referred to the direct issue of salt as part salary to Roman soldiers.

With its antiseptic qualities, salt had been widely used in preserving food, particularly the curing of fish. But for cured fish and meat, sailors on long voyage would have been starved of proteins.

Yet, salt's current levels of consumption are caught in a controversy. The prevalence of high blood pressure (hypertension) is largely attributed to the stepped up salt consumption. To prove the point, there are primitive societies that hardly have access to salt, such as the Yanomamo Indians in Brazil or Solomon Islanders. Researchers find little incidence of high blood pressure among them.

The exact mechanism whereby the kidneys' difficulty to excrete salt raises the blood pressure is not yet known. But enough evidence is there to link high blood pressure with excess salt intake, often combined with some kidney abnormality. And dangers of high blood pressure, especially to older people, are too well understood to merit enumeration.

It has been clearly demonstrated that in, patients with mild to moderate hypertension, a reduction in salt intake from approximately 10-12 g to 5-6 g induced a marked fall in blood pressure equivalent to that experienced with a beta blocker pill. Perhaps of equal importance to the effect of salt restriction on its own is the recent finding that the efficacy of most blood pressure lowering drugs is enhanced by salt reduction.

Of course there are quite a few people with hypertension who are known to be salt resistant. Lowering their salt intake would evidently not benefit them. With simple tests a doctor can find out whether a particular person is salt resistant or not.

And there is evidence that apart from raising blood pressure, the present high consumption of salt, is responsible for, or aggravates, osteoporosis, kidney stones, enlargement of the heart, and stomach cancer.

Incidentally a popular notion persists that in a hot environment you need more of salt as there is a large continuing loss of salt in the sweat. This isn't exactly true. Many studies have now shown that the body adjusts the amount of salt in the sweat in the same way as it does in the urine and the saliva, so that on a low salt intake there is little salt in the sweat. Our kidneys are highly resourceful when it comes to preserving salt in the body. The less salt we eat, the more they will hang on to what we have.

Once you concede that a reduction in salt intake is good for you, how best to set about it? All the more compelling if you're getting on the wrong side of sixty.

It is true that the body needs a small amount of sodium, the main active part of salt. But the FDA (USA) points out, it would be almost impossible to eat no salt, because it occurs naturally in many foods. The recommended healthy intake (inclusive of what obtains in foods) is 5g or 6g—equivalent to one teaspoon.

A major step is to cut down on processed foods, such as sausages, bacon, ready-made soups, potato chips, wafers, pickles, samosas, and other salty snacks. These commonly contain 2 to 2.5 gram of salt in 100 grams of food. Most fast-foods such as pizzas and hamburgers also contain large amounts of salt—a slice of pizza as much as 3.5 g. Corn flakes, with no hint of salt in their taste, contain half a gram of salt in a bowl of flakes. Even commercial bread contains something like half a gram of salt in a slice weighing 40 grams. We have this advantage; salt is rarely added to atta for our rotis.

Industry uses salt liberally as a preservative, and to improve the taste—let alone a means of masking inadequacies of ingredients. Salt also increases the weight of the food at very little cost. For instance, if the salt content of sausages is increased from 0.5 per cent to 2.5 per cent, which is the normal concentration of salt in sausages, their water content can also be increased by approximately 20 per cent—salt helps retain water. Another commercial reason for the high salt content; salt increases thirst. It is not surprising that in pubs there are free supplies of salted peanuts and crisps; it makes people drink more. And soft drinks sell better with highly salted chips.

Laws in most countries now require that processed food in packs should carry labels giving the nutritional facts, including percentage of salt. But manufacturers, in a bid to minimize the presence of salt, often give only in terms of sodium. You have to multiply the sodium percentage by 2.5 to arrive at the quantum of salt. Campaigners for salt reduction advocate putting greater pressure on industry to cut down on salt in processed foods.

As against processed foods, fresh foods have remarkably low levels of salt. For instance, fresh meat and fish contain only 0.1 g salt in 100 grams. And fresh fruits and vegetables have as little as 0.04 g salt in 100 grams. That makes an overwhelming case for using fresh foods instead of processed ones if you want to keep your salt intake down.

Another approach is to add no salt at the table. For many people, adding salt at the table is a routine—this automatic habit of adding salt to food even before it has been tasted as seen in restaurants and canteens. A good strategy at home is to have the saltshaker removed.

Most of us can't visualize cooking without salt. Yet the flavour of food can be enhanced by reducing the use of salt if fresh ingredients are used. Again salt can be largely replaced by herbs, lemon juice, onions, garlic, pepper, chillies, and other condiments. Over time, one can get adjusted to cooking with little salt, the way people get acclimatized to tea without sugar. Many of our present day ailments can be traced to excessive consumption of the two; sugar and salt.

It is important to remember that any change in one's diet takes time to get used to and this particularly applies when reducing the intake of salt. The salt taste receptors will take at least a month to adjust to a lower salt concentration.

For most of us, reduced salt intake should make for better health and a longer life span.

The Coffee Health Check

> Caffeine is a little like a criminal suspect who's repeatedly pulled in for questioning, with the evidence always too short to indict, but usually substantial enough to justify continued surveillance.
>
> *Consumer Reports*

No substance has been the subject of more health bulletins—mostly contradictory—than coffee. Over the years, countless researchers have declared coffee bad for virtually every part of the human system. People eagerly consume these reports along with their morning coffee.

On the other hand, reports routinely surface up which rate this bean—the second most actively traded commodity on the planet, after crude oil—as downright beneficial and healthful. Among the benefits listed: increases energy and endurance, staving off exhaustion; keeps workers alert at night, especially those driving at night; gives the brain a boost, the beneficial effect of coffee on mental output more marked with older people than the young; reduces depression and suicide risk; even helps colds. Caffeine makes us feel alert because it blocks the receptors for a brain chemical called adenosine, which normally dampens the activity of other neurotransmitters. Blocking adenosine boosts brain activity.

Anyway it's made out that coffee poses no risk to your heart or general health if taken in moderation—"moderation" defined by experts as an intake of 500-600 gm of caffeine per day, the equivalent of about five coffee cups of average strength.

"So don't panic when the health police knock at your door. Offer them a cup of coffee instead," say the brew's backers.

Many studies published in the 1970s and early 1980s seemed to implicate coffee in everything from bladder, pancreatic and breast cancer, and high cholesterol to increased heart attacks, premature births and low birth weights. Further research revealed, however, that the listed factors of heavy coffee drinkers frequently included unhealthy behaviour such as cigarette smoking, which was often later found to be the chief culprit.

Coffee's role in raising cholesterol has been linked not to the caffeine itself but to the oil from the coffee beans. Using paper filters reduces the problem because the bean oils get trapped in the filter as the coffee passes through it. French presses don't use paper filters but then they produce better-tasting coffee.

Some findings have shown that caffeine in four or five cups of coffee can raise blood pressure by about five points. Yet there is no hard evidence that coffee incurs any added cardiac risk for drinkers who consume fewer than five cups a day, except for the elderly.

Female coffee drinkers will be relieved to hear that no studies have confirmed relationship between coffee and breast cancer. Yet women who drink caffeine lose more calcium in their urine (coffee, a diuretic, produces more urine). Thus they may end up having less dense bones than do non-consumers. Calcium loss makes them more susceptible to bone fracture; quite a common occurrence in the elderly. However, a recent study demonstrated that drinking just one glass of milk can offset the calcium loss induced by two cups of coffee.

There is then the finding that drinking more than three cups of coffee a day lowers a woman's chances of conception by a third. And excessive caffeine consumption has been linked to miscarriages and low birth weight. Caffeine passes easily through the placenta to the foetus, and through the mother's milk to the breast-fed baby.

A 1981 study had concluded that coffee was a major cause of pancreatic cancer. The same now stands discredited.

And caffeine's role as an anti-depressant is gaining greater recognition 2-3 cups a day containing around 300 milligrams of caffeine can even have the effect of preventing suicides in certain cases.

Coffee, as everybody knows, prevents sleep (the Arabic word *qahwa* literally means "one that prevents sleep"). And the effects of coffee last far longer than what people commonly assume—it takes the body three to six hours to get rid of half the caffeine consumed. Even after you've dozed off to sleep, coffee taken at dinnertime can interfere with REM cycles, making sleep less restful.

Coffee is a colonic stimulant, which means it causes the stomach to empty faster without effecting the rate of digestion. Current medical opinion does not rate it a health hazard.

Is caffeine addictive? Those accustomed to but deprived of it, report irritability, nervousness, restlessness, and inability to work well. A common complaint is headache; dull or severe, short-lived or persisting over the day. And this headache eases with the intake of caffeine. No wonder so many headache remedies include caffeine.

Caffeine use seems to fit several parameters of drug addiction: compulsion to continue use, tolerance for the drug, and the withdrawal syndrome. And this withdrawal can occur in people who have as little as 200 milligram of caffeine a day, about the caffeine in two cups of instant coffee.

Too much coffee brings on "caffeinism", a condition characterized by anxiety, irritability, nervousness, lightheadedness, and even diarrhea (coffee is a mild laxative). Caffeine dependence makes drinkers rely on a regular fix to ward off fatigue and headaches and to increase concentration. Kicking a coffee habit can be hard for heavy consumers—in the worst cases it can cause withdrawal symptoms similar (though less severe) to those from quitting more serious addictions.

If caffeine is addictive, coffee drinkers still have a route open to them, and that is of the decaffeinated coffee. Now more than 20 per cent of the coffee consumed in USA is decaffeinated. It's another matter, most of the decafs taste terrible. The industry is now coming up with chemical processes that leave the decaf with a more acceptable taste, such as the chemical process of methylene chloride or the latest one of using supercritical carbon dioxide.

On the other hand, coffee is making inroads into ice creams, yoghurt and confectionery. More and more concoctions come laced with coffee.

Mankind's love affair with coffee seems set to continue, notwithstanding all those debates on the health risks involved. Indeed a new coffee chic is developing: fancy coffee bars, impressive coffee-making machines, and the rising demand for pricey coffees.

The Tea Chic

The 1980s saw the rise of coffee chic. Pricey coffee bars began replacing cheap coffee counters. Starbucks, the most prominent of the coffee chains now expanding all over, not only reinvented coffee, it reinvented the café.

Coffee is considered conducive to productivity: people drinking more and stronger coffee putting in bursts of caffeine energy into work. The urban workday economy is almost unthinkable without coffee.

Now it seems it's the turn of tea. Some serious marketing effort is afoot to impart a new chic to tea. "We want to contemporise tea for a younger generation," explains Mr Hill-Norton, the new business director for Whittard of London, a traditional British tea merchant that just declared war against the gourmet-coffee invasion of Britain.

The company has set up the first t-bar to rival trendy coffee bars. Stainless steel counters, wood floors and mellow jazz music; a relaxed atmosphere with moody lighting. Sofas invite lounging. Curiously shaped chrome-and-glass designer teapots and cups have been introduced. The staff sports polo shirts emblazoned with steaming teacups.

And an astonishing choice of exotic teas and different flavours are on offer: from Darjeeling First Flush to Cinnamon Early Grey, English Breakfast, Japanese Green, Lapsong Souchong, Spice Imperial, Assam, Ceylon. And exotic varieties like Apple Crumble, Jasmine Pearls, Formosa Oolong, Gunpowder.

A few tea-bars have even put up replicas of Japanese teahouse. This is usually a 9-ft square room with an alcove, and emphasis on refined simplicity in build and furnishings.

Separately, the benefits of drinking tea are being highlighted through articles by food writers in various magazines and newspapers. People are told, tea can protect them against heart disease and cancer, lower blood pressure, and relieve migraine.

We are a tea drinking country. We like tea. And the tea industry is now claiming quite a few health benefits of drinking tea.

The Cheer of Chocolate

Chocolate isn't just another sweet. It holds an extraordinary attraction for millions, some to the point of addiction. Ads promote it variously as a stimulant, comforter, or one that makes an ideal present.

What actually accounts for the cheer of chocolate? Some scientists believe it is a sex substitute because every 100 grams contains up to 660 milligrams of phenylethylamine, a stimulant closely related to the body's own dopamine and adrenaline. It induces a high; similar in kind if not in intensity to that experienced in sexual activity. No wonder, chocolate ads in some countries often show a young man or woman happily alone with a bar of chocolate.

Chocolate is surely a stimulant, like coffee or tea. Every 100 grams of it contains 5 milligrams of methylxanthine and 160 grams of theobromine. Both are caffeine-like substances. They stimulate kidneys rather than the brain. One reason why cocoa makes a good bedtime drink. However if taken in large quantities, these chemicals can induce nausea and vomiting. It happens to children who have gorged themselves on chocolate.

Is it a comforter? Chocolate consumption is known to go up in affluent countries in times of economic recession and unemployment. Apparently the increased stress and depression makes people seek some comfort in chocolate.

And, of course, chocolate has food value. It is rich in carbohydrate and thus an excellent source of quick energy. Soldiers carry a bar or two in their knapsack and so also high-altitude mountaineers.

Fortunately for chocolate lovers, it has little effect on serum cholesterol levels. Cocoa butter—the fat squeezed out of cocoa beans and then added to impart chocolate its unique qualities—behaves differently from other fats. Cocoa butter, despite being one of the most saturated fats known, has this property of getting poorly absorbed in the system. That way, cocoa butter can be viewed as a "good" dietary fat. It's another matter, this butter is too expensive for everyday use.

Much of the pleasure of chocolate is derived from its quality of melting in the mouth. That's the property of cocoa butter; solid up to 31 Celsius but melts at body heat of 37°C. And in the process of melting in the mouth, heat is absorbed from the lining of the mouth, giving the eater a nice sensation.

Admittedly chocolate encounters a problem in hot countries like ours; it can become a sticky mess when room temperatures rise to 37°C and beyond. Our manufacturers get around it by adding hydrogenated vegetable oil—also much cheaper than cocoa butter. The nickel in vegetable oil acts as a coagulant. But then nickel poses its own health hazards. And the product tastes different.

Some believe chocolate's attraction is largely psychological, rather than from any magic chemicals. According to them, people from their childhood get emotionally and socially conditioned to regard chocolate as a coveted reward or gift. They start liking chocolate not only for the taste and caloric value but also because of the situation in which chocolates are given. People eat chocolate even when full, more as an indulgence than food.

Chocolate as we commonly see now—a solid sweet melt-in-the-mouth snack—is only a hundred years old. Yet cocoa itself has been there for centuries. The Mayan Indians were using cocoa around AD600. And Aztecs in Mexico made a bitter, spicy cold drink from it. The Spanish conqueror Cortes introduced cocoa beans into Spain. By the 17th century, cocoa became a high class drink in Europe. Chillies were replaced with sugar and it was usually drunk warm. In Britain, several Quaker businessmen—the Cadburys, Frys and Rowntrees—promoted it as an alternative to alcoholic drinks, and made fortunes in the bargain.

Towards the close of the 19th century, a process was developed to extract the fat from cocoa beans—the bean is over half fat. The extracted cocoa butter when added back to the cocoa liquor, enables plain chocolate to be set into moulds easily. In many brands of chocolate, milk is added and so also nuts.

Milk anyway contains an element called casein phospho-peptide which can fight tooth decay. To that extent a milk chocolate should be less injurious to the eater's teeth.

Worldwide chocolate is big business. Germans are currently the most avid consumers, averaging around 18 kg per person per year. In affluent countries chocolates are eaten equally by adults and children. In fact, in UK women consume 39 per cent of all chocolates, children 35 per cent and men 26 per cent.

French are known to make the world's best chocolates. Their umpteen small manufacturers pack chocolate with cocoa solids, displaying this percentage prominently on the wrapper. And no vegetable fat is ever added. Continentals tend to deride the British product with its small percentage of vegetable fat as "vegelate", not chocolate.

The ambience of a top notch French chocolate shop, with its discrete lighting and beautifully displayed products, is more of a jeweller's gallery than a food store. Some exotic gift wraps even come with a thermometer so that you can check your chocolates are being kept at the optimum temperature (between 15 and 22 degrees).

And they have Chocoholics Unanimous—an appreciation society rather than a self-help group. One of its lady enthusiasts says, "You could leave me in a room quite safely with your husband, your tiara or your cheque book, but not with your open box of chocolates." And Caroline Sarll, the founder of Chocoholics Unanimous remarks, "I've been known to eat a two-pound box at one sitting. The uneaten ones wink at me until I've finished the whole lot."

"The best time to taste chocolate, " says one expert, "is at 11 in the morning or between five and six in the afternoon. You need to be a little hungry so that your taste-buds can get to work properly."

And the society's recommended technique for eating quality chocolate:

1. Let it melt in your mouth for a few seconds so that you can detect the basic aromas and flavours.
2. Crunch it between five and six times. This allows access to secondary aromas.
3. Then let it melt slowly while you rub it gently across your palate.

Chillies: Friendly Fire

Many of us are astonished, even express disbelief, when told that chillies didn't exist in ancient India. Hard to envisage that in this land of spices, people weren't eating chillies in King Ashoka's time.

The Capsicum plant probably originated in Bolivia; the hunt for the mother plant still goes on. Chillies were in common use in Mexico for at least 8000 years, both as food and medicine. These were even used in defence; Incas burning dried red chillies in the path of invading Spaniards.

Columbus brought the plant to the Old World, and later the Portuguese to India. And in the mistaken belief that he had reached India, Columbus called it pepper. The name stuck on; in the West they continue to call it pepper, or chilli pepper to distinguish it from black pepper. By now, chillies are grown extensively in many countries. And they form a regular part of the diet of over a quarter of the earth's inhabitants.

The mankind's affair with chillies is odd. Humans are programmed to stay clear of things that hurt. And yet they have embraced this fruit that has the unique characteristic of biting back.

It seems, once the first bite is endured, a certain pleasing sensation flows back. One theory holds that capsaicin (the extract from capsicum), by triggering pain receptors, prompts the release of endorphins—those feel-good natural opiates in the brain. This evidently makes the eater take another bite, and so on. Indeed it's hard to overestimate the passion millions have for the eye-watering, mouth-searing, tongue-numbing, lip-burning, sweat-inducing hot chillies.

Perhaps the world can be divided into two groups: those who relish chillies and those who don't, with few occupying the middle ground.

And amongst those who relish chillies, there are its fans to whom a meal is really not complete without its side-complement of sharp green chillies; food seasoned with chillies is one thing, eating raw chillies alongwith is another. In the latter event, you—not the cook—retain control over how much pungency you want and at what points in your meal.

Chillies have since evolved into a bewildering number of varieties. Some of the better known of pungent chillies are: Mexican habanero, jalapeno, tabasco (from which the famous Tabasco Pepper Sauce is made by an American company), birdeye, serrano, piquin, cayenne, Japanese santaka and hontaka, Indian Sannam, Mundu, Coimbatore, Bombay cherries, and Chinese tianin. All these vary widely in shape, size, colour, flavour, and pungency.

Generally speaking, chillies grown in hot climates are hotter than those grown in milder climates. And the smaller varieties are usually sharper than the ones bigger in size. Interestingly enough, people living in southern parts eat hotter food than their northern counterparts. This rule, without exception, applies in the context of continents and countries.

On an economic-culinary pattern, the poor eat more hot chillies than those who are well off. Our labourers and peasants are wont to make their dry bread or plain rice palatable with pungent chillies. That way, chillies are also instrumental in masking the taste of food.

While Hungarians prize flavour in their mild paprika and Mexicans prize both heat and flavour in their habanero, we generally prize heat more than flavour in chillies. A small purple-black chilli in Bihar is simply called *ake lota mirch,* because it requires one tumbler of water to combat its heat. Guntur is the chilli capital of India. Such vast quantities of chillies come there for trading that the bazaar air is full of chilli dust—like the whisky whiff in some Scottish glens.

At times an argument would arise as to how hot a variety of chilli was. Again, firms making chilli sauces or pickles or other products with chillies as an important ingredient, wanted to make sure their product met the preset levels of pungency. Anything too hot or too mild could alienate the consumer.

In 1912 Wilbur L.Scoville, an American pharmacist, invented a scale of pungency. He would dilute with sugared water the chilli juice of the tested variety, till a distinct but weak pungency was barely perceptible on his tongue. The volume of sweetened water needed to accomplish that stage became the Scoville measure. This ranges between 0 for the bell pepper to 3,50,00 for habanero, the hottest chilli in the world. Birdeye from India measures between 1,00,000 and 1,25,000. Now computerized machines have taken over the measuring, yet the unit of pungency is still Scoville.

Chillies not only vary in their pungency, but also affect the eater in their own specific ways. For instance, habanero offers a sharp, violent bite but then it disappears quickly, leaving behind a soothing, aromatic sensation. Thin and small chillies from India and Thailand have bites that linger long in the mouth, sending even the most hardened chilli eater to reach for a glass of water. Some chillies produce irritation more towards the back of the mouth than front, others burn lips more than the tongue, and some sting only the tongue. It all depends upon how capsaicin, the chemical found in chillies—surprisingly found in no other plant—behaves in a particular variety.

Nobody really knows why capsaicin is there in peppers. Perhaps nature intended to protect the fruit of this knee-high plant from its predators. Rabbits, deer, squirrels don't like chillies. And dogs, too—postmen in some countries carry a protective spray that contains chillies. But then rodents attack chillies and birds don't seem bothered by capsaicin's heat. And goats can get addicted to it.

Chillies are a part of the nightshade family which includes tomatoes and potatoes. Chillies horticulturally are fruit, though botanists call them berries. And they are commonly known as vegetables but are spice when dried.

What about the health aspect of chillies? Chillies have a whole history of medicinal use. Long before they reached Europe and Asia, chillies were already in wide use in the New World as medicine. The Maya Indians rubbed on the gum to relieve toothache. The Aztecs employed chillies against cramps or diarrhoea.

Spanish sailors ate chillies on their voyages, believing it helped their eyesight. In Malaysia chillies are used to treat digestive problems, in Indonesia to stimulate childbirth, and in Philippines as poultices. In the Indian *Materia Medica*, chillies and hot water make a beneficial gargle for sore throat.

And these days a few modern doctors are recommending the use of chillies as a treatment for cold, flu and bronchitis; anyway it has no side effects unlike antibiotics. The idea is that hot chillies help dislodge mucus in the chest when the body is afflicted with cold and fever.

In early 1994, a team of Yale scientists came up with the disturbing news that hot chillies could be causing stomach cancer. This was based on a study of a thousand persons who had either described themselves as "heavy pepper-eaters" and those who took chillies rarely. Laboratory experiments lent support that capsaicin could cause mutations in bacterial cells.

The scare has since subsided. The researchers themselves admit they needed more studies. In fact, Mexicans or Thais or Indians who consume far more chillies than the Europeans have actually lower rates of stomach cancer than the people of Europe. Indeed, a view is being advanced that the fire in the chillies may well be protecting against cancer. Capsaicin being an antioxidant, can interrupt harmful reactions.

The popular apprehension that chillies exacerbated peptic ulcers while bland foods like milk and bananas helped, is again under question. Researchers are finding out that by stimulating the flow of digestive juices, capsaicin could be shielding the stomach lining against damage from acids and alcohol.

And it is common knowledge that chillies are brimming with important vitamins. A paprika, for example, contains five to six times more of vitamin C than an orange or lemon. And carrots, believed to be full of carotene (converted by the liver into vitamin A), contain only a fraction of what chillies contain.

Chillies are now coming under increasing scientific scrutiny. Japanese researchers have reported that the heat element in hot chillies could prevent obesity because it promoted metabolism of the fat. Some researchers in Thailand make out that there is evidence of chillies reducing blood-clot formation. "The daily stimulation of fibrinolytic activity is perhaps sufficient to prevent thromboembolism," the group concludes.

Of course, a whole lot of people stay wary of hot chillies. They fear its fire and the complication the morning after. Yet it is essentially friendly fire; the health benefits of chillies seem to outweigh any potential risks. But what really matters to its patrons is the taste, or what can be termed the cheer of chillies.

That the chilli lends "mouth feel" to plain food explains its great popularity among the poor whose fare is mostly dull and bland. "... when the tongue rebels against plain boiled rice, desiring ghee and salt and spices which one cannot afford, the sharp bite of a chilli renders even plain rice palatable," says Kamala Markandaya in *Nectar in a Sieve.*

The chilli acts in another way to enhance food's acceptability: by producing saliva. The constant production of saliva helps move the food down the throat. And the gut, which is also activated by capsaicin, digests faster. No wonder, people who eat chillies often complain of overeating.

Chillies are fiery things. Yet their fire is largely friendly.

Index

B

C